Praise for *Critical Mental Health Nursing: c*

This is a timely and much-needed publication, the first of its kind I believe in which the central argument is put forward that mental health nursing should subject itself to its own critical scrutiny.

Some of the chapters are likely to frustrate, infuriate, startle, confuse, provoke anger, confront, unsettle and challenge the reader. I hope, though, that the book will also encourage critical reflection and debate and lead ultimately to real and lasting change.

Until my recent retirement, I taught a module centred around engaging undergraduate and postgraduate mental health nursing students in critical debate about issues of concern in the mental health field, including examining the role and position of mental health nurses. This did not always go down well with the students, who felt I was undermining the profession. This text would have been very helpful in exploring mental health nursing in its various forms and settings in much further depth than I did at the time.

I would like to thank the editors for having produced this first critical text on and around mental health nursing, which will hopefully be used and worked with in practice and education settings alike.

Harry Gijbels PhD, retired senior lecturer in mental health nursing; co-founder of the Critical Voices Network Ireland; co-organiser of the annual Critical Perspectives Conference, Cork, Ireland

A critique of psychiatry and related biomedicine is timely in a neoconservative and neoliberal era where mental health services are increasingly privatised to address long waiting lists for specialist care and talking therapies. Practices to address human suffering are constrained by specific legal frameworks while functioning in a marketplace with firm links to profit-generating industries such as psychopharmacology. This text troubles the relationship between psychiatry and mental health nursing.

What can mental health nursing become to speak to the politics of social justice? Much work is needed to reduce the health and social inequalities that are seen in the material hardship of those in mental distress. This text provides helpful insights of a potential future where people hold ownership of their own life stories, where they are heard by others and treated with kindness and respect.

Dr Laetitia Zeeman, Principal Lecturer in Mental Health, University of Brighton

CRITICAL MENTAL HEALTH NURSING

OBSERVATIONS FROM THE INSIDE

Edited by
PETE BULL, JONATHAN GADSBY
AND STEPHEN WILLIAMS

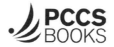

First published 2018

PCCS Books Ltd
Wyastone Business Park
Wyastone Leys
Monmouth
NP25 3SR
contact@pccs-books.co.uk
www.pccs-books.co.uk

Critical Mental Health Nursing:
observations from the inside

British Library Cataloguing in Publication data: a catalogue record for this book is
available from the British Library.

ISBN 978 1 910919 40 8

Front cover illustration by Jason Anscomb
Typeset in-house by PCCS Books using Minion Pro and Myriad Pro
Printed by Short Run Press, Exeter, UK

Contents

Acknowledgements

We would like to thank a number of people.

We would like to thank Mick McKeown, Alec Grant and Jim Chapman, for their energy, warmth and support of the Critical Mental Health Nurses' Network from its earliest days, and Lucy Johnstone for inspiration in the past and the present. We would particularly like to acknowledge Sean Walton for his help editing some early chapter drafts.

Our thanks to Catherine Jackson (Commissioning Editor, PCCS Books), for her understanding, support and enthusiasm for the project, especially in the face of the significant editorial challenges.

Jonathan would also like to thank Mervyn Morris for a unique array of skills and kindnesses, Joachim Schnackenberg (no nurse should say something is impossible without meeting Joachim first), and his own sister, Joanna Page, who always makes writing seem more possible.

Pete Bull would like to thank his wife, Felicity, and his boys, Henry and Wilfie, for putting up with him not being around so that he could help with this book. He would also like to thank his fellow editors Stephen Williams and Jonathan Gadsby for making it all a fun experience. He'd also like to thank his team at work in Brighton for supporting him to have unpaid leave so that he could finish the book off!

Stephen Williams would like to thank his co-editors for the sterling work they have undertaken in this collaborative volume. Without them, the idea of the book would never have transformed into the eclectic, thought-provoking volume that lies in your hands. He'd also like to thank Alec Grant for his ongoing inspirational writing and furtherance of the autoethnographical approach to mental health discourse that has been a key influence on his own writing development. Stephen would also like to thank his co-author Steve Prosser for taking up the challenge of writing about his experience and helping bring their chapter into being.

To all the contributors – especially acknowledging those whose work didn't make it into the final volume – thanks for rising to the challenge and working with us to make a special experience and a book of many rich shades and stimulating hues.

Our apology

The Editors

We, the three registered mental health nurses and editors of this book, apologise to you, the recipient of or carer for a recipient of mental health nursing care in the UK, for the many historical and present ways in which mental health nurses have contributed to your distress and disempowerment. We dedicate ourselves to your future.

Background

The world is a troubling place and it is our belief that to be engaged with it, to know it, experience it, to try to get one's needs and hopes met within it, to achieve within it or to try to change it will all lead a reflective person to be troubled. It would be foolish for a mental health nurse to try to apologise for the precariousness of life, the degradation of the environment, the inequalities that lead to much suffering and the operations of what may be referred to as a 'military-industrial complex' of corporate power, exploitation and war. In many ways, nurses' work is defined and made difficult as much by these things as by anything and anybody else.

However, mental health services in the UK fall seriously short of all that they should be, that people who use services deserve and that should be afforded to them, as a human right. This is not a new phenomenon; it has been the case throughout our history. We recognise a profound and deeply saddening gap between that to which many mental health nurses aspire and much of what we actually do. We recognise that we are the largest professional group in a service that many find reductionist, invalidating, self-serving, drug-pushing and re-traumatising. Above all, every single aspect of it is tinged with coercion. This coercion takes many forms and is not simply a feature of the lives of people detained on locked wards and subjected to forced treatment. It permeates all that we do; it even hangs over shared cups of tea in a person's own home.

We understand that mental health nursing has gradually evolved this culture of coercion, from its role as untrained attendant in pauper lunatic asylums to today's qualified professional. As the profession has supported the growth of psychiatry's coercive practices, through the administration of the law and delivery of psychiatric treatments, so must we own the legacy of having participated in some of the greatest untold human rights abuses of the 19th, 20th and 21st centuries. In the asylums, in the hospitals and in the community, mental health nurses have restrained and assaulted people who use services, as a part of everyday practice. Mental health nurses have enabled and carried out the forced drugging of people who use services; we have inflicted and assisted incarceration, electroshock treatment and its ensuing brain damage, lobotomisation and insulin comas. Aside from continuing to detain and restrain people, mental health nurses, through the administration of antipsychotic depot medications, continue to collude in the wholesale tranquillisation of people who use services without ever obtaining proper consent by candid disclosure of everything we know about what these drugs do to people over the longer term. The profession uses the ethics of 'best interests' to excuse, condone and perpetuate these practices. We candidly acknowledge the violence, the silence that permeates both the establishing and existence of our profession: it is part of who we have become.

There are many ways to try to explain (or explain away) the gap between what you need and what we give. It is true that mental health services in the UK have become smaller and more coercive over the last decade and this is probably best understood as driven by decisions made in Westminster rather than in the ward round. It is probably also true that society remains mostly unskilled and prejudiced when it comes to acknowledging and helping people in distress, those who have unusual thoughts and beliefs and those whose behaviour falls outside of expected norms. The design of mental health services has always reflected what society wants them to be – a place of incarceration and exclusion for people who are different, under a 'care' narrative, rather than the promotion of mental health. It would probably be valid to argue that mental health services mainly exist to treat the anxieties of all the people who are *not* using them.

The basis of our apology

Yet, despite a context over which we have limited power, mental health nurses have for a very long time claimed to offer much more than a vehicle for the whims and priorities of society about people it deems 'mad'; we have claimed expertise. In the last three decades, mental health nursing has become a university degree course and our catch-phrase for that drive has been 'a profession in our own right'. While nurses have always been accountable to codes of conduct, this 'coming to university' seems a meaningful entry point for new kinds of responsibility, new standards of accountability. We believe that a 'profession in our own right' is exactly what we have not been. Instead, we have continued to be the custodians of an ever-more coercive practice, mostly following other professions whose reductive knowledge base is aggressively and effectively critiqued across many faculties in the universities to which we now belong. We have spoken lazily about 'holistic care' but have not sought to understand and change all that undermines it.

We cannot think of a new knowledge, approach, skill or kind of empowerment that nurses have themselves forged as a 'profession in our own right' from which our service users have identifiably benefited. The best that we can claim is that we have occasionally, to limited extents and with limited understanding of their wider meanings, allowed ourselves to be influenced by survivor knowledges and by some aspects of psychology.

Instead, as a 'profession in our own right', we have presided over an increase in use of detention. In our actions we have put most of our hope in whatever the doctor believes; people who use services are still dying young of preventable physical health problems. Despite two decades of university education, every day in the UK mental health nurses make statements such as 'You have a chemical imbalance in your brain'; this is wholly without credible science to support it. We are conduits for the continued cultural practices of institutions and uncritical recipients of others' perspectives and values. We have allowed the contradictions of our practice to continue at university, creating curricula that are full of unexplored conflicts, so that first-year mental health nurses write charming essays about Carl Rogers, but third years write about 'psychoeducation' and 'adherence' and uncritically about 'schizophrenia' as a brain-based disorder, and frequently leave the course still unsure what a mental health nurse is.

This lack of critical thinking about what we do and who we are is inexcusable. For more than two decades student nurses' academic work has been assessed under university marking schemes that prize critical thinking beyond all other attributes. No one should be able to graduate under such a marking scheme if their standard practice is to unreflectively follow orders or continue culturally received views. It is as if we have allowed ourselves to develop two standards of 'critical'; too often we critique the internal validity of research (by using critical appraisal tools, for example) but neglect the context of a highly contested field and political concerns that would be needed to explore the external validity. In short, we frequently operate in an echo chamber of our own making. This should be impossible at a university.

So many mental health nurses ache for much better services but our lack of direction means that, even in large numbers, we experience little collective power. Being a mental health nurse and a critical thinker is frequently a lonely experience, even when close colleagues may say that they agree. Once again, this seems to point the finger back at universities. If ever there was a profession in need of well-articulated and decisive unifying initiatives, it is mental health nursing.

Our collective failure has cost us dearly. Perhaps more than ever before, the aspirations we have for helping others must find expression in the diminishing gaps between bureaucratic demands and other professions' agendas, with models of delivery driven more by spreadsheets than any nursing vision. At a time when we should have been reaching towards new concepts and new leaders, we have allowed much of our work to be downgraded to tasks to be done by less qualified staff. In our distress, we tell ourselves that we are the victims of the system of which we are the key facilitators – a statement we would be quick to label 'personality disordered' in others. Instead of reaching for a new empowerment, we are now losing hold of the profession as a distinct branch of nursing, as nurse education swings back to the generic. University mental health nursing tutors are even now meeting with their counterparts in the adult, child and learning disability fields to try to find a role for themselves in new 'integrated' curricula. Yet in truth, the legacy of mental health nursing as a distinct field of nursing is difficult to defend.

However, while as a profession we have experienced the results of our deficiencies and face a very uncertain future, it has been the people who use our services who have suffered most from our lack of direction and continuing facilitation of coercive practices.

Not all mental health nurses will want us to apologise on their behalf and some may be angered. Some may feel that they stepped up to help and they have worked hard – so when did it all become their responsibility? This argument tempts us, too. However, we want to recognise that this ability to distance oneself from other nurses of whom we may feel critical partly protects the status quo and our lack of coherent direction as a group. For us to make this apology is therefore partly a recommitment to mental health nursing and a demonstration that a critical mental health nurse is not someone who slings mud from a distance.

Equally, not all people who use services may feel that we have a right to make this apology. Some may feel we have inadequately acknowledged their experiences, or that we simply do not have enough influence to make this apology meaningful to them. If a fellow nurse says to us that we should not criticise unless we can say how we would do things better, we feel confident that we can show them how quickly that argument falls apart. However, if people who use our services, on reading this apology, were to feel the same, it would be hard for us to disagree, because we do feel that we owe them that better service.

For the three of us, our rededication to the profession of mental health nursing is a commitment to work towards an unashamedly and unflinchingly critical nurse education and greater collaboration with survivor groups, whose vital contributions we gratefully acknowledge.

Stephen Williams, Jonathan Gadsby and Pete Bull, July 2018

Introduction

Pete Bull, Jonathan Gadsby and
Stephen Williams

Thank you for browsing, borrowing or buying this book. It is an eclectic collection
of academic writing that we hope will provide stimulation, challenge and joy.
Over the course of a year and a half, we three editors have worked hard to support
our authors in bringing their work to fruition and we are now ready to share the
bounties of their harvest with all of you. We want to change minds and engage
people in thinking.

We think that it is helpful to provide background, synopsis and history of
the book, in order to position the various texts among other writings that you
know. With this in mind, we have written a bit about the impetus for the book
and the formation of the Critical Mental Health Nurses' Network (CMHNN), a
frank account of the process of editing and a summary of the chapters themselves.
Finally, we talk about coercion.

The impetus for the book and the Critical Mental Health Nurses' Network

One way to view this book is as part of a process that began in 2013, when 10
qualified and student mental health nurses began to meet to talk about the possibility
of a network of critically minded nurses. Several of these nurses were connected
with universities in the UK, several had found connection and inspiration in the
Hearing Voices Movement and three were students who were struggling to know if
they really wanted to qualify. The group did not know exactly what the purpose of
the network would be. Several of the bi-monthly meetings began with asking each
other how they were feeling and sometimes got stalled (productively) with that.

Several in the group were struggling with work situations they found immoral and the formation of the CMHNN is due in no small part to the integrity of those who explored and expressed their inner conflicts in those meetings.

Further impetus was found at the 2014 Intervoice annual congress, in Thessaloniki, where an experienced mental health nurse from Bradford and a student nurse at Canterbury University ran a workshop attended by some 80 voice-hearers and professionals about being a registered mental health nurse (RMN) *and* part of the Hearing Voices Movement. Also at the event was one of the leaders of the 'Hearing the Voice' project at Durham University, who offered support. In early 2015 the CMHNN was launched at a conference at Durham. Later that same year, there was a second conference at Birmingham City University.

Much of the early work of the CMHNN was focused on creating and editing a website. This website began to get some fairly heavy traffic, particularly from the UK, Australia, Canada and the US, and from over 30 countries in total. Some visitors sent emails of support. Three of the chapters in this book were written by people who initially contacted the CMHNN via the website to identify themselves as allies.

Yet to say that this book is a *product* of the CMHNN is wrong. Two of the editors had little active involvement with the formation of the CMHNN (although both were invited to early meetings in Bradford); they represent the fact that, actually, mental health nurses have been interested in thinking critically about their roles for a long time before 2014. In fact, healthy scepticism has been present as part of mental health nurses' professional identity for decades. It is questionable whether the CMHNN has or will produce much in the way of entirely new knowledge. Instead, if it has a value, it is hoped that, through it, the term 'critical mental health nurse' will become a stronger identity and a locus of shared experience, replacing the more negative labels that have been used to isolate those with questioning minds, such as the one with the 'wacky ideas' or the one with 'problems with authority'. To be a critical mental health nurse is to be open to the complexity of the world, not to be content with the lazy simplicity of the single explanations and single solutions that are so often used to tidy up real experience for the benefit of those most able to have their preferred simplicities accepted.

'Critical' is not a particular stance but a profound interest in stances. Once again, there is nothing new about this. 'Critical' is the key word that adorns university marking schemes in every discipline. To be *trained* is to be encultured, socialised and disciplined; to be *educated* is to become critical. The CMHNN and this book are both part of the inevitable consequence of nurses aspiring to be more educated over the past three decades. We view the CMHNN as consistent with the openly stated mainstream educational goals of our profession, and if such education leads nurses to ask very difficult questions about our own profession and its context, that is only right.

Originally this book was going to be entirely different. One of us, Stephen, was working up a book proposal titled *A Handbook of Recovery-Oriented Mental Health Nursing*, and was looking for collaborators to produce a practice-focused guide to fill what he perceived to be a gap in the market for nursing texts. After conversations between the three of us, it became apparent that the book should have a strong critical focus on recovery, as there is a highly critical dialogue around that subject, mainly through survivor/user groups on Facebook and Twitter. Having learned that another book that sat in that niche was close to publication and that this was likely to be singularly uncritical, the focus of the book radically changed.

There is already plenty of critique of psychiatry, and a Critical Psychiatry Network; these do not need to be duplicated. The CMHNN has the special remit of critiquing our own profession. Sometimes mental health nurses say that 'critical' does not feel like the right word for them; they would prefer words that express some of their values of pragmatic, hopeful and relational ways of working. Perhaps 'critical' feels negative. We can only respond by saying that 'critical' is, for us, both practical and interpersonal; it speaks of engagement and dialogue, shared and alternative perspectives, advocacy and respect for individuality. A student nurse at one of our institutions, in a class discussion about understanding research, observed that the skills needed to explore ideas from several angles, to ask whom they suit and why (some hallmarks of critical writing), have strong parallels with empathy, which is a much less controversial core nursing skill and one that many see as key to our identity. This is another reason why we contend that being a critical mental health nurse is to be deliberate and rigorous about being a practical and positive mental health nurse.

However, we are not naïve. Critical thinkers of every discipline, from the natural sciences to the arts and humanities, always become interested in how *dominance* is built and how it is maintained. Such questions are seldom popular with those who benefit from that dominance. Therefore, in addition to having a very natural relationship with education, the CMHNN is also a refuge and a source of solidarity for those with unpopular and 'subversive' questions. We know this because of our own experiences and because the most common emails sent to the CMHNN express relief and gratitude and often describe the loneliness – and, indeed, the professional dangers – of being a critical mental health nurse.

The editorial process

While it is hoped that this book will provide a sense of 'what is out there' – an introduction to the kinds of topics and interests that concern mental health nurses when thinking critically – the chapters are not a purposeful selection or a representative sample of ideas associated with critical mental health nursing. What we have here is simply the result of a process, begun by sending out, via emails, Facebook posts and Twitter, invitations to people we knew and people that we didn't know, inviting them to contribute chapters towards a critical mental health nursing book. It would be 'a critical, poly-paradigmatic, pluralistic approach to mental health nursing as an anthology of lightly edited chapters'. It would 'introduce and bring alive the value of autoethnography as a means of challenging "othering" practices, fostering empathy and reflexivity of the challenges, strengths and weaknesses in current UK and international mental health nursing practice'. It would also 'give space and value to different kinds of philosophical analysis – those that centre around themes or disciplines of power, identity, organisational, cultural, intersectional, post-modernist, post-structuralist, empirical, connectionist, and so forth'. Whether we have succeeded in this endeavour, you, the reader, can judge.

Twenty chapters were submitted, and we have ended up with 13 chapters by 15 authors, excluding our own introduction. This in no way represents all possible views or even properly reflects a diversity of authors; these are simply the chapters that survived the creative and editorial process – products of the relationship between us, as editors, our contributors and the world we inhabit. Our ambition to produce a book that properly reflects a diversity of authors has, for us, at this time, been impossible to realise. All three of us gave our time to this book for free, although one of us was able to use short periods of university-funded writing time to complete some tasks. We were limited in the amount of time we were able to give to those who would have needed more help to get their chapters to a place where they met the publishing standards of academia. Not all authors submitted work that really met our brief, although, as we read all of the submissions, we were moved by a sense of their value. We rejected five chapters, after a process of consultation with the authors, either because they did not substantiate their claims in ways that academic writing demands or they required too much prior knowledge on the part of our readers, or we felt the writing was too sophisticated and scholarly to be easily accessible to our readership.

Perhaps unsurprisingly, 11 of our authors are white men who are older than middle age and 12 are employed by universities or self-identify as independent scholars. Each decision to reject was made with extreme difficulty, especially as every rejection reduced the diversity of the authors. The decisions felt academically right but morally wrong and did not sit easily with us. Two of us regularly mark essays written by mental health nursing students, in which well-referenced paragraphs may obscure a naïve lack of critical engagement with their subject (a criticism that arguably can be levelled generally at mental health nurse education in the UK, despite our profession's move to degree status). Yet here we were, rejecting chapters that articulated critical perspectives with which we had a strong affinity, on the basis that they were too poorly referenced – oh, the irony of our own 'narrative entrapment' (Grant, 2013; Grant et al, 2015)! However, we believe academia to mean critical thinking and *vice versa*, and we wanted that to be evident in every chapter.

There are other, no less telling questions to which we have had to find answers. Is this an academic book or a nursing book? What does this question reveal about (self-) perceptions of nursing as a body of knowledge and/or a practical discipline? What is the relationship between critical mental health nursing and the increasingly well-organised and well-articulated body of survivor scholarship/critique? Does 'academic' writing, because it conforms to certain institutional standards, *de facto* make a work part of the establishment, and can it from that position critique established concepts and structures with any credibility? All three of us have been driven towards academia by our contact with survivor movements, some of whose members may retain strong reservations about the value of the academy, while others have embraced it. 'What use is it to voice hearers that you get these letters after your name?' is a question asked of one of us that he will never forget.

In inviting autoethnographic contributions, we consciously hoped to meet some of these difficulties head on and to promote a form of academic work that undermines some of the empiricist assumptions in mental health that may drive practices of which there is cause to be very critical. We feel a great sense of privilege in being able to present these chapters to you. There are some very special writers here, some who have been widely published elsewhere and some who have never been published before. All of these chapters have value, and several are all that we hoped for: simultaneously academic, intellectually challenging, generously personal and deeply moving.

Summary of the chapters

We start with our apology. We felt that we wanted to offer this as part of this book because there is so much to be sorry for in the history of the profession and how we practise now. We would like things to be better than they are. While we recognise that there are many individual nurses doing fantastic work in poorly paid and difficult situations, we all, as a profession, need to be more honest, more candid about what we have been and what we are now and what we need to become. We must acknowledge that our situations at work and how we are equipped to deal with the problems we face need more thoughtful consideration, at the very least, if not some concerted action.

Jonathan Gadsby's first chapter exemplifies this honesty with its admission to the violence that is intrinsic to mental health nursing. He is now a university research fellow but worked for many years as a mental health nurse in the NHS. Writing autoethnographically, he discusses issues to do with control and restraint and his own experience of a client taking his own life, before going on to discuss how some of the narratives used by nurses shape experience.

We decided to put this chapter first because of its explicit naming of the violence inherent within the role of the mental health nurse. Whether we like it or not, as trained professionals with a code of conduct (Nursing & Midwifery Council, 2015), as public servants or employees of large corporations who recommend and dispense the drugs produced by large pharmaceutical companies, we are purveyors of ideology. The ideological violence we participate in is both relational and physical. Mental health nurses must own this responsibly if we are to be candid in encounters with others. Reading Jonathan's chapter is a good starting point for discussions about the nature of nursing violence. It runs through the fabric of who we are, in every role, and to pretend otherwise is to be naïve. How will/do you restrain? How will/do you inject with antipsychotics? How will/do you contribute at Mental Health Act tribunals?

Next, Alec Grant has produced a masterful 'critical meta-autoethnographic performance' in 'Moving around the hyphens', drawing on his Dr Grant–Alec Grant–ex-cognitive behavioural therapist–ex-mental health nurse–ex-service user-survivor of the institutional psychiatric system–narrative researcher identity. He is a recently retired lecturer who has worked with mental health discourses since the 1970s. He recounts four separate encounters from various times in his career and uses what was said to uncover the contradictions between the rhetoric and reality of mental health nursing education and practice. He highlights the gaps between how mental health nurses and patients are talked about and the reality of experience for both groups. He makes us think about how we talk about these matters. He calls out stupidity, obedience and uncritical thinking. As mental health nurses, don't we often do what we believe is required, without question? Is that right?

In Chapter 3, Stephen Williams and Steven Prosser grapple with identity issues that emerged when they were both involved in the Recovery College in Bradford. Stephen discusses being the college's clinical academic lead when he was also a recently-incarcerated mental patient; Steven describes deteriorating into 'the Beast', which manifested in depression, and then enrolling at the college, which ultimately led to his becoming a mindfulness practitioner. By writing together, they expose the transience of identity, reflecting on the literature around 'illness', psychosis and consciousness as they do so.

From a critical mental health nursing perspective, we understand that the self is not fixed; our identity is constantly in flux. We know how easily mental health nurses can adopt diagnostic terminology without thinking, as a form of professional shorthand that speeds up communication and learning. Stephen and Steven's chapter demonstrates the richness of human experience: how can the singular narrative identities in which both authors were trapped adequately reflect the multiple realities of their existence that they describe?

Darren Mills is a mental health occupational therapist and lecturer in New Zealand. In Chapter 4, 'A balancing act', he picks out the weaknesses of that country's mental health system through an autoethnographic account of an encounter with a Māori family seeking the help of the crisis team where he worked. He interweaves the story with statistical data, contemporary news stories, official reports, opinion pieces and academic material. The story moves from the relational moment to the objective fact, each informing the other. The chapter powerfully captures what it is like to work within a poorly resourced system that is alien to the culture that it encounters. It vividly illustrates how we mental health nurses can struggle to make sense of data, how difficult it is to negotiate differences in cultures and languages, how we often find ourselves at the complex intersection between numerous competing interests and ways of understanding situations.

Next, in 'Power at play: the Doctor–Nurse Game in acute mental health care' (Chapter 5), Anne Felton and Gemma Stacey re-analyse data taken from a previously published study (Stacey et al, 2016) to explore power, positioning, performance and hierarchy within decision-making forums such as acute mental health admissions unit ward rounds. Using the rules of the Doctor-Nurse Game (Stein, 1967) as a critical deductive framework, they unpick the data to show how mental health nurses get caught up in this game with medical professionals, although they also discover some interesting subtleties in the details of the game and the justification for the rules. Anne and Gemma's chapter provokes us into questioning the continuing status-quo in the doctor-nurse relationship. What is the justification for the socially legitimised role of psychiatrists and the level of pay they receive – up to five times greater than the basic nursing salary – for carrying out tasks that could be done by a mental health nurse, including Mental Health Act assessments and prescribing drugs from the British National Formulary? Can we call this out as a professional group or in our individual practice, or will we remain forever entrenched within the Victorian hierarchies that still determine the responsibilities each professional group is willing to take for their work within the mental health services? Will we mental health nurses cling onto our 'professional inferiority complex' (Nolan, 2012) in cherishing our role as the psychiatrist's handmaiden?

In Chapter 6, 'Colluding with prejudice? mental health nurses and the Mental Health Act', Gary Sidley argues that, by its very existence, the Act legalises discrimination and so makes mental health professionals, including mental health nurses, responsible for delivering discriminatory practices. He outlines the evolution of the legislation, rails against community treatment orders and deconstructs the concepts of 'mental disorder' and 'risk assessment'. He questions the role of preventative detention and the increasing use of coercion and asks why mental health nurses continue to work with the Mental Health Act in its current form. At the time of writing, the Act is yet again under review. What should be our position on this issue? What are the alternatives? What is legal and what is moral should, in the best of possible worlds, at least overlap, but they are not always the same thing. What does our collective failure to object to the Act's everyday use say about our individual and collective moralities? Is this an issue on which we, as a profession, need to take collective action and advocate for change?

Next, Marc Roberts moves the book into a more philosophical space with 'The development of a critically orientated mental health nursing practice: Michel Foucault's history of the present' (Chapter 7). Marc draws on Foucault and his methodological framework of the 'history of the present' to argue that we need to understand our past in order to better interrogate and make sense of the concepts and shared assumptions that dictate how we practise today. Mental health nurses commonly use terms such as 'schizophrenia' or 'bipolar disorder' as if they were real, obvious and their meaning universally understood and agreed. By both becoming more aware of the instability of the evidence around these ideas and understanding more clearly how such concepts have emerged over time, we are better placed to think critically about if and how we work with them now. This disruption and critical thinking are surely what we ask the people who use our services to do when we demand that they speak about their history in therapy, or expect them to change. Do we in fact conceptualise reality in ways that can be just as rigid and concrete as the thinking of the people we work with and for? Isn't all the knowledge that we use of its time and sanctioned by institutions and government? Does this mean that we can never be objective?

In 'The ideology of recovery in contemporary mental health care' (Chapter 8), Alastair Morgan critiques the concept of recovery using a Marxist definition of ideology. By unpicking assumptions about different definitions of recovery and pointing out how recovery functions as a discourse and what it conceals, he throws light on the political nature of the concept and the interests it serves. Alastair challenges us to consider if recovery is even possible while coercion exists – this is not about recovery from some constructed 'mental illness' but the recovery of our lives. Does the incoherent, individualised, mystifying notion of recovery propagated by mental health services effectively stymy people's attempts to find ways of living less problematically? As critical mental health nurses, how can we avoid perpetuating unkindness and serving the interests of a government intent on saving money?

Continuing the recovery theme, in 'Ackin' it back t'brick with autoethnography, reflective practice and mental health recovery research' (Chapter 9), Tony Sparkes explores his experiences of becoming and working as a mental health social worker and the link between autoethnography and reflective practice. He problematises the way services changed to becoming 'recovery-oriented', shines light on how people are actually treated in those services and presents conversations with colleagues and descriptions of encounters with people who use services, to draw attention to the conflicts inherent within the recovery model. His chapter raises yet more questions for critical mental health nurses: do we need to resist and oppose changes that we perceive to be harmful to the people we care for? What is the ethical mental health nursing response to top-down change? How ought we to mobilise our shared concern for people who may become further disadvantaged by the actions of national and local government?

Mick McKeown's chapter, 'Mental health workforce and survivor alliances: a personal story of possibilities, perils and pratfalls', picks up the theme of challenging change. Mick draws on his own past experience to explore the potential for creating and sustaining solidarity between social movement activists concerned with mental health and mental health services. Might different ways of organising, relating and dialoguing bring new potential to these kinds of encounter? The chapter encourages us to consider the potential in uniting with people who use services to bring about sustainable change. Do we not both receive money from the government as a consequence of how we live? Are we not caught together in situations where we must share space and where we are both subject to the law? Can we develop a shared understanding of the politics of mental health? Could this be a psychotherapy in which we are both patients? As mental health nurses, are we able to acknowledge our work is political? It seems clear that, borrowing from Hanisch (1970), it is important to recognise that the 'professional is political'.

Next, Benny Goodman offers a personal account and autoethnographic analysis of how health and wealth can protect against becoming a mental health patient. 'Standing at the cliff edge but very safely belayed' explores Benny's own masculinity through the lens of the concepts of health assets, self-policing, the value we accord personal action and experience and how structures in our culture can shape these. Models for change certainly have to go beyond individualised, psychiatric, biomedical understandings of health and illness; education is not a universal panacea. This chapter encourages us to look at ourselves, to consider what we bring to encounters with others, to own our own ways of self-policing and to appreciate our own health assets. Can critical mental health nurses see the relevance of the social and political contexts of people's lives when trying to help them? Does that not mean we should think carefully about how we talk about them and their problems, as well as consider how we talk about our own?

In Chapter 12, writing from Houston, Texas, Erica Fletcher offers an autoethnographic, non-linear account of her unfolding relationship with her sister, her understandings of their family, their shared history, their relationships with the cultural contexts in which they have found themselves and how she copes with her sister's descent into and emergence from madness and the Houston public mental health system. It is a 'messy text' that calls into question the significance and usefulness of culturally acceptable forms of meaning-making. It speaks honestly of Erica's own attempts to straddle the growing gap between what she believes in – her values and politics and her sister's wishes – and the realities of caring for someone in acute mental breakdown. It takes us to an uncomfortable place. In our work, we daily listen to voices from different places and aspire to accept complexity, nuance, sophistication and creativity and hold lightly the technical way of speaking that we have developed in training. Are we prepared to hear and work with the voices of service users and carers and their different understandings of experience? How easily do we leave our own values and politics outside the ward door when presented with expediency and organisational expectations?

Finally, in 'Mental health nursing as a therapy', Tony McSherry explores how mental health nursing could craft an identity and function as a discipline separate from psychiatry. Drawing on his own experience and existential, phenomenological and psychoanalytic literature, Tony takes us to a new place of understanding of the possibilities in mental health nursing. His chapter encourages us to be optimistic about who we can become, as well as be honest and responsible. Dare we move away from technical understandings of what it means to be human and into a messier, more confusing space? Can we embrace the shadowy, complex, ambiguous and difficult, which we, as critical mental health nurses, should surely prefer? McSherry suggests we should call ourselves social therapists. As mental health nurses, we might reject this notion, but there is clearly a need for reconsidering and rearticulating who we are as a distinct profession, separate from psychiatry and the traditional subservient role, in order to claim our expertise in the very specific, non-technical realm of relational therapy.

Readers will notice recurring themes throughout the varied chapters presented here. For us, an outstanding theme is concern about the ubiquity and depth of coercion within mental health nursing work – a concern equally evident in the contributions and correspondence on the CMHNN website. There seems little doubt that mental health nurses today are delivering, facilitating and witnessing deeply coercive practices. It may not be possible to have a mental health service without a Mental Health Act (we do not know), and yet as a profession we are a very long way from being accused of that kind of idealism. This is a conversation that we must continue to progress. In 1998, Arundhati Roy wrote an essay deploring India's becoming one of the small group of countries in possession of nuclear weapons. She titled it *The End of Imagination* (Roy, 1998). Her argument is that, with such a power, the Indian government would not need to use any creativity to engage with its own people or other nations to gain respect; they would possess a weapon that would command a respect born of fear. When a nuclear bomb is brought to the negotiating table, not many genuine negotiations take place. Likewise, the omnipresence of the Mental Health Act, and perhaps especially community treatment orders, makes us mental health nurses unimaginative, uncreative, de-skilled and unaware of our own potential and the potential of those we hope to help. Many nurses have never witnessed non-coercive relationships and skills and do not glimpse what could be achieved if they built alliances with people who use their services. Most seem to believe that 'psychosis' is the dead end of interpersonal possibilities and understanding. The Mental Health Act prevents our profession's growth. Its ubiquity means that the best we can be for many of the people who use our services is kind but untrustworthy. It is chilling to wonder if, when they like us, it is more Stockholm syndrome than therapeutic alliance. To trust a nurse with one's inner self is to put one's freedom in their hands and so the people who use services must, at times, take great care of *our* 'mental state'.

If we are going to ever be a profession in our own right, we need to debate this issue, share our experiences and fears with honesty and, above all, look to all of the places in which imagination has been ignited before we proclaim 'There is no alternative'. *We look to a time in which the presence of a mental health nurse in the room can be said to open up new possibilities that make coercive options fall away.*

Awareness of coercion must also extend to the conversations we have with people who use services, not just in relation to the use of the Mental Health Act and the law. Coercion is expressed in the very language that we use and the way we relate with people who use services. We must endeavour to become more aware of the ways that we commit violence in all our relationships (both at work and at home) and in how we talk to one another. This includes acknowledging that mere presence can be violent, that silence can be violent and that no conversation or encounter or therapy session can take place without a multiplicity of shared or unshared assumptions that may impact on what unfolds between people. There is always, already, a relationship between us and the people who use services that is structured around differing manifestations of power. The words we use within that relationship can impact on people's experience of reality and their capacity to survive. We are responsible; is our own survival more important than that of the other?

We hope you will enjoy this book.
Pete Bull, Jonathan Gadsby and Stephen Williams

References

Grant A (2013). Writing, teaching and survival in mental health: a discordant quintet for one. In: Short N, Turner L, Grant A (eds). *Contemporary British Autoethnography*. Rotterdam: Sense Publishers (pp33–48).

Grant A, Leigh-Phippard H, Short N (2015). Re-storying narrative identity: a dialogical study of mental health recovery and survival. *Journal of Psychiatric and Mental Health Nursing 22*(4): 278–286.

Hanisch C (1970). *The personal is political.* [Online.] www.carolhanisch.org/CHwritings/PIP.html (accessed 7 June 2018).

Nolan P (2012). Nursing: the heart of mental healthcare. *British Journal of Mental Health Nursing 1*(1): 8–11.

Nursing and Midwifery Council (2015). *The Code: professional standards of practice and behaviour for nurses and midwives.* London: Nursing and Midwifery Council.

Roy A (1998). *The End of Imagination.* Kottayam: DC Books.

Stacey G, Felton A, Morgan A, Stickley T, Willis M, Diamond B, Houghton P, Johnson B, Dumanya J (2016). A critical narrative analysis of shared decision-making in acute inpatient mental health care. *Journal of Interprofessional Care 30*(1): 35–41.

Stein LI (1967). The Doctor-Nurse Game. *Archives of General Psychiatry 16*(6): 699–703.

1 | Nursing violence, nursing violence

Jonathan Gadsby

I began attending a Quaker meeting when I saw that to be peaceful I needed new kinds of conversations about violence. Public perception may be that Quakers are joined to one particular kind of pacifism, but in fact they have always held a variety of beliefs about the possibility of a genuinely peaceful world; mostly their commitment is to maintain unresolvable questions about violence, rather than a blanket idealism. They concede to the charge of utopianism: a society without violence is utopian but so too is the notion of violence as problem solver, whether in the arena of international war, in intimate relationships or in one's relationship with oneself. Within these unresolvable questions, they suggest that one can either engage with (and be continually troubled by) issues of violence or choose to avoid them (The Religious Society of Friends, 2013: chap 24). I want to responsibly raise trouble rather than to irresponsibly resolve or avoid it (Frank, 2012).

I believe that mental health nursing is wrapped up with violence. Since my first experiences of that violence, I have been trying to distance myself from it, only to discover that each successive role I take has been equally part of it, though perhaps in more subtle ways. Anarchist economist David Graeber describes debt as violence, noting that the further down the socio-economic strata one goes, the more debt violence takes physical form (Graeber, 2014). If that is true, then my nursing experience is similar: moving from staff nurse to community nurse to research fellow, I have seen violence shift from the grotesquely physical to the more abstract or ideological, but the two permeate each other – both are violence, just as a mortgage, or even just the expectation of ownership, has as much power over a person as a crowbarred midnight eviction.

I want to illustrate that violence – from the direct and shocking moments of ward 'restraint' incidents, with their pleading, their shouted obscenities and weeping (the moment when I chased a terrified young woman through a carpark and caught her) to the violence found, for example, deep within *The Origins of*

Happiness (Clark et al, 2018) (see Gadsby (2017) for further discussion). In telling the story of my relationship with a man I will call John, I will show that even my attempts at 'working to change the system from within' contained awful violence.

I do not like to say, as some critics do, that reform of mental health nursing is impossible; I think of good moments and good colleagues and feel it betrays them. I worry that this chapter will feel that way too. But here is my truth, and perhaps it is theirs: almost every truly uplifting or liberating moment I experience with a 'mad' person is a moment in which psychiatry and the mental health system is subverted, usually explicitly. Therefore, this chapter is also violent. Some of what I write may be hurtful, especially to nurses. Maybe I never wanted to be that person; perhaps I always have been; I get tired of trying to know. But exercising power for ends that I hope are liberating is still a form of force, and when I helped the Critical Mental Health Nurses' Network into being it was not so we could merely be another psychiatry-bashing organisation; it was because I wanted to critically think about nursing and its context. I take comfort in this; the world of mental health is one of many competing 'monologues', and dialogue refuses what monologue aspires to (Frank, 2012). However much those recruited by monologues – stories that can only work if they are able to aggressively remove or discount others' views – may dislike dialogue, it is monologues that are the real source or conduit of violence. So writing that attempts to show alternative perspectives is never as violent as writing that excludes them.

Is this autoethnography? When writing this chapter, I repeatedly found that the philosophical arguments here are my personal identity and the personal stories are forms of argument. I think this is the result of the many beliefs expressed here about the storied nature of self and of nursing and a product of years of trying to view myself and the world as storied and inter-permeated, leaving me sometimes present to the world and yet also unable to point at much and call it 'me' – a sort of dispersed self. I write about what it is like finding within oneself the intersections of others' stories.

Three conversations

This need to write about violence I owe to three sets of conversations. The first two were interviews, held in 2014, with participants in my doctoral research. The two people, different and with differing experiences of mental health nurses (MHNs), were able to describe precisely their experiences of several kinds of violence and the untrustworthiness of MHNs.

For one of them, the violence was the full spectrum of everything permitted under the Mental Health Act (MHA): detention, forced polypharmacy (with highly undesirable effects) and community treatment orders, and also all the less visible forms of violence that are frequently part of mental health services, not least a wholly prejudicial set of diminished expectations about her future, bringing new forms of vulnerability.

For the other, the violence was a kind of isolation: his remarkable mental journeys had to be kept hidden from nurses. While MHNs 'monitored for symptoms' and even widened this to promote aspects of 'wellbeing' – supporting retention of involvement in higher education, physical activities and social opportunities – he continued, companionless, on a breath-taking and creative exploration with his voices and emotions, unaware that his questions and revelations were the stuff of international congresses, university philosophy departments, academic papers and impassioned debate. Although he considered MHNs to be nice people, he soon recognised that sharing this journey with them would lead to disaster, that complexity in his mind would equate with illness to them, and that coercion and loss of his future would be the likely result. *He* took care of *their* mental state. I have come to believe that this is common; our simplistic stories leave our service users having to channel their real lives into fairly useless false binaries and sanitised, dishonest versions of their actual experiences, in order to gain or retain any power. This has been going on a long time:

> What I am is a heretic who's recanted, and hereby in everyone's eyes saved his soul. Everyone's eyes but one, who knows deep down inside that all he has saved is his skin. I survive mainly by pleasing others. You do that to get out. To get out you figure out what they want you to say and then you say it with as much skill and originality as possible. (Pirsig, 1974)

Both interviewees exhibited remarkable courage. Their accounts of interactions with MHNs showed in-depth analysis of the systems of thought and organisation from which MHNs operate. Between them, their diagnoses described them in terms of faulty genes, faulty brain chemistry, poor choices, being manipulative and uncooperative and perhaps being incapable of genuine friendship. Meeting them as a researcher rather than a nurse contributed greatly to my growing realisation that MHNs are untrustworthy conduits of violence and that I have been this, too. Quite simply, they told me things they would not have told me as a nurse and these turned out to be very important things.

The final set of conversations followed a moment in June 2016 when, in a post to a Facebook mental health nursing group, a student MHN described their encounter with a ward 'control and restraint incident'. They had found it upsetting. Similar posts had been made before and responses to it were predictable: that this was a necessary but sad part of the job, an action of 'last resort'; that often service users were grateful afterwards and it was 'in their best interests' (about half the comments used this phrase). A few comments could be summarised as, 'If you can't take the heat, get out of the kitchen.' However, it was the *rate* of responses that was striking: at the time there were more than 13,000 people in the group,[1] and comments came at a rate of two a second. Although there was not much originality, there was a great need to speak out.

---

1. I have since been banned, with no apparent awareness of the irony, for raising issues over censorship.

I then had an extended conversation with about 15 members of the survivor and activist group, Recovery in the Bin. Many had experienced nursing violence first-hand, and some found it impossible to describe, explaining that both restraint and its constant threat were now only understandable to them as a form of torture from which they had not fully escaped. The group provided a nuanced discussion that helped me recognise that, within nursing violence (I promised I would use that term), there are perhaps three related areas to discuss:

1. a few bad apples?
2. 'genre violence'
3. the world is violent.

With reference to the first, conversations with service recipients, nurses and university tutors in charge of student placements lead me to believe that there are nurses who seek out violent roles and situations, perhaps to form machismo cultures that they find energising and enjoyable in some way, and even sexually arousing (I am afraid that this was reported by female 'patients' in more than one testimony of control and restraint, when they were aware that a 'restrainer' had an erection). One MHN from my own control and restraint training (in 2001) seemed over-excited and did not understand that the group agreed to be practised on in various scenarios but not during the coffee break; he was asked to leave. The frequency with which one finds these aspects reported in survivor groups and staff groups is not reflected in the literature about nursing and violence.

There are serious questions to be asked about how people who may be attracted to the direct experience of conflict find themselves a place in the MHN profession, but it is not my intention to explore this first aspect of nursing violence, despite its alarming nature. I could write as if violence were intrinsic to these MHNs, and that contradicts my beliefs and much of this chapter. I am glad that I will not be focusing on this question. Of course, I want to say that not all nurses are like this, but in fact 'not all nurses' was precisely the title that a member of our conversation gave to the manner in which this theme is generally downplayed.

Instead, I want to explore the second and third categories, hoping to illustrate their interwoven nature. To begin, I will introduce John, whose story is central to this chapter.

John

It was my first community job, with my first caseload, in 2004. I was taken to meet John by his previous community MHN. The MHN parked the car facing away from the flats, telling me this was a necessary precaution because John had once chased him. He told me that my job with John was simple: I was to see him every week and make sure he was taking his lithium. At the first sign that John was becoming unwell, I was to arrange to have him detained. 'Don't fuck about,' he said. I heard this, but I was *working to change the system from within*. I had a new manager, a social worker, who told me that she 'lived for social inclusion'. The anti-medical stance that I began to favour at university was being bolstered by early contact with the Hearing Voices Network; the word 'recovery' was in the air and I thought this was the revolution I was waiting for.

I went to see John every week and spent hours with him. Although very different, we hit it off. I am good at that. Yes, I cared for him, and looked forward to seeing him. We built a trusting relationship. We laughed together, listened to music, drank tea. He showed me his UV cupboard of cannabis plants and I told him I would pretend I hadn't seen it.[2] I wasn't just there to 'monitor for signs of relapse'; I was *in the recovery business*. I didn't badger him about meds. We had a few ups and downs, but his mental health seemed to me to be improving and his psychiatrist agreed. This is not a story about my naïvety leading to not taking a 'genuine illness' seriously enough. I got his medication reduced slightly, with hopes for more reductions in the future; I helped him see his GP for some other health issues; we did some budgeting work. Gradually, we started to talk more about what he did with his time, about his skills. He was adamant that he would not do volunteer work. If he was going to work, he would be paid. We went to the job centre.

It was my first time in a job centre. Despite his habitual bravado, John seemed vulnerable and nervous. I helped him talk with an advisor. It was absolutely hopeless. Even though he had a good practical skill that is normally well paid, if he got any work he would be financially worse off than on benefits. I felt deflated.

After that, John didn't want to talk about work, but in the following weeks he suddenly started talking about his ex-partner and children, with whom he was not allowed contact. He told me he thought about his children constantly. I supported him to visit a building society where, I discovered, he had put aside nearly £100,000 from years of Disability Living Allowance (and drug-dealing) for his children. Just before I went on a week's annual leave, we started talking about family mediation. John was thoughtful but positive; it felt hopeful. But three days later, while I was on holiday, John killed himself.

I grieved for John. I will never forget sitting at his funeral, wishing I was someone else. Part of my sadness was that I had not been able to prevent what had happened. I also just missed him. All my reports over nearly two years of visits were examined and I was interviewed as part of an 'unexpected death audit'. My work was described as 'exemplary' and John's consultant told me I had helped improve the last period of his life. Over the next couple of weeks, I was frequently tearful in the office. I felt a little resentful when colleagues told me I should go home, but mostly everyone did their best to support me. They said I should not blame myself,

---

2. At the time I had a motorbike and years later I got another one. I had kept the same helmet, the one that had sat next to me on John's sofa a decade before. The first time I rode the new bike, the wind blew through the helmet's air vents and filled my head with the potent smell of John's home-grown 'Christmas Trees'.

that John had never been thought to be a high risk of suicide. His mother told me that no one could have done more for him.

After a few weeks, I felt I needed to go to a cathedral I had once visited; I hoped for some kind of resolution. I sat in an empty side chapel for a long time, before speaking John's name out loud. I hoped that act would leave him there, but it didn't. Years passed. Not long ago I told someone else about John, and I think it was then that I began to understand something new about his story.

I thought that John's recovery would be found in helping him see that he could make positive changes in his life, and that much of his so-called 'mental illness' was really about sitting around believing himself to be unwell (fully understandable, given the efforts taken to persuade him of this), and not doing things that contribute to mental wellbeing. I thought that, if he had something valuable to do, became more organised, managed his finances, ate more healthily and used fewer drugs, he would be on the way to getting better. In one sense I was right: when he killed himself, everyone agreed he was the best he had been for years.

Before describing ways in which I feel I was naïve, I want to restate that people around me did not think so. I also want to affirm that it is not wrong to support someone to try to make positive changes in their life. Five years on from John's death, I was asked to speak at my trust-wide nursing conference about using the Recovery Star (Triangle, undated), of which I was an early adopter. I was essentially acting as a life-coach, and others seemed impressed: *de-medicalised, de-institutionalised, recovery-orientated nursing.* A senior manager came up to me with tears in her eyes and told me how brilliant she thought my presentation was. If I had been asked about John at that moment, I would have said that hope is sometimes dangerous, but did people really want to work in ways that did not promote it?

Genre violence

Many terms are used to describe and define 'narrative', often rather loosely. For my purposes, I follow Arthur Frank (2012) in using 'story' as a temporal explanation of particular circumstances that are often imbued with the workings of wider narratives, which often exist more at a cultural level. The phrase 'genre violence' is one I have adapted from the work of historian Philip Smith (2010), and here, one could say, he uses 'genre' to try to categorise and understand the workings of narratives. A war historian, he shows that, prior to military engagement, there are 'genre wars', in which certain forms of narrative (he focuses especially on the narratives invoked by national newspapers) are inflated or deflated. He offers a diagram to show what might be taking place:

Figure 1.1: The structural model of genre (Smith, 2010)

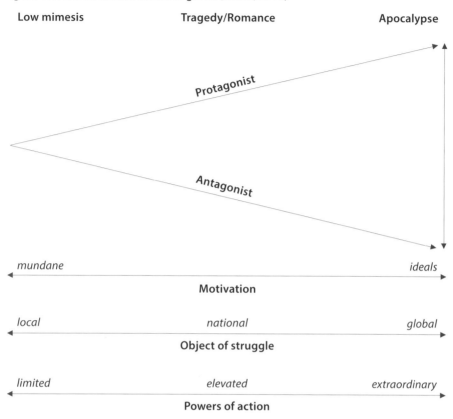

For Smith, an apocalyptic genre is required for a democracy to go to war; for me, something at least approaching this is required for nurses to be violent (although within such genres the word 'violence' is seldom used). Exactly what are the blows struck by MHNs engaged in 'genre violence'? Perhaps that is the least helpful way of articulating the question; the powers that come from inflating or deflating genres through connection to certain narratives are a wider issue that concerns the very nature of self, agency and power in society. I hope that what follows will show why the sense that many MHNs have, that their daily struggle is to weigh up best interests against self-determination , is not an adequate understanding of the powers at play.

MHNs, like everyone else, do not simply 'wield' narratives 'at' people; they become connected to them or are recruited by them, are conduits for them, are employed by them; they are even constituted of them, as well as, at times, deliberately performing them for a purpose. This is why the three headings identified in my conversation cannot really be held apart. Many of these narratives begin and end elsewhere and, since we all have this kind of three-fold relationship with narratives, it could not be otherwise. In fact, it is this idea that really forms the essence of my argument about 'genre violence'; it is frequently the case that the stories many

MHNs perform *hide or deny* the three-fold nature of service recipients'[3] experience of violence. Others recognise this same three-fold relationship: for example, Galtung's conflict triangle, which divides violence into 'direct', 'cultural' and 'structural' forms, each reinforcing the other (Galtung, 1969).

Within the narratives that meet in the role of the MHN is the legitimation of extraordinary powers of action: the MHA and more. This includes enforced drugs, control and restraint, control and restraint with 'stress positions', locked units and seclusion, and the coercion that is either direct or more cultural/structural in all of the above over all service recipients, regardless of their 'MHA status'. As one might have predicted from the volume of responses on the Facebook page, most of these activities are present in nursing literature, but there nurses are rarely considered to be the instigator: they are the regretful responder, creating safety and care, not danger and aggression, acting as a last resort, perhaps even heroically, within Smith's tragic/romantic genre.

Although there is an increasingly well-articulated critique of the MHA as a form of legalised discrimination (Sapey, 2018; Sidley, 2015), it is not present in nursing literature about 'restraint', in which illness models dominate; the efficacy of treatments is taken for granted, and the morality of the law itself is largely unquestioned. It seems to me that MHNs should maintain a flexible relationship with the belief systems of psychiatry, but unquestionably they find their strongest and simplest faith at those times in which they are violent; just as in Smith's diagram, they need to become connected to its moral polarisation, idealistic drive, global reach and powers of action. Violence and nursing seem so far apart conceptually that we must be interested in all stories that nurses use (or that use nurses) to understand and process their violent actions. Biomedical narratives play a part and we should allow that overlap to inform us about the philosophical work of biomedicine for nurses, but the narratives are wider.

It is not merely that narratives permit, enable, justify or even valorise violence; they are also violent themselves. Smith's work is about how wars may be initiated by democracies, and one can see that genres must be connected to violence because they have such bearing on agency – not only on how much agency is available, but to whom.[4]

Simple stories may do a lot of this work. I once explained to a student nurse that it was best to say (about a service recipient), 'They have become upset,' rather than, 'I have upset them.' This took the narrative from being about protagonists and antagonists, located within at least two people in a set of particular circumstances, and *deflated the genre* (towards the left of Smith's diagram), making the emotions the

---

3. Here I am executing a narrative move of my own – an act of rebellion against the story 'service user'. 'Service user' connects to narratives of certain kinds of agency, 'service recipient' to different ones. Neither is neutral and both do the typical work of narratives of altering who or what may be considered responsible (Frank, 2012). Just as Smith shows, agency and morality are at stake.

4. Agency, according to many philosophers post-Anscombe (2000), is not a property of individuals but a part of descriptions and narratives. There is a very long line of philosophy surrounding this idea, with its own contested areas. I have been most heavily influenced by Ian Hacking, Michael White and Arthur Frank. Each owes much to the work of Anscombe, Michel Foucault and Mikhail Bakhtin.

property of the individual and not the result of the interaction. In so doing, it made the emotions mundane, suitable for reclassification as personal pathology, limited the sense of morality and the powers of action available and so made it less possible to hold the nurse accountable for the person becoming upset.[5] The localisation of 'They have become upset' makes it more difficult to consider whether this is something about hospitals, cultures or the world, and to make connections with the past or the future, because that would risk inflating the genre with new players and moral questions. Imagine me knocking quietly on the bedroom door, an hour later. I say, with my caring voice and concerned face, 'I noticed you became upset this afternoon and I wonder if there is anything I can do to help?' Is that not a scene of violence? I like to think I would have been genuinely caring, but can a compassionate outlook mitigate such violence? Or does it make it yet harder to resist?

My caring manner did its work on John. The stories I used similarly all worked to change responsibility. The key realisation for me now is this: I suspect that John had an accurate understanding of the way that society viewed him and his future, while I believed some kind of fantasy. Apart from the one he was already taking, there are not many viable roles for someone like John in our society: single, male, middle-aged, unemployed, subject to a court injunction, on high doses of medication, with a history of detained admissions and an extensive criminal record. I may have been right that his problems did not have to be medicalised, that a medical view was disabling him, damaging his health and keeping him locked in an endless pattern. After years of further study, I am surer than ever that it is contentious (scientifically, ethically) to say that the differences between John and me were driven by biology, even if they were sometimes experienced in the body.

I was 'doing recovery', promoting a 'healthy lifestyle', trying to 'instil hope'; I was using 'motivational interviewing' and ideas from 'solution-focused therapy', promoting an 'internal locus of control'. But I think I achieved several toxic things, exacerbated by my good relationship with John; the fact that my fantasy was so reasonably and amicably expressed just made it harder to resist. In essence, I was trying to generate recovery from within the body, thoughts, feelings, habits and decision-making of John. I more or less assumed that John had the same experience of power in society as I did; that society was a level playing field, that life is a blank slate.[6] I recreated the differences between us into things for which

---

5. Arguably, for all characters. However, once thus storied, the service user can be subject to other stories that give mental health professionals extraordinary powers.

6. Years later, after completing my master's degree, I was unemployed for six months. I never expected this as a nurse, but I was new to the area and the economic climate meant that all local vacancies were subject to internal redeployment. Agency nursing roles were few and, as well as having moral concerns about them, I felt low in confidence. As time went by, I realised I would have to consider taking Job Seekers Allowance, or think more radically. When I left my previous nursing role, I told my colleagues I would work at a supermarket if I had to, but they were now only taking people unpaid, under the government's 'workfare' scheme. The JobCentre Plus website claimed to have thousands of jobs. I entered my details, my posh school grades, my university degrees. The top match was 'cornrow technician'. I never even go to the hairdresser, just buzz-cut it all off, that's my level. It was terrifying. I had to use every trick I knew to keep myself positive, yet I think three days out of seven were just awful.

he could (and ought to) take responsibility. In fact, my work contained precisely the aspects identified by Harper and Speed in their critique of 'recovery': the individualisation and obscuring of social problems and a model still based on personal deficits. I think I can agree with them that my work was 'founded on a model of identity politics which displaces and marginalises the need for social, political and economic redistribution to address many of the underlying causes of emotional distress' (Harper & Speed, 2012: 9). Arguably my recovery-orientated practice contained one-to-one neoliberal propaganda. It now feels far too simple to say that I was working to promote hope, since I was a conduit for ideas that John saw to be hopeless.

Later, I worked in early intervention services, hoping of course that, by meeting people before they had got into the 'John' kind of patterns, I would have more chance of promoting recovery. I was not wholly wrong, but I still believed in a conceited version of individual autonomy and I can see now that all my efforts showed I thought that autonomy and health were the same thing and that both were personal attributes.

Many nursing stories about service recipients are stories of 'low mimesis'. We could use Smith's chart to explore any number of nursing stories and discover that narratives available to service recipients that begin in the middle or to the right of the chart are often shifted to the left by MHNs. We speak of 'behaviour', rather than 'action'; we discourage narrativity with CBT; we try to promote personal resilience instead of societal justice (social injustice being a synonym for Galtung's structural violence), for – a key point – 'mental health' itself is already a very low mimesis narrative among the set of narratives about distress in society. It supports MHNs to use stories such as 'best interests' and its many supporting assumptions, or what might be called stories of mythologised future gratitude: the person will eventually thank the nurses for that which they may currently detest. By contrast, many stories we have about ourselves are towards the right of Smith's chart, imbued with wider purpose and inner morality. It all smacks of Orwell's famous quote, perhaps the pithiest statement about narratives and power: 'Who controls the past controls the future. Who controls the present controls the past' (Orwell, 2004/1949).

The powerful decide the genre in which stories may be performed and this is the source of their continuing power and the expression of it.

The narrative I invested in most heavily is another with a sleight-of-hand effect on responsibility, but less immediately obvious: *working to change the system from within*. This is a story to which many nurses with critical perspectives are attracted. On a daily basis, it has been highly motivating and certainly created moments when I felt I did some good work, which are terribly important if you retain strong reservations about the helpfulness of the mental health system as a whole. Yet, viewed across two nearly decades as an MHN, it appears mostly to be a self-protective story in which all the things I do that are good are because *I am good* and all the things I do that are against my values are because *others are bad*. This is one of the reasons why it is important to write this chapter from the position of one who is also its target; otherwise I would be writing to distance myself from violence in the same way once more. That I *do* want to distance myself from many nursing narratives and practices is therefore confessional rather than merely critical.

These stories are in addition to the ones that Bonnie Burstow describes in her institutional ethnography, one of the most notable of which is the notion of psychiatry being perpetually on the cusp of a humane scientific breakthrough, a breakthrough making the violence of the present excusable because it already belongs to the past (Burstow, 2015). I teach psychiatrists about the critical ideas that surround their profession, about which they are, in my experience, strikingly ignorant. Confirming Burstow's finding, their strongest sense is that those who criticise psychiatry do so because they do not realise that the profession has *moved on*.

Hui's research into violence in a secure mental health setting finds nurses engaged in a variety of narratives that create cultures in which no one is allowed to dissent from or avoid this violence. She describes nurses undertaking hard emotional labour to be able to continue with what they view as contradictory to their motivations for joining the profession and hiding this aspect of their work from friends and family, while knowing that it is plain frightening but nevertheless something they had to force themselves to get used to (Hui, 2016). Throughout, Hui's moving work conveys the sense that nurses choose this kind of numbing or 'unstorying' (dissociation?) in order to continue to do this work, and that it is also one of the achievements of the 'They have become upset' story.

All such narratives are vital for MHNs in order for them to maintain the belief that they are nice people. I expect this chapter to generate numerous negative responses: that it is somehow not nice, that nurses are only trying to help, that they are being pragmatic and caring and that they are acting in good faith. Collectively upholding those stories is part of our violence. This is just the beginning. I have witnessed many kinds of conversations by nurses about the word 'care'. Some insist that there is a crucial difference between 'caring about' and 'caring for' others; that being *the caring profession* is our very identity. If I get branded as being uncaring I can be dismissed, I am no longer one of us, not a real nurse. We have *models of care*, we *provide care*, and nurses, according to the findings of the inquiry into the Mid-Staffordshire Hospital (Francis, 2013), *failed* to care.[7]

These phrases feature heavily in our textbooks and training. I know MHNs who feel that we should speak more openly about *love* and, while I find I often appreciate their motives, I agree with Thomas Foth (2013) that we will never address our capacity for harm while we speak of 'care' in this way. 'Love', like 'care', is too depoliticised. For Foth, we neglect to realise that care contains an asymmetrical power relationship. Nurses assisting the deaths of those described as having a 'life unworthy of living' during Germany's Third Reich felt this was part of nursing work

---

7. This is not to say that this is the only pertinent finding of the report, which viewed the problems as being as much structural and cultural as direct, to put it in Galtung's language. It should not surprise us that those elements have been neglected in nurse training; one of the 'six Cs' should undoubtedly be 'capitalism'.

and consistent with caring; they quite literally held people's heads while they were killed (Foth, 2013: 284). Readers who now find themselves shaking their heads at the thought of *those* nurses are 'othering' in the way Foth describes; they should instead notice the dark possibilities of care narratives.

It's not uncommon to find mental health nursing described as a complex balancing act between caring and controlling, advocacy and correction (although not many nurses use the word 'correction'), between a role for the person and a role for the state. MHNs clearly understand something of the conflicts within ourselves, yet these distinctions fall down and continue to make our violence more difficult to understand: nice people doing nasty things. Foth shows that those killed during the Nazi regime often became invisible months or even years before their deaths, disappearing from the records – a chilling example of Arthur Frank's assertion that 'a life that is not fully narratable is vulnerable to devaluation' (Frank, 2012: 75). Within the Hearing Voices Movement, it is repeatedly reported that people can spend years in the care of nurses without ever being asked about their actual experiences, without their lives becoming narratable. Violence that is not fully narratable is liable to be called something else; it is not really nursing, not really *us,* and a caring core of us remains unchanged by it; the violence is not part of our story. This is not to argue that correction or control is *always* undesirable (that is another question), but it suggests that having it carried out by teams of people recruited into self-serving *decontesting* ideologies,[8] *being the caring profession*, is dangerous. John did not live under the Nazis. John lived and died under 'the recovery model'.

MHNs and other professionals are socialised into ways of relating to ourselves and others that create the kind of deep irony I first read about in the work of Lisa Blackman (2015): we always accuse the 'mentally ill' of errors at the interface between body and world. We do this in many ways: saying that inner states are *incongruent* with outside events; that voices heard are mistaken for external ones but are really internal; that the past or future somehow permeate the present wrongly; that external events are perceived as relevant or symbolic in incorrect ways; that the main issue is that the person fails to accept that they are responsible for their own inner world and their actions.

We also find that their behaviours may be *splitting* (by which we mean they are using stories for sanctifying some and vilifying others for a purpose). However, our own errors in each of these regards are so grievous that, in fact, it is really *we* who most consistently exhibit all that of which we accuse others – of a deep confusion and twisted sense of 'individual autonomy' leading to scientifically bizarre and dehumanising reductionism of others' distress (on the one hand) and a 'personality disordered' inability to take responsibility for the system of which we may claim to be victims but of which we are the largest facilitators (on the other).

---

8. That is, ideologies that contain within them aspects that attempt to inoculate themselves from contest, a key part of the work on ideology of political philosopher Michael Freeden (eg. Freeden, 1994).

We frequently work within models that fail to make sense of connections between inner and outer experience, past, present and future, not just accidentally but as the very basis of their appeal. The 'psychotic symptom' of 'depersonalisation' is clearly found in narratives we rely on to make our violent action possible; the sinister story that might be called 'This isn't them'. We can thus be violent towards an 'it' (illness), not a person, with 'treatments' being a sort of contemporary exorcism.

'This isn't them' is frequently used in meetings to make decisions about prescriptions and about the MHA. It is internalised by service recipients as 'This isn't me', or even just 'the illness'. We strongly encourage this, calling it 'insight', although for other service recipients (or the same ones but at a later stage in our relationship) we may describe it as a failure to take responsibility: an externalised locus of control. For recipients of mental health services, responsibility is an unwinnable game. We are the smiling face of the violence of mental health services, the very essence of duplicity, the often well-meaning employees of a system that raises some profoundly disturbing questions about its political affiliations. Yet we so often decide that it is those we nurse who are incapable of 'true' friendship; that they choose only to be nice when they feel they will gain from it. By the time we have convinced ourselves that we are working to change the system from within, we can be part of things we know to be wrong and shrug them off, facilitating the continuation of that system better than anyone.

Yet in all of this I run the risk of grouping MHNs together in ways that are themselves violent. There have always been nurses who have resisted these ways of thinking. Some of them, like me, have responded by putting themselves into roles where other nurses do the directly violent bits. At some point we have to acknowledge who we are as a whole profession (we do, after all, take the money).

The world is violent

Contributors to the Recovery in the Bin conversation were more generous in describing nurses as (like themselves) caught up in forms of structural violence that they mirror or pass on to service recipients, and in this we are not so clearly responsible. If the above section feels uncomfortably damning, here at least might be our momentary reprieve. This was the much broader understanding within the conversation: that the violence found within and produced by certain ideologies may begin far beyond the narrow world of 'mental health'. David Smail labels this 'distal power', 'over the power horizon'. He would have seen the above paragraphs as reflecting the 'illusion' that proximal experiences and interactions are the most causal in our experience (Smail, 2001: 228). One member of the conversation said:

> Nursing is a feminised labour, and so both sides are oppressed, but the
> cared-for are the oppressed of the oppressed when they are subject to
> violent restraint.

Similarly, Alec Grant, a mental health nurse, writes that:

> … institutional psychiatric treatment spaces create possibilities for already damaged bodies to perpetuate unkindness on other bodies. Mental health nurses and other state psychiatric workers are systematically stripped of their capacities to be kind through, among other things, being neoliberalised, classed, gendered, Psydisciplined and socialised to institutional psychiatric custom and practice. (Grant, 2015)

One of the first conversations reported in this chapter (my research participant who had to hide his real thoughts from nurses who were nice yet untrustworthy) illustrates that violence that begins elsewhere may either be passed on through nurses or, should a nurse perhaps be more reflective, be caught in the body of the nurse. Nurses are made untrustworthy by the conceptual conflicts of the multi-storied worlds in which they operate. For example, they must report to others what is told to them in confidence, and those others may re-interpret complexity as more illness, often causing further losses of autonomy. Service recipients soon learn this. The interfaces between conflicting narratives can be embodied in the nurse, sometimes surfacing as the personal duplicity I describe above, and perhaps they are not necessarily our personal attributes at all. As a nurse, I often choose to act duplicitously towards colleagues rather than service recipients, hiding my real relationships with service recipients. The genre violence is then held or role-played between myself and colleagues. This has fed my 'working to change the system from within' story and a certain amount of paranoia, but it suggests to me that the duplicity is not exactly mine but something inherent in the systems of thought I work within. Violence could become focused into me more directly (disciplinary actions?), were the extent of my collaboration with service recipients known, yet I cannot help but seek this collaboration; it is what supportive exploration between equals demands.

Nowhere have I found this theme more evident than at Hearing Voices Movement congresses. I have cried until my eyes felt damaged. Powerful stories of recovery – even the sense of guilt I might feel as a professional at such a meeting – do not explain the extent of my emotions. I think it is that I experience a few golden moments of the explanatory power of a single story[9] and the conflict is temporarily clearly outside of my body. The feeling is religious.[10]

---

9. It is not right to say that the Hearing Voices Movement presents a 'single story'. The one I respond to most in this way is the perspective that voice hearing is a 'common human variation', subject to pathologisation in a similar way that homosexuality has been.

10. I do mean religious and there are voice-hearers who convert and then lose the faith, as I do a little on my return home and as I have got to know more details (it is always details that puncture the elevated genres found on the right of Smith's diagram). If that sounds very critical, I hope it is clear from much of what else I write that I view medical psychiatry much less respectfully, as much easier to puncture with details. The academic world knows psychiatry is a normalising ideology and not a medical science, and is laughing at it (see Kriss, 2013).

There is nothing unique about mental health services or the bodies of nurses. Genre violence pervades the world; we must ask if all this violence within us is merely a symptom of wider conflict, exploitation and 'othering'. In critical literature in the UK, the most common means to lay out such an argument would be through showing that psychiatry is a practice of normalisation dressed as medicine (a Foucauldian stance taken up by many), wrapped in neoliberal economics (eg. Metzl & Kirkland, 2010;[11] McKeown, Wright & Mercer, 2017) and unsupportable notions of autonomy and individuality. Such arguments are of crucial importance. They suggest that the practice of MHNs, far from being 'autonomously professional', with our own 'evidence base', is a reflection of the politics of the state. It seems to me that generally MHNs have become bored with that accusation, without ever seriously engaging with it. They just tell themselves they mean well. In Grant's words above, there is an implication that MHNs and the recipients of nursing are locked together in some way, that the only release will be a collective one. There is also the implication that MHNs are significantly unaware of the meaning and context of their work (McKeown, Wright & Mercer, 2017). This is transparently clear in my story about John; I had no idea of the politics of my perspectives, the neoliberal selfhood, and nor did anyone else.

Medication in the sacrifice zones

For me, the writer who most effectively links the smallest scale human ability to 'other' people (like my 'They became upset' story, 'This isn't them' and 'Not all nurses') with massive global consequences (and vice versa) is Naomi Klein. She writes about a world of sacrificial people and sacrificial places required to continue the unsustainable 'extractivist' needs of free-market capitalism (Klein, 2015). The sacrifice zones, she says, are expanding. Just as US drone strikes in Syria map uncannily onto changing lines of aridity (Klein, 2016), so I want to say that 'neuroleptic bombing' maps onto the impoverished land and most densely urbanised and otherwise marginalised people: medication in the sacrifice zones. Psychology is not necessarily to be preferred (Coles, Keenan & Diamond, 2013: 114).

I have already made the claim that MHNs often promote low-mimesis genres, the left of Smith's chart. This suits the status quo that Klein shows us *must* be challenged, and 'evidence-based practice' and 'mental health' are low-mimesis stories. It is the genre that wants us to imagine business as usual, that recreates distress as individual, 'efficient' 'interventions' 'delivered' to promote distraction and 'coping', painting health as if separate from morality, facts as if separate from values. Keep calm and carry on. This low-mimesis storying sees experience as driven from the inside outwards (because it makes distress a plotless happening),

11. In the US, critical literature is rather different, and part of the reason I go on to focus on the work of Naomi Klein and climate change is that it suggests reasons why some of the right-wing libertarian critical psychiatry in the US is unlikely to bring the emancipation required.

a perfect match for the ever-present bio-determinism of psychiatry and the promotion of right-wing notions of freedom.

For Klein, it is time to see all these as linked issues with the same root causes and the same beneficiaries. Climate change is the crisis of militarism, industrialisation and neoliberalism and is forcing all of us to fight 'genre wars'. When looked at through this lens, mental health services play an important role in these genre wars and they thrive in the sacrifice zones. History is unlikely to view us as the good guys. I feel awful about describing the sum of our actions in this way, effectively placing us within the industrial-military complex. Once again, I think of some great colleagues working with sincerity, perseverance, humour and courage, and I know they would want to point, as I am tempted, to other moments that felt like breakthroughs. I know too that members of my conversation with Recovery in the Bin, even people who have felt tortured by nurses, would not wish there to be no nurses, only that they would be different. We need to find a collective voice to say that we are being asked to bomb lines of aridity. We need to see the emancipation of ourselves and of those we nurse as the same project and to understand that, since all stories suit someone, they are inherently political. We need to understand the work of stories in new ways.

What should I have done differently with John? Now, I would try to spend more time talking with him about his past and his family much earlier on. I would try to work with an appreciation that the differences between us are more about society than bodies; to try to 'externalise the problem narrative', 'bringing the world into therapy' (White & Epston, 1990: 50). I would allow and encourage talking about problems for a long time before engaging in bright conversation about possible futures. I would hope to find ways to connect John with other people with similar experiences. I do not know that I would have been successful, whether that would have made John feel less alone and more able to access a different future. Possibly, he would have merely gone from being a victim of his body to a victim of society. Fundamentally, I now feel that, by the time I sat talking with John, most of the important things were already beyond Smail's power horizon. Writing this chapter is what I would have done differently about John.

References

Anscombe GEM (2000). *Intention* (2nd ed). Cambridge, MA: Harvard University Press.

Blackman L (2015). Affective politics, debility and hearing voices: towards a feminist politics of ordinary suffering. *Feminist Review 111*(1): 25–41.

Burstow B (2015). *Psychiatry and the Business of Madness: an ethical and epistemological accounting.* Basingstoke: Palgrave Macmillan.

Clark AE, Flèche S, Layard R, Powdthavee N, Ward G (2018). *The Origins of Happiness: the science of well-being over the life course.* Princeton, NJ: Princeton University Press.

Coles S, Keenan S, Diamond B (eds) 2013. *Madness Contested: power and practice.* Ross-on-Wye: PCCS Books.

Foth T (2013). Understanding 'caring' through biopolitics: the case of nurses under the Nazi regime. *Nursing Philosophy* 14(4): 284–294.

Francis R (Chair) (2013). *Report of the Mid Staffordshire NHS Foundation Trust Public Inquiry*. London: the Stationery Office.

Frank AW (2012). *Letting Stories Breathe: a socio-narratology*. Chicago, IL: University of Chicago Press.

Freeden M (1994). Political concepts and ideological morphology. *Journal of Political Philosophy* 2(2): 140–164.

Gadsby J (2017). *The Layard Report*. [Blog.] The Critical Mental Health Nurses' Network. https://criticalmhnursing.org/2017/01/23/the-layard-report (accessed 7 June 2018).

Galtung J (1969). Violence, peace and peace research. *Journal of Peace Research* 6(3): 167–191.

Graeber D (2014). *Debt: the first 5,000 years*. Brooklyn, NY: Melville House.

Grant A (2015). *Perpetuating Unkindness*. [Blog.] Critical Mental Health Nurses' Network. https://criticalmhnursing.org/2015/06/25/perpetuating-unkindness (accessed 25 June 2018).

Harper D, Speed E (2012). Uncovering recovery: the resistible rise of recovery and resilience. *Studies in Social Justice* 6(1): 9–25.

Hui A (2016). Mental health workers' experiences of using coercive measures: 'You can't tell people who don't understand'. In: Vollm B, Nedopil N (eds). *The Use of Coercive Measures in Forensic Psychiatric Care: legal, ethical and practical challenges*. London: Springer (pp241–254).

Klein N (2016). Let them drown. *London Review of Books* 38(11): 11–14.

Klein N (2015). *This Changes Everything: capitalism vs the climate*. London: Penguin.

Kriss S (2013). *The Book of Lamentations*. [Online.] The New Inquiry; 18 October. http://thenewinquiry.com/essays/book-of-lamentations (accessed 20 January 2014).

McKeown M, Wright K, Mercer D (2017). Care planning: a neoliberal three card trick. *Journal of Psychiatric and Mental Health Nursing* 24(6): 451–460.

Metzl JM, Kirkland A (2010). *Against Health: how health became the new morality*. New York, NY: University Press.

Orwell G (2004/1949). *1984*. Harmondsworth: Penguin Classics.

Pirsig R (1974). *Zen and the Art of Motorcycle Maintenance: an inquiry into values*. London: Vintage Classics.

Sapey B (2018). Madness and the law. In: Wright K, McKeown M (eds). *Essentials of Mental Health Nursing*. London: Sage (pp138–149).

Sidley G (2015). *Tales from the Madhouse: an insider critique of psychiatric services*. Ross-on-Wye: PCCS Books.

Smail DJ (2001). *The Nature of Unhappiness*. London: Robinson.

Smith P (2010). *Why War? The cultural logic of Iraq, the Gulf War and Suez*. Chicago, IL: University of Chicago Press.

The Religious Society of Friends (2013). *Quaker Faith & Practice* (5th ed). London: Quakers in Britain.

Triangle (undated). *The Outcomes Star for Adults Managing their Mental Health*. [Online.] Triangle. www.outcomesstar.org.uk/mental-health (accessed 5 October 2016).

White M, Epston D (1990). *Narrative Means to Therapeutic Ends*. New York: WW Norton & Co.

2 | Moving around the hyphens: a critical meta-autoethnographic performance

Alec Grant

The important question

A classroom in a university in the south of England in 2016. Thirty-six BSc mental health nurse students in the last months of their final year. Dr Grant, their teacher for the afternoon. The topic: Working in Partnership.

Alec: Okay, let me ask you a question. A very important question. In my view, the most important question. What is your understanding of the following social psychological phenomena: confirmation bias, fundamental attribution error, and actor-observer effect?

Feeling a little nervous, I pace around with a hint of a smile on my face. Most of them won't know the answer to this question. They never do.

Students: (…)

Oh Christ, here we go again. The only thing I can hear is my own breathing and footsteps. Surely one of them must have an inkling.

Alec: Can anyone have a stab at answering this question? Come on, don't be shy.

Students: (…)

Right, get it together, Dr Grant. Be nice. Not their fault. Don't swear.

Alec: Have you heard of these terms? In any of your lectures or reading or practice placements over the last three years?

Students: (…)

What the fuck do they teach them? They're mostly bright kids. I know they are.

Alec: Okay, let me explain.

Moving into fourth gear. Hope I take some of them with me.

Alec: When mental health workers act on the basis of confirmation bias, they selectively attend to the people they are supposed to be caring for in response to what these people do and say. This enables mental health workers to develop theories about these people – about who they are, and why they are who they are. Many mental health workers will then in a circular way interpret what these people subsequently do and say on the basis of these theories. These theories usually coincide with, or are informed by, the functional psychiatric diagnoses of institutional psychiatry, which turn the extremes of human misery into 'mental illnesses'.

However, functional psychiatric diagnoses are about as real as fairies. There are no fairies. There are no mental illnesses (Grant, 2015a; Smith & Grant, 2016).

When mental health workers act on the basis of fundamental attribution error, they assume that the way the people they are supposed to be caring for act – in acute ward and other environments – is typical of the way they always act, how they have always acted and, frequently, how they are likely to act in the future. This confirms the institutional psychiatric theories of who these people are. Mental health workers discount situational factors that might explain their behaviour – such as being in an acute ward or having lived with people and places that make their lives a misery or the fact that they are experiencing a major interruption of their life stories (Frank, 2011; Grant, 2013; Grant & Leigh-Phippard, 2014; Short, 2011).

When mental health workers act on the basis of actor-observer effect, they tend to excuse away their own behaviour, even though this may be frequently bad towards the people they are supposed to be caring for (Grant, Biley & Walker, 2011). If those people act in a way that annoys mental health workers, however, their behaviour will be explained in accordance with the theory of who they are, who they always have been and who they are always likely to be. This theory is frequently likely be based on non-existent 'mental illnesses' (Grant, 2015a; Smith & Grant, 2016), and also may be overlain with moral judgments about their character – for example, 'attention seeking' or 'manipulative' (Grant & Leigh Phippard, 2014; Grant, Leigh-Phippard & Short, 2015; Short, 2011).

Confirmation bias, fundamental attribution error and actor-observer effect can all be seen in action in the classic and seminal experiment conducted by Rosenhan (1973) and his colleagues, which some of you might have heard of or read about?

A couple are nodding their heads in slow recognition. Good.

Alec: Okay, what do you think the relevance is of these concepts for your own practice as mental health nurses?

Student (Ben): We might keep people locked into a kind of forced identity or something?

Good. At least a few are on board. Breathing slowing down.

Alec: We call that 'narrative entrapment' (Grant, 2013; Grant, Leigh-Phippard & Short, 2015). How would you like someone to do that to you, Ben?

Ben: It would be horrible.

Student (Lucy): But surely this happens less in community mental health, Alec?

Alec: Maybe, but it still happens. A mental health nurse might get a referral from a GP that describes the person referred as 'having agoraphobia'. Now, many GPs and other referrers don't know 'agoraphobics' from aardvarks. Despite this, community nurses often take the description of the person being referred at face value, and then act towards them from that point on as though this definition is absolutely true.

Or one group in a mental health service – say, a day hospital – might refer a person for specialist, cognitive behavioural help, on the basis of problems that are often assumed rather than accurate. This example demonstrates how narrative entrapment can result from what Bach and Grant (2015: 145) call poor 'referral etiquette'.

In spite of all the rhetoric about collaboration in mental health work, both of these examples, and others like them, often happen as a result of the opposite. Mental health workers and others with the power to refer often don't talk with the users of mental health services sufficiently seriously, respectfully and in the depth needed to adequately understand not just their difficulties but the contexts of those difficulties (Grant 2015a; Smith & Grant, 2016). This points up in turn the bigger problem of a relative lack of narrative competence among health and mental health workers (Corbally & Grant, 2016).

Lucy: Seems so obvious, but why does it keep happening?

Ben: Power.

Alec: Yes. I think the power phenomenon that plays a major part in keeping this happening is built into institutional psychiatry – mainstream psychiatric business as usual – as a normative, self-perpetuating phenomenon. Has been down the decades.

Ben: How do you change this?

Lucy: How can we change this while still working with our colleagues who still think and talk in terms of 'mental illness', 'burnt-out schizophrenia', 'borderline personality disorder' and so on?

Fair questions. These come up again and again.

Alec: I'm not sure if your question implies a kind of impossibility of changing things? Or maybe it signals another question that people often ask me: 'What's the alternative, Alec?' – as if there wasn't one; as if this is the natural way of things.

Some are looking uncomfortable now. Good.

Alec: If any of you really want to promote change, maybe 'How do you change this?' is the wrong question. 'How can I contribute towards changing this?' is a better one, perhaps? I don't think that, as individuals on your own, you can do much to change the power of institutional psychiatry that's in constant cahoots with Big Pharma. My advice is to join forces with the critical mental health communities, as I have done and do in a lot of my writing, networking and, obviously, teaching practice. You can do this too by reading a lot and making international connections and/or doing postgraduate work.

Doing some or all of this will help increase your levels of confidence to routinely challenge immoral and unscientific institutional psychiatric practice (see, for example, Grant, 2015a; Kinderman, 2014; Rapley, Moncrieff & Dillon, 2011; Smith & Grant, 2016). It will also help you become more aware of, and challenge, contradictions between the rhetoric and reality of mental health practice (Klevan et al, 2018).

You will be better able to promote the local development of community-based and psychosocial interventions, in the context of re-envisioning mental health recovery more explicitly located as psychosocial rather than biomedical provision (Kinderman, 2014). These interventions include cognitive behavioural approaches (Grant, 2010a; Grant et al, 2008, 2010); formulation as intervention and alternative to diagnosis (Grant et al, 2008; Johnstone & Dallos, 2013), and peer support (Flegg, Gordon-Walker & Maguire, 2015), which all complement Open Dialogue and Hearing Voices Network recovery work (Read & Dillon, 2013; Thomas, 2014). At a more fundamental level, all of these approaches to recovery need to co-exist with what my esteemed colleague, the Norwegian scholar-practitioner Trude Klevan calls 'helpful help' (Klevan et al, 2016, 2018).

These psychosocial approaches have more than sufficient respectable evidence behind them (Read & Dillon 2013; Thomas, 2014). However, the combined power of institutional psychiatry and the global pharmaceutical industry tends to constantly marginalise and trivialise this body of evidence and thus puts its transfer to practice in perpetual deferral. You will not be at all surprised to hear that!

Laughter. Good.

Alec: One of the first things I think you need to square up to is that there are at least three curricula. The first two are mutually contradictory. There's the university curriculum – all the modules you've done in the last three years, rubber-stamped and validated by the Nursing and Midwifery Council (NMC). Then there's the alternative practice or service curriculum – 'the way things are done around here/forget all that shit they teach you in the uni' curriculum. Finally, there's the less apparent critical curriculum, which I represent as an occasional teacher. From a critical perspective, Mark Radcliffe and I recently wrote about the ways in which the need for the 'competencies' deemed important for the wards (including risk management practices, medication and administration) is always in danger of trumping what we described as the thoughtful practice of 'professional artistry'. Performing professional artistry would make reflexive awareness of confirmation bias and the related concepts always uppermost in people's minds (Grant & Radcliffe, 2015).

The question is: which curriculum is most valued. And by whom?

How many of them will they remember this session in years to come?

Moving around the hyphens

Who am I as a mental health nurse educator? That depends on who is asking, what I'm talking about and who my real and imagined audiences are. With postgraduate qualifications in psychotherapy and three decades of practice as a therapist turned academic-practitioner (Grant, 2010a; Grant et al, 2008, 2010), I was much, much more a cognitive behavioural psychotherapist (CBP) than I ever was a nurse.

Including RMN training, my incarnation as a mental health nurse – psychiatric nurse in those days – lasted from 1974 to 1983. I didn't really get much out of being one because it was tedious a lot of the time, and I could see then that it was more about social control than caring and help, which is why I jumped ship into CBP.

And then I was a 'service user'. I've written fairly extensively about this (Grant, 2006, 2010b, 2010c, 2011, 2016b; Grant & Zeeman, 2012; Short, Grant & Clarke, 2007). This gave me first-hand experience of the other side of the fence – or, more importantly, it showed me that there is no fence; that it's an imaginary one (Short & Grant, 2016).

So maybe a better question is, why am I a mental health nurse educator – albeit an occasional one? As far as I'm aware, the only person that asks this question about me is me. And for me, the best thing about me teaching student mental health nurses is that I can be:

> Dr Grant–Alec Grant–ex-cognitive behavioural therapist–ex-mental health
> nurse–ex-service user–survivor of the institutional psychiatric system–
> narrative researcher.

And all other possible permutations created by moving those identity descriptors around the hyphens.

I think that student mental health nurses get a good deal from this. But only a few of them realise this, maybe?

The debating society

An office in a university school of nursing and midwifery. A deputy head of school, in charge of the delivery of the nursing curricula across all branches. And Dr Grant.

Deputy head: You have an idea, Alec?

Alec: Debating societies.

Deputy head: Where?

Alec: Here?

Deputy head: Why?

> *Oh God…*

Alec: Nurses don't do formal debate, irrespective of what branch they're in. Nurses can't debate. Nor can they critique. They think critique and debate amount to being nasty. They confuse debate and critique, in person or in writing, with *ad hominem* attack.

Deputy head: They're encouraged to debate in teachings sessions and critique in their essays.

> *I hate nursing and nurse educators.*

Alec: You think so?

Deputy head: You clearly don't. So how do you propose we move forward?

Alec: Debating societies.

Deputy head: How would they change things?

Alec: Have you by any chance seen the 2007 Denzel Washington film, *The Great Debaters*?

Deputy head: Yes. How's that relevant?

Alec: Emancipation of an historically under-valued cultural group? Academic confidence-building through preparing to defend your ground and principles in formal debate in front of an audience? Couple of wee things, maybe? And it would help reduce the contradictions between what we practise and preach.

Deputy head: What contradictions?

Alec: The ones that are always apparent.

Deputy head: (…)

Alec: (…)

> *But not to you.*

Deputy head: I suppose I can put a call out in the next school magazine to see if there're any students who are interested in forming one.

Big of you.

Alec: Right. A couple of points. There needs to be more than one group in order to have a debating society.

Deputy head: I know that. I'm well aware of that.

Alec: And we need to role model it.

Deputy head: We?

Alec: Us. Academics. This being a university and all.

Deputy head: Don't think so.

Alec: Why not?

Deputy head: Well, it's easy for you. You always teach from your published work and research.

Alec: Isn't that what we're all supposed to do? Research-based pedagogy rather than knowledge always coming in from some mystical and mythical outside?

Deputy head: People are afraid of you.

Alec: I'm a pussycat. What are they afraid of?

Deputy head: Your knowledge. Your confidence.

Alec: Shouldn't we practise what we preach? Wouldn't doing so help in the development of knowledge, confidence and standpoint positions among our colleagues?

Deputy head: (…)

Oh… bugger.

Alec: Look, tell you what. I'll start the ball rolling. There are guidelines in print for setting debating societies up. It's straightforward. You and I can do the first one? It'll be fun.

For me. In more ways than one.

Deputy head: Let me think about it.

Months pass and months turn into years. Every so often along the way, prior to their retirement, Alec reminds the deputy head of school about the idea and they, generously, never stop thinking about it. The deputy head's successors think about it a lot too, say they love the sound of it and, as of 2017, have great ideas about key people other than themselves and their academic colleagues who might be interested in getting this initiative off the ground.

And in his 65th year, Alec looks forward to his impending retirement.

Colours that always fade

Mental health nursing is an absence. Liberal-humanist ideologies of care try to rectify this absence at theoretical, research and practice levels, while ignoring the lived social, psychological and material circumstances of nurses and those in their 'care' (Grant 2014a; 2016a).

In the film *The Pervert's Guide to Ideology*, the public intellectual and philosopher Slavoj Žižek (2012) argues that, in our engagement with the world, we are always in 'the trashcan of ideology'. By this, he means that we can never occupy a position in the world that is ideologically neutral, if 'ideology' is regarded as the time- and place-bound meanings that are given to things in the world. So, these things – including people, events, institutions and cultural and professional groups – are always already and inevitably inscribed within ideology.

It is important to stress that ideologies are arbitrary. People, events, institutions and cultural and professional groups don't have single immutable meanings that coincide with their essential, foundational and timeless reality and moral purpose. The definitive meaning of events, things, institutions and professional groups is culturally contingent or exists in specific contexts. Meanings change over time as a result of economic, socio-cultural and other circumstances. In this regard, ideologies are always political, since contingent meanings always serve the interests of the people and groups who invest in them. That being the case, contingent meanings are equally always likely to be contested by other people and groups who see flaws in them, whose needs don't coincide with them and who refuse them.

An enduring ideology held by mental health nurse academics and practitioners is of the human and caring nurse who offers the gift of self and time in a view of nursing as an activity that is fundamentally human. This idea of what it means to be a mental health nurse is, arguably, a bourgeois conceit and fantasy that does not stand up well to critical scrutiny (Ducey, 2007). It romanticises the job of mental health nursing and conceals its banalities. These include the fact that nursing is waged labour that generally always serves the interests of Big Pharma-supported institutional psychiatry (Grant, 2015a; Smith & Grant, 2016).

In its specific form as the 'Tidal model', for example (see, for example, Buchanan-Barker, 2009; Ellis, 2009; Simpson, 2009), this ideological take on mental health nursing is palimpsest- and medieval dye-like. It is difficult to see how it can stand up to the rough emotional and social control climate of the average busy acute ward, and when it fades in impact and function, the enduring colours of mental health nursing are always likely to appear. In the mainstream institutional psychiatric inpatient context, mental health nursing is condemned to be the constant administrative and social policing arm of institutional psychiatry (Grant, 2014b).

What does not fade is the eternal picture of sometimes insidious, sometimes stark, damaging social control masquerading as help and care (Grant, Leigh-Phippard & Short, 2015; Short & Grant, 2016). Stories of 'care' and 'treatment' are always undermined by various forms of institutional and narrative violence (Grant, 2013; Grant, 2016b; Grant & Leigh-Phippard, 2014; Grant, Leigh-Phippard & Short, 2015).

In June 2015, I wrote a blogpost titled 'Perpetuating unkindness' for the Critical Mental Health Nurses' Network website (Grant, 2015b). In it, I asserted that 'institutional psychiatric treatment spaces create possibilities for already damaged bodies to perpetuate unkindness on other bodies'. I was alluding to the hybrid nature of mental health nurses who are always, already 'the other'. This is an issue that, with rare exceptions, including my own co-written work (Grant & Barlow, 2016; Grant, Leigh-Phippard & Short, 2015; Short & Grant, 2016), is not formally acknowledged in the mainstream mental health nursing literature.

'I agree with what you've said, but I don't like the way you've said it'

A classroom in a university in the south of England in 2015. Seventeen master of research postgraduate students. Dr Grant, their teacher for the afternoon. The topic: Narrative Inquiry and Critical Autoethnography.

Alec: Okay, you've all read *Restorying Narrative Identity* (Grant, Leigh-Phippard & Short, 2015). I wonder what you make of it?

Student (Sue): I'm with you in what you've said, Alec, but I wish you'd said it differently.

Alec: Okay Sue, before we discuss this, can you remind us all what your professional role is?

Sue: I'm a mental health trust lead for research and development with a mental health nurse background.

Alec: Right, thanks. So, tell us a bit more.

Sue: Okay, so the paper dealt with the specifics of how two people were treated badly on acute wards, and how writing their stories has helped them in their own recovery process, independent of the mainstream mental health system.

Alec: Yes, that's a fair summary of the paper's autoethnographic content, outside of the narrative theory parts. Can you talk more about the problem you have between what was said and the way it was said?

Sue: Well, the paper highlighted difficulties in the mental health system in terms of acute care, but I think this could have been done in a more tactful, less critical way.

And you're a trust research lead. Typical! Speaks volumes.

Alec: For what reasons?

Sue: Well, it would have made the story more palatable.

Alec: Palatable for whom?

Sue: Just generally palatable.

> *Right. That's cleared that one up then.*

Alec: Can I ask you how you felt when you were reading it?

Sue: A mixture of emotions. I felt upset when I read what the two people had experienced. There again, I felt angry about the criticisms of mental health care.

Alec: How could it have been written differently to make it better, do you think?

Sue: If the language was gentler throughout, in the literature review and narrative theory as well as the stories, making it fairer. Less strident maybe. More balanced.

> *Here we go again... the old mantra: fair and balanced, fair and balanced.*

Alec: Yes, okay. However, the paper is explicitly written from a critical standpoint position. It uses storytelling as a method for challenging dominant and oppressive power structures. In the case of our paper, we were critical of institutional psychiatry practice in locations involving mental health nurses – specifically acute wards. So, in the literature review, to set the scene for the stories, we took issue with the then current Department of Health review of mental health nursing in England because, quoting from our paper:

> … from a critical social and human science perspective… and in line with the thrust of this paper, it remains arguably neglectful of important aspects of the complexities of lived experience of many individuals who have used mental health services. (Grant, Leigh-Phippard & Short, 2015: 279)

We wanted to show in stark, concrete detail how these complexities were not captured in the review, which from our reading of it:

> … constructs gender-neutral, homogenized and compliant users, excised from much of their life contexts. As a relatively power-silent story, it fails to acknowledge the potential for… the ways in which people often oppose the power structures they are caught up in. (Grant, Leigh-Phippard & Short, 2015: 279)

So, we wanted to use the stories to illustrate such opposition.

Sue: Okay, but I still think this could have been done in a gentler way.

> *Starting to feeling irritated. Must handle this reasonably.*

Alec: For whose benefit?

Sue: What do you mean?

Alec: Would it have benefited the two people writing the stories to have done it differently, in the way you suggest?

Sue: (…)

Alec: Would it have been better for me as lead on the paper to have written, structured and presented it differently, in the way you suggest?

Sue: I suppose not.

Alec: So, who would it have benefited? Whose lives would have been made better from, if I've got you right, writing a critical standpoint paper in a less critical way?

Reader response theory

People often experience the stories they read in ways that jar with their implicitly held world views. Reader-response theory is helpful in making sense of this state of affairs (Tyson, 2015). The theory holds that readers actively construct meaning from texts in a range of different ways, as opposed to simply passively consuming them. Tyson argues that readers are often likely to react to texts, including autoethnographic work, by using the well-rehearsed responses they bring to bear on other aspects of their lives. The way that such work is read, or rather interpreted, may thus be mediated by individual reactions, fears and defences that are more or less unconscious. The goal of such interpretation for readers is to fulfil psychological needs and desires in the effort to restore psychological equilibrium.

So, for example, readers may experience autoethnographic work as personally, professionally and culturally threatening, and may in consequence read it in a defensive way. Moreover, Tyson argues that individual responses to a text often reflect the interpretive communities to which readers belong. Interpretive communities draw on shared sets of assumptions and vary from one another in relative levels of sophistication, with relatively more sophisticated communities likely to exercise and display greater levels of critical consciousness (Freire, 1970/1993; Mills, 1959/2000).

Tyson asserts that interpretive community readings happen at conscious and unconscious levels and readers can belong to several intersecting communities simultaneously. In this regard, autoethnographic texts can be read on the basis of a multiplicity of communal authorities. It is likely that mental health worker readings will be variously informed by a mixture of professional, disciplinary, institutional and lay community perspectives.

Working in the paraversity, paid by the university

Alec's home study, winter 2016. Dr Roman Imyata, an independent scholar, friend and muse, in conversation with Alec.

Roman: I read what you said in your *Nurse Education Today* article about how you think the neoliberal agenda has saturated university life internationally, with specific reference to your own institution (Grant, 2014c).

Alec: Yep, Roman. I think, along with many other people, that the neoliberal discourse is about getting academics to work harder, in unquestioning ways, in line with national and international economic objectives. Everything's joined up.

Everything's sewn up!

Roman: What do you think the ideology is behind this, then, Alec?

Alec: These objectives are portrayed as 'naturally' coinciding with institutional professional and academic responses to public need and are reflected in professional and educational policy. This makes it understandably hard for mental health nurse academics to question them. Unfortunately, the net result of this state of affairs is that mental health nursing knowledge is packaged and transmitted as a commodity – a fact that is not generally acknowledged by academics, their students or those in practice. This reflects a training rather than an educational agenda, where what is commodified are sets of competencies that nurses are perceived to need in order to qualify for, and contribute to, the mental health labour market.

Roman: Training masquerading as education can keep nobody happy, I'm thinking.

Alec: Yep. This is a big, under-acknowledged contradiction at the heart of the interface between mental health nurse education and practice. The annual UK National Student Survey (www.thestudentsurvey.com) captures student satisfaction with their teaching and learning experiences. Some students and those academics who teach them who want an easy ride might be content with unchallenging curricula. The cognoscenti among both groups are less likely to be happy with this.

Roman: Can you expand on that point?

Alec: Well, nursing competencies are informed by what Schön (1987) described as 'technical rational' assumptions. He critiqued an aspect of technical rationality central to the world of professional education and practice – the idea of discrete, context-neutral problems requiring specific techniques, strategies and algorithms to solve them. With regard to mental health nursing knowledge and practice, such a model of 'professionalism' is overly simplistic and one-dimensional in paying insufficient attention to the messy relational and material contexts in which problems occur, and the broader contexts of power that inform mental health work, notably including the de-medicalisation agenda (Grant, 2015a; Smith & Grant, 2016).

With regard to mental health nursing, a technical rational training, as opposed to education curricula, fails to adequately address the skilled, multicontextual knowledge and skills needed by students to help them engage in the unruly and complex identities, relationships and life and treatment environments of contemporary mental health service users (Grant, 2015c).

Moreover, they are ill prepared to deal with the relational and identity political fallout that's occurring more and more as mental health users, survivors, their relatives and friends and mental health workers question mainstream institutional psychiatric approaches. By default, this is mostly all that is on offer for them a lot of the time (Grant, 2015a; Smith & Grant, 2016). That's even before we consider the demands on them to recognise and engage with gender and sexual politics and how this impacts on the lives of people involved in mental health services – both users and workers (Naish, Grant & Zeeman, 2016).

Earlier this year, we put forward the argument that such engagement requires an explicit, un-apologetic educational curriculum (Grant & Radcliffe, 2015). This would promote what Polanyi (1967) and Schön (1987) described as 'professional artistry'. In practice, professional artistry requires increasing levels of critically reflexive organisational and political awareness. This is because, in all of its aspects, mental health nursing practice is political, historically contingent and socially and environmentally contextual. It is political because it takes place within power relationships. It is historically contingent because it happens at particular points in time, with guidelines and expectations around how mental health nursing is perceived and practised, determined by associated policy and public perception. It is socially and environmentally contextual because it occurs within specific configurations of relationships, events and work and material settings.

Roman: If there's a knowledge deficit that needs rectifying to enable the development of professional artistry, what is it then, Alec?

Alec: I think that – in my own institution and perhaps more generally – the technical rational training agenda in mental health nursing marginalises and silences knowledge I've been alluding to – narratives based on lived experience. These are often relegated to the status of non-evidence-based knowledge and dismissed as 'anecdata' (Bach & Grant, 2015). This is lamentable since this is the very stuff that nurses need to get to read and grapple with.

A few years back, although we were by no means the first to do this, colleagues and I used such narratives – stories from lived experience, provided by service-user and other contributors from both sides of the Atlantic – to expose abusive experiences perpetrated in the name of institutional psychiatric treatment and care (Grant, Biley & Walker, 2011). We then produced a book of suicide narratives a couple of years later (Grant, Haire & Stone, 2013). This was soon followed by one of narratives of self-harm (Baker, Shaw & Biley, 2013), and most recently, one of stories by the victims of stalking (Taylor, Grant & Leigh-Phippard, 2018). Among lots of other things, each of these books documents narrative abuse, or what I prefer in my work to call narrative violence. This refers to health and mental health workers, and other people and statutory service groups, writing and talking people into entrapment within pejorative identities.

Our work gives the lie to assumptions of mainstream mental health environments as neutral, unproblematic backdrops to mental health nursing practice, as conveyed in many mainstream professional and educational texts. Moreover, these mainstream texts, and related mental health nurse educational curricula, do not up to this point in time seem to value multi-faceted lived experience knowledge written by 'hybrid' narrative researchers who are simultaneously mental health academics and survivors of the institutional psychiatric system (Grant, Leigh-Phippard & Short, 2015; Short & Grant, 2016).

Roman: All well and good, but from previous conversations (Grant, 2013), your problem always seems to be that these ideas don't go down too well in your own institution.

Alec: Yep! This is a perpetual source of regret and frustration, and that's putting it mildly. My concerns are not often acknowledged, or indeed recognised, by many of my local colleagues.

Roman: How do you live with that?

Alec: Good question. Well, as with many things that trouble me, I take intellectual, and I think emotional, refuge in theory. I made theoretical sense of this local lack of acknowledgement, validation and recognition using Alvesson and Spicer's (2012) functional stupidity theory of organisations (Grant & Radcliffe, 2015).

Roman: Tell me more about this.

Alec: Alvesson and Spicer describe functional stupidity as a cognitively- and affectively-informed unwillingness or inability to employ reflexivity, justification and substantive reasoning in work organisations. In this context, reflexivity refers to the active questioning of organisational knowledge claims and norms by organisational members. Justification entails that these members routinely both demand and provide reasons and explanations for decisions made within organisations that impact on professional practice. Substantive reasoning constitutes the act of engaging thinking as broadly as possible in relation to professional practice and related work problems. This contrasts with applying thinking myopically about practices and problems, in technical rational ways that pay insufficient regard to their contextual bases and referents.

Roman: Okay. So, you experience this as going on. How have you coped with it?

Alec: It's been difficult. Acknowledging that this might well sound arrogant and superior on my part, what I see around me in mainstream mental health nurse education is organisational functional stupidity in action. The fact that I try to do organisational reflexivity, in terms of recognising, writing and teaching uncomfortable issues, means that I constantly cross the Rubicon into that which is usually ignored, passed over, dismissed, not attended to or even recognised as problematic by many of my colleagues. This invites censure, the 'othering' that I often write about, and, at worst, unpleasant, defensive negative labelling from colleagues in mental health nurse education and practice, in my own institution and beyond.

I feel that I am constantly walking a path between two mutually antagonistic worlds. One is the world that I work in and contribute to, according to my critically reflexive sensibilities, along with a very few other allies in mental health nurse higher education. In the other world are the education and practice colleagues who often seem to express the caring qualities of mental health nursing in glowing terms from insufficiently scrutinised humanistic perspectives, as self-evident truth rather than ideology. This allows academics and practitioners inhabiting this world to over-invest in success stories, including stories about how nurses turn people's lives around for the better. These abound in the mental health nursing literature.

An ideological function of these stories is of course to either minimise or ignore the contextual features of institutional psychiatry that lead to abusive rather than success experiences for both mental health service users and nurses. From my position in the critically reflexive world, I do the opposite. I constantly engage in difficult and uncomfortable teaching and writing on these ideologically challenging issues. I believe that this rescues them from being constantly ignored or left to languish in the curricular margins.

Roman: Why do you think organisational reflexivity is not practised, though? The concept of the un-reflexive university would seem strange to a lot of folk. It sounds like an oxymoron, a self-contradictory concept.

Alec: Yes, it does seem deeply strange. Functional stupidity theory casts light on the nature of organisations where critical reflexivity is regarded as an anathema and threatening. I think it helps explain why many, maybe most, colleagues make sense of their lives according to the dominant ideologies of the organisations and wider cultural institutions within which they are positioned. Teaching and writing activities that do not fit with these are likely to be neutralised in various ways. As a general example of this, Mark Radcliffe and I described the negative, trivialising and dismissive response of academics in our organisation to his championing fiction as methodology, and my own championing of autoethnography (Grant & Radcliffe, 2015). Sometimes this makes me feel like Lear's Fool in my own institution, in spite of the esteem held for me outside of it.

I think this is why many of my nursing and mental health nursing academic colleagues won't seriously read or engage with my autoethnographic and lived-experience narrative work. To illustrate this, a few years back I was asked by a nursing academic colleague, who had previously published quantitative research on suicide, what my latest writing project was. I told her that I was collecting and analysing narratives for the book *Our Encounters with Suicide* (Grant, Haire & Stone, 2013). She instantly physically recoiled about two feet back from where she'd been standing. Realising what she'd done, she tried to make light of it, saying, 'Oh, that'll make good bedtime reading then, ha ha.' This made her actions worse, of course.

I've also witnessed a grudging, reluctant and qualified acknowledgement of the relevance and simultaneous dismissal of critical pedagogy for the mental health nursing curriculum. In regard to the content of my teaching, for example, I often hear statements from my nurse academic colleagues and managers along the lines of, 'Very interesting, Alec, but the students aren't ready for it. This is postgraduate level work.' I often hear equivalent comments expressed about its relevance for postgraduate study, which to me reflects a state of perpetual deferral of the relevance of my work at all levels. I believe that what all of this really signifies is that it's the academics, as opposed to the students, who aren't ready for it.

It's tempting to extrapolate from this state of affairs beyond my own institution. It seems to me that an implicit curricular rule may always be operative in many mental health nursing and, I suspect, other higher educational disciplinary cultures in the UK, and possibly elsewhere. This rule can be expressed as: 'If it don't fit, it don't exist.' This arguably results in a form of enforced invisibility imposed on knowledge areas and sources that challenge and threaten mainstream assumptions – a kind of curricular NIMBYism.

Roman: Not in my curricular back yard. Why should this be so?

Alec: It seems to me that such knowledge is excluded precisely because it challenges taken-for-granted assumptions and policy- and professional-led principles that inform dominant curricula. This is certainly the case with regard to the mental health nursing programme in my own institution. On the basis of my international peer review, external examiner and consultancy work, and international discussions resulting from my Mad in America blogposts, it seems also to be a feature of mental health nursing curricula internationally – at least in the US and the Antipodes. As an example of what's excluded, take what Nigel Short and I described as 'hybrid pedagogy' (Short & Grant, 2016). We used this term to refer to teaching on the basis of prose and poetic autoethnographic narratives of lived experience provided by mental health nurse educators who have also been mental health service users. This does not as yet have an established place in mental health nursing knowledge and practice. I think this is because of a policy- and discipline-sanctioned need to maintain the clear cultural demarcation between mental health nursing 'professionals' and 'mentally ill' patients.

Roman: I can't help thinking that it must be difficult – dangerous maybe – for you to maintain your critical educator position? I can see the payoff, but what about the costs?

Alec: Good question, Roman! I agonise about the relative success of my 'ideology-busting' scholarship and teaching in the total scheme of things. I also feel constantly troubled and somewhat paranoid, although much less so now, with retirement looming, about the tensions between what I teach on the basis of my scholarship and lived experiences and what my managers would prefer me to teach. One of the things at stake here in my own institution is the perceived threats that my work constitutes to the so-called 'partnership' relationship between the nursing academy and local nursing practice organisations, within which it's arguably politic to not be seen to be too critical. I know this to be a fact, since I have in the past been explicitly warned off writing critical mental health autoethnography by senior colleagues.

Roman: Really?

Alec: Yep. They said things like, 'Stick to the straight stuff, Alec, like the cognitive behavioural stuff you write about, otherwise it'll be bad for your career. And besides, at our partnership meetings, our colleagues in the trusts are clear about what they want, and it's not autoethnography.'

Roman: What was your reaction?

Alec: I instantly thought, 'Right. This is what I need to do – write more and more autoethnography!'

Roman: They represented negative role models for you?

Alec: Nail on the head, Roman! To me, some of them perfectly embody the academic organisational 'artificial persons' described by my autoethnographic colleague Brett Smith (2013) – educational policy-delivering civil servants masquerading as 'academics'.

Roman: There's lots of them around these days!

Alec: Yeah, and in spite of its obvious benefits, I think this encounter highlights what Andrew Sparkes (2018) describes as a major risk of autoethnography, especially for younger academics who turn their research gaze to their own organisations. In his view, the audit culture and the infusion of neoliberal ideologies in the academy increases the risk of potential punitive consequences for autoethnographers who are 'out' about their academic organisational and practice experiences. That said, in line with the writing of Denzin (2010) and Denzin and Giardina (2016), it is precisely because of the existence of these oppressive practices and ideologies that Sparkes equally advocates autoethnography as part of a critical, collective act of resistance.

I think Sparkes and Denzin and Giardina are absolutely right. I argued a few years back that subjectivity is a great ethical and methodological resistance resource, in spite of its being traditionally regarded as an irritant (Grant, Short & Turner, 2013). This has broader implications. As Trude Klevan (2017) recently asked me, 'Why do we think that displaying vulnerability is unprofessional? How do we think that we can offer humanising services without being human? Why do we find it unprofessional to feel?' I think her questions apply equally to doing both mental health nurse practice and mental health nurse higher education.

Roman: Easy for you to say, though, Alec, with you just about to retire from university life!

Alec: Yeah, tell me about it! This is a valedictory chapter. I feel easier about writing all of this stuff because I'm formally retiring from my university on my 65th birthday, in May 2017. By the time this chapter and book are published I'll be long gone.

But I'll still be writing. To borrow a concept from Mark Radcliffe (Grant & Radcliffe, 2015), I'm not going to be leaving the 'ideas garden' any time soon. Nor am I going to relinquish my place in the paraversity.

Roman: So how would you like to be remembered when you eventually hang up your hat?

Alec: If I was remembered as an old grouch who had lots to say about things that desperately needed saying, I'd be pleased. A Victor Meldrew of mental health/nurse education, with a justifiable axe to grind would do me very nicely!

Acknowledgements

I would like to thank Trude Klevan, Benny Goodman, and Drs Helen Leigh-Phippard, Nigel Short and Mark Radcliffe for their helpful critical readings of this chapter in its development.

References

Alvesson M, Spicer A (2012). A stupidity-based theory of organizations. *Journal of Management Studies* 49(7): 1194-1220.

Bach S, Grant A (2015). *Communication and Interpersonal Skills in Nursing* (3rd ed). London: Sage Publications.

Baker C, Shaw C, Biley F (eds) (2013). *Our Encounters with Self-Harm*. Ross-on-Wye: PCCS Books.

Buchanan-Barker P (2009). Reclamation: beyond recovery. In: Barker P (ed). *Psychiatric and Mental Health Nursing: the craft of recovery*. London: Hodder Arnold (pp681–689).

Corbally M, Grant A (2016). Narrative competence: a neglected area in undergraduate curricula. *Nurse Education Today 36*: 7–9.

Denzin N (2010). *The Qualitative Manifesto: a call to arms*. Walnut Creek, CA: Left Coast Press Inc.

Denzin NK, Giardina MG (2016). *Qualitative Inquiry Through a Critical Lens*. New York, NY: Routledge.

Ducey A (2007). More than a job: meaning, affect and training health care workers. In: Clough PT, Halley J (eds). *The Affective Turn: theorizing the social*. Durham/London: Duke University Press (pp187–208).

Ellis D (2009). Nursing diagnosis. In: Barker P (ed). *Psychiatric and Mental Health Nursing: the craft of recovery*. London: Hodder Arnold (pp141–148).

Flegg N, Gordon-Walker M, Maguire S (2015). Peer-to-peer mental health: a community evaluation case study. *Journal of Mental Health Training, Education and Practice 10*(5): 282–293.

Frank AW (2011). Foreword. In: Grant A, Biley F, Walker H (eds) (2011). *Our Encounters with Madness*. Ross-on-Wye: PCCS Books (ppviii-x).

Freire P (1970/1993). *Pedagogy of the Oppressed*. London: Penguin Books.

Grant A (2016a). Storying the world: a posthumanist critique of phenomenological-humanist representational practices in mental health nurse qualitative inquiry. *Nursing Philosophy 17*(4): 290–297.

Grant A (2016b). Living my narrative: storying dishonesty and deception in mental health nursing. *Nursing Philosophy 17*(3): 194–201.

Grant A (2015a). Demedicalizing misery: welcoming the human paradigm in mental health nurse education. *Nurse Education Today 35*(9): e50–e53.

Grant A (2015b). *Perpetuating unkindness*. [Blog.] Critical Mental Health Nurses' Network. http://criticalmhnursing.org/2015/06/25/perpetuating-unkindness (accessed 5 July 2018).

Grant A (2015c). Beyond technique. In: Bach S, Grant A. *Communication and Interpersonal Skills in Nursing* (3rd ed). London: Sage/Learning Matters (pp165–173).

Grant A (2014a). Troubling 'lived experience': a poststructural critique of mental health nursing qualitative research assumptions. *Journal of Psychiatric and Mental Health Nursing 21*(6): 544–549.

Grant A (2014b). Breaking the grip: a critical insider account of representational practices in cognitive behavioural psychotherapy and mental health nursing. In: Zeeman L, Aranda K, Grant A (eds). *Queering Health: critical challenges to normative health and healthcare*. Ross-on-Wye: PCCS Books (pp116–133).

Grant A (2014c). Neoliberal higher education and nursing scholarship: power, subjectification, threats and resistance. *Nurse Education Today 34*(10): 1280–1282.

Grant A (2013). Writing teaching and survival in mental health: a discordant quintet for one. In: Short N, Turner L, Grant A (eds). *Contemporary British Autoethnography*. Rotterdam: Sense Publishers (pp33–48).

Grant A (2011). Performing the room. In: Grant A, Biley F, Walker H (eds). *Our Encounters with Madness*. Ross-on-Wye: PCCS Books (pp131–138).

Grant A (ed) (2010a). *Cognitive Behavioural Interventions for Mental Health Practitioners*. Exeter: Learning Matters.

Grant A (2010b). Autoethnographic ethics and re-writing the fragmented self. *Journal of Psychiatric and Mental Health Nursing 17*(2): 111–116.

Grant A (2010c). Writing the reflexive self: an autoethnography of alcoholism and the impact of psychotherapy culture. *Journal of Psychiatric and Mental Health Nursing 17*(7): 577–582.

Grant A (2006). Testimony. God and aeroplanes: my experience of breakdown and recovery. *Journal of Psychiatric and Mental Health Nursing 13*(4): 456–457.

Grant A, Barlow A (2016). The practitioner/survivor hybrid: an emerging anti-stigmatising resource in mental health care. *Mental Health Practice 20*(1): 33–37.

Grant A, Leigh-Phippard H (2014). Troubling the normative mental health recovery project: the silent resistance of a disappearing doctor. In: Zeeman L, Aranda K, Grant A (eds). *Queering Health: critical challenges to normative health and healthcare.* Ross-on-Wye: PCCS Books (pp100–115).

Grant A, Radcliffe M (2015). Resisting technical rationality in mental health nurse higher education: a duoethnography. *The Qualitative Report 20*(6): 815–825.

Grant A, Zeeman L (2012). Whose story is it? An autoethnography concerning narrative identity. *The Qualitative Report 17*(72): 1–12.

Grant A, Biley F, Walker H (eds) (2011). *Our Encounters with Madness.* Ross-on-Wye: PCCS Books.

Grant A, Haire J, Stone B (eds) (2013). *Our Encounters with Suicide.* Ross-on-Wye: PCCS Books.

Grant A, Leigh-Phippard H, Short N (2015). Re-storying narrative identity: a dialogical study of mental health recovery and survival. *Journal of Psychiatric and Mental Health Nursing 22*(4): 278–286.

Grant A, Short NP, Turner L (2013). Introduction: storying life and lives. In: Short N, Turner L, Grant A (eds). *Contemporary British Autoethnography.* Rotterdam: Sense Publishers (pp1–16).

Grant A, Townend M, Mills J, Cockx A (2008). *Assessment and Case Formulation in Cognitive Behavioural Psychotherapy.* London: Sage Publications.

Grant A, Townend M, Mulhern R, Short N (eds) (2010). *Cognitive Behavioural Therapy in Mental Health Care* (2nd ed). London: Sage Publications.

Johnstone L, Dallos R (2013). *Formulation in Psychology and Psychotherapy: making sense of people's problems* (2nd ed). London: Routledge.

Kinderman P (2014). *A Prescription for Psychiatry.* Basingstoke: Palgrave Macmillan.

Klevan T (2017). Personal communication.

Klevan T, Davidson L, Ruud T, Karlsson B (2016). 'We are different people': a narrative analysis of carers' experiences with mental health crisis and support from crisis resolution teams. *Social Work in Mental Health 14*(6): 658–675.

Klevan T, Karlsson B, Ness O, Grant A, Ruud T (2018). Between a rock and a softer place: a discourse analysis of helping cultures in crisis resolution teams. *Qualitative Social Work 17*(2): 167–170.

Mills CW (1959/2000). *The Sociological Imagination.* New York, NY/Oxford: Oxford University Press.

Naish J, Grant A, Zeeman L (2016). Depathologizing sexualities. *Mental Health Practice 19*(7): 26–31.

Polanyi M (1967). *The Tacit Dimension.* New York, NY: Doubleday

Rapley M, Moncrieff J, Dillon J (eds) (2011). *De-Medicalizing Misery: psychiatry, psychology and the human condition.* Basingstoke: Palgrave Macmillan.

Read J, Dillon J (2013). *Models of Madness* (2nd ed). London: Routledge.

Rosenhan DL (1973). On being sane in insane places. *Science 179*(4070): 250–258.

Schön D (1987). *Educating the Reflective Practitioner: toward a new design for teaching and learning in the professions.* San Francisco, CA: Jossey-Bass.

Short NP (2011). Freeze-frame: reflections on being in hospital. In: Grant A, Biley F, Walker H (eds). *Our Encounters with Madness.* Ross-on-Wye: PCCS Books (pp131–138).

Short N, Grant A (2016). Poetry as hybrid pedagogy in mental health nurse education. *Nurse Education Today 43:* 60–63.

Short N, Grant A, Clarke L (2007). Living in the Borderlands; writing in the margins: an autoethnographic tale. *Journal of Psychiatric and Mental Health Nursing 14*(8): 771–782.

Simpson A (2009). The acute care setting. In: In Barker P (ed). *Psychiatric and Mental Health Nursing: the craft of recovery.* London: Hodder Arnold (pp403–409).

Smith B (2013). Artificial persons and the academy: a story. In: Short N, Turner L, Grant A (eds). *Contemporary British Autoethnography.* Rotterdam: Sense Publishers (pp187–202).

Smith S, Grant A (2016). The corporate construction of psychosis and the rise of the psychosocial paradigm: emerging implications for mental health nurse education. *Nurse Education Today 39*(April): 22–25.

Sparkes AC (2018). Autoethnography comes of age: consequences, comforts, and concerns. In: Beach D, Bagley C, Marques da Silva S (eds). *Handbook of Ethnography of Education.* London: Wiley Blackwell (pp479–499).

Taylor S, Grant A, Leigh-Phippard H (eds) (2018). *Our Encounters with Stalking.* Monmouth: PCCS Books.

Thomas P (2014). *Psychiatry in Context: experience, meaning & communities.* Monmouth: PCCS Books.

Tyson L (2015). *Critical Theory Today: a user-friendly guide* (3rd ed). London: Routledge.

Žižek S (2012). *The Pervert's Guide to Ideology* (S Fiennes dir). New York, NY: Zeitgeist Films.

3 Tales of leadership and studentship: a duoethnography of a nurse-led recovery college

Stephen Williams and Steven Prosser

In the summer of 2016, I (SW) launched a recovery college summer school at the University of Bradford, in partnership with primary and secondary care colleagues from the local mental health trust and third-sector mental health organisations. Recovery colleges are envisaged as educationally based, situated co-productions that include service users as peer-professionals in the development of group psychoeducational programmes in illness management and wellbeing-focused psychosocial interventions (see also Williams, 2016). Recovery colleges emerged through Implementing Recovery Organisational Change (ImROC). This is a national programme, originally launched by the Department of Health and now hosted by Nottinghamshire Healthcare NHS Foundation Trust, that seeks to address the organisational challenges of implementing recovery practice in the UK (Perkins & Slade, 2012).

While I am well aware of arguments against 'personal recovery' (see Chapter 8), forming an open 'learning community' in education (rather than one that is co-opted into the NHS healthcare/medical context) remains appealing to me. Of course, this could become another form of co-option itself, and being 'in charge', as the 'clinical-academic lead', for such an endeavour, has troubled me throughout the three-year process of forming partnerships and running the pilot summer school. It does so still, as I sit writing this chapter. This affected me during the delivery of the College and, in the spirit of narrative inquiry, I and Steve, my co-author, set out to write this duoethnography (Short, Turner & Grant, 2013) to trouble these feelings further, see where they led and unpick the aspects of identity politics with which we grappled from our different perspectives as leader and student.

To this end, we wrote our sections independently and agreed to reflect on each other's writing after we had reached a fairly stable draft. We then agreed any further changes together, but favoured leaving texts as unchanged as possible, warts and all, to reduce censorship and aspects of bias in our reflections. We then constructed from a videonetnographic dialogue our joint 'conclusion'.[1]

We start with my perspective.

Part 1: On becoming what I hate the most – a 'clinical academic leader'

Scene 1: Open induction session one, May 2016
Recovery College seminar room, University of Bradford

I'm sat nervously awaiting the arrival of anybody to the first session of the university's Recovery College, a project I'd conceived, developed, organised and now was on the cusp of delivering. Of course, I wasn't alone in all this, but I very much felt the heavy weight of responsibility as the author of it all. Not only that, but to be seriously in the running for an NIHR clinical academic fellowship the following year, I had to demonstrate that I had the required clinical leadership acumen when I made the application. So, a lot was riding on this. Meanwhile, the clock ticked inexorably towards 10am and the new building and room were as empty as they had been when I arrived to set up, ridiculously early, at 8:30am.

My thoughts:

> Is anybody going to come to this? We only had a month to promote it and I don't know if this is going to be a success or not. What will my colleagues sat with me think if we get a bad turnout? We have four of these introductory sessions – it could be a disaster.
>
> Applying the cognitive-behavioural therapy model of social anxiety to myself right now, I recognise that these are thoughts that mix a fear of failure with a fear of negative judgment by others. That much is pedestrianly obvious to me, and predictable. I also perceive an undercurrent of wanting to do well and to offer up a 'shared endeavour' to others and not a rehash of mental health treatment options as I experienced them years ago when I was stuck in a mental hospital getting the treatment-de-jour of that time.

When I strive to understand where my revulsion for taking on the mantle for leadership comes from, I tap into predictable worries and anxieties that are readily elicited through the application of cognitive-behavioural therapeutic principles. The memory frequently disturbed in so doing is that of the extra-care unit and being incarcerated at Her Majesty's displeasure for 28 days all those years ago. It remains an experience that for years begged to dominate my identity and being.

---

1. The unedited version of this discussion can be found in the accompanying online materials at http://mhnurselecturer.co.uk/?page_id=229

Figure 3.1: A cognitive-behavioural formulation of my experience on the first induction session (adapted from Clark & Wells, 1995)

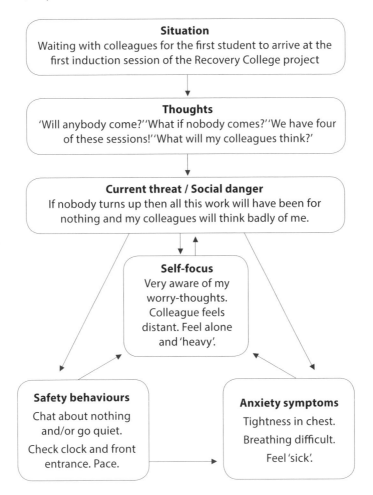

Scene 2: The inpatient lounge of doom

'Everyone ends up here, either working, visiting someone or being a patient.'
(A common local saying about the psychiatric hospital in Worthing)

The shared lounge of the extra-care area of Homefield (high-risk, acute psychiatric, mixed, inpatient ward) Hospital was cramped. A ring of worn-out armchairs encircling a threadbare blue carpet; the television, mounted high on the wall in the corner, blaring inanely away. I lay on the sofa with my cast-bound leg propped up on the other arm of the sofa. I was having a difficult day with the world. Everything seemed to have a peculiar significance – people were being handed things that were of vast importance to them and to me and my future. Letters, envelopes, photographs, circulating from person to person, chair to chair, in an Escher chain of causal power. I couldn't fathom it, or what I had to do to escape this inexorable chain – imprisoned, like my leg in the cast, in the inpatient ward, with 28 days to endure. No matter what I did or said, I had no power or control, freedom or rights.

Figure 3.2: My recollection of the shared lounge, provoked by my ongoing reflexivity

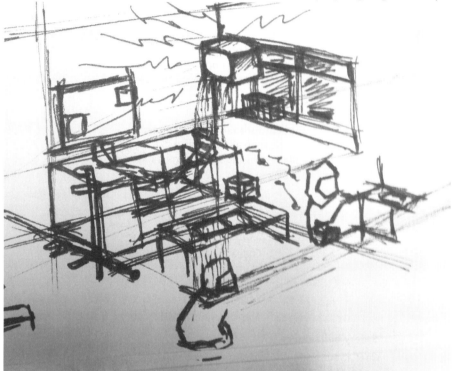

Who was I? I was an incarcerated mental patient. How must I act? I did not view myself as a mental patient at the time and I can recall times (as time is something you are replete with while sat or, in my case, mostly lying down as a mental patient) when I found myself actively pondering 'Is there such a thing as a mental illness?' while actively being observed by others to assess and determine their consensus, truth-value perspective of that very thing. What kind of philosophically and pragmatically ludicrous act is that? To cast judgment (while labouring under the flawed nature of one's own self) over the veridicality, validity and verisimilitude of a person's perspective on themselves, others and the world.

I did then, as I do now, reject as philosophically and logically flawed the notion of 'mental illness' as a narrowly constrained, mental, pathological disease. All that aside, this internal metaphysical quandary made no difference to my circumstances or status. I was seen as a 'mental patient' by those at large – friends, family, casual visitors, professionals and other inmates. At times they confirmed this to me verbally, and on occasion I received written confirmation through the professionals' statutory missives. And yet I continued to reject this notion. I was forced through circumstance to act in that role: escape from the ward was not possible, as was made evident to me when a fellow inmate was tackled to the carpet as he made a sprint for the closing self-locking ward door. If I refused medication at the hatch during the prescribed times, I found myself running the risk of receiving it anyway through forcible injections. I never did refuse, as I recall, but that didn't stop the nurses from giving me forcible injections anyway – other excuses were found. Better to avoid those that you could and submit to the double-bind. Free will may well be illusory; indeed, leading influential philosophers of science such as Dennett (1991) maintain academically and in the broadsheet press that consciousness itself is nothing more than a bag of tricks and not all that it is cracked up to be. However, in that place, exercising this illusory free will (ie. saying 'not today, thanks') in certain circumstances, was met with harsh punishment – and that was far from illusory. In summary, I had no choice but to act as if I were 'a mental patient'; whether or not that was a conscious or non-conscious action is a moot question when one is cast in the role, with all the trappings, setting and supporting cast of a thousand nurses and nursing assistants barely able to spend time with you if you even wished it. All the while I found myself secretly nursing the belief that I was no such bloody thing, thank you very much. I wrote down who and what I was – my name and qualification, if I recall correctly – the first night of my incarceration, having been transferred there from A&E, in felt-tip pen on the wall under my bed, where I knew it was written but others couldn't see it.

> My name is Stephen Williams and I have a first-class degree in Experimental Psychology.

It was a delicious repudiation of the circumstances I found myself in at the time. Secret graffiti. I remember writing this to affirm to myself who I was and the importance and status and significance I had to my world when all about me seemed intent on taking this power and control from me.

Of course, if I apply here an analytical lens to my reflection, I can pick out some highly ironic and empirically validated themes. First, we know very well that we are poor at distinguishing reliably between those who are 'sane' and those who are not (Rosenhan, 1973). This is no doubt compounded by the empirical finding that psychotic states can be transient in nature (Singh et al, 2004). In addition to that, as Rosenhan (1973) discusses in his seminal study, clinicians are heavily biased towards 'Type II' errors – that is, being more likely to mistakenly judge someone who is healthy as sick rather than mistaking someone sick as healthy (which is a 'Type I' error).

The current trend in psychology with respect to 'psychosis' is to contend that the difficulties contained beneath that umbrella exist on a spectrum or continuum of difficulties, and this contention works hand in hand with a normative and normalising agenda. Critiques of this approach, such as James Coyne in his critique of the recent BPS *Understanding Psychosis and Schizophrenia* report (Cooke, 2017) are that this risks 'romanticising' psychosis and down-playing the severity of suffering and degree of risk (of death and harm to others) associated with this condition (Rhodes, 2015). People resisting ideas of recovery complain similarly of feeling forced to recover and oppressed by the implicit toxic assumptions that recovery should be 'obtained by all' (Harper & Speed, 2014).

The traps in continuum approaches might be summarised as falsely equating less distressing experiences with those that are both distressing and life threatening and giving hope for recovery that becomes oppressive. There is perhaps a 'banality of hope' akin to Arendt's banality of evil (Arendt, 1963). Aligning experiences of psychosis unthinkingly along a spectrum of the normal to build hope that we aren't so bloody strange after all is potentially plain disrespectful to some. If anything, my own experiences of psychosis have been weird, odd, disruptive and crazy. They strike me as weird and typically strike others as the same – and they call me that too. That others can't apprehend and comprehend them is, in a sense, unique to me but is also not uncommon to the human condition – it is an oppositional paradox. It is a form of oppression to have the peculiarity and uniqueness of one's experience obliterated under the response, 'Well, anybody could be weird like you if they tried hard enough or had a miserable life like yours, you know', which the tarring brush of normalisation can do, particularly through processes of formulation and diagnosis. Normalisation seeks to make us feel like we are 'all in this together' but plainly we are not, so maybe we shouldn't pretend we are. It's an act of psychopolitical ignorance and harmful as a result. Spectrums can be just as major a hindrance and just as harmful and 'other-reinforcing' as binary distinctions, the one being presaged from the other. More nuanced combinations are demanded. Other logical conjunctions – but-for, not-and, exclusive-or – exist to describe contradictory and juxtapositional states and this is where the approaches adopted in connectionist and computational approaches to mentation can lend us a hand to escape these binary and spectrum malassumptions.

I am with Grant (2016) and Butler (1990), who argue that it is a trap to think that 'identity' is some kind of proscribed, constraint-free, essential quality of personhood. We are neither free from culture nor imbued with inherent agency (Zelazo, Astington & Olson, 1999). My mental health status is perhaps rather more like Grant's (2016) description of a 'performed activity reinforced through repeated action and conformity or resistance to culture pressures'. It could be argued that we would be better served focusing on 'subjectivity' over identity if we follow Butler's (1990) thoughts. However, I would argue that we should continue to focus on identity and necessarily embrace subjectivity as an integral constituent thereof (Zelazo, Astington & Olson, 1999). This is something inherently acknowledged in the theoretical work on the nature of the self that follows Bahktin (1929/1985), which positions the 'self' as inherently 'dialogical'. That is, as Lysaker and Lysaker (2001) put it in their case-study exploration of psychosis and self-structure, that the self is the product of 'ongoing dialogue within the individual and between the individual and others' (p25). It is also pertinent to reflect that, in this reading of the self, it is not an 'awareness of a single-perspective' but rather a dynamic, multi-component collection of sometimes complementary but also contradictory views, beliefs and voices (Lysaker & Lysaker, 2001).

While even in what psychiatry terms 'psychosis' – that is, caught in the midst of world reality-bending perceptual disruption (Williams, 2016) – my identity and status were still things I strove to cling onto while seemingly all those about me were either deliberately or unintentionally stripping them away. By this I mean that it was frequently assumed I had no 'insight' into my own condition and thus no expertise to bring to bear upon myself. As a result, I was no longer able to attend my course or go home without sanctioned leave and official negotiation.

At times I couldn't go out of the ward without being accompanied, and sometimes, because there was no one suitable to accompany me, not even then. I had at times very little contact or opportunities for contact with friends or, indeed, anybody, apart from my fellow inmates (and in this I include 'patients' and 'staff'). Of course, this was not true all the time or for all things. However, the burden of proof was high and showing any signs of being disrupted by a vision or having wild, exciting or disturbing, impossible ideas did lead to a 'You can't go on leave and you must stay'. Even just giggling out loud could lead to that if the staff deemed it was 'inappropriate'. I did have some money in my bank account but getting to a cash machine unimpeded was a challenge.

There is a wealth of literature and research that identifies the important role of structural threats to our health and wellbeing. Consider income inequality as one such structural threat. A raft of studies and papers have found that so-called mental illness is more common in societies that are more unequal, and that specific forms – ie. depression, schizophrenia and psychotic symptoms – are all more common in more unequal societies (Burns, Tomita & Kapadia, 2014; Messias, Eaton & Grooms, 2011; Pickett, James & Wilkinson, 2006; Pickett & Wilkinson, 2010). A psychosocial explanation of the effect of income inequality on health is consistent with the biology of chronic stress; it impairs memory and increases the risk of depression (Sapolsky, 2005). Threats to self-esteem are linked with cortisol responses (Dickerson & Kemeny, 2004); neuroimaging studies show that the social pain of exclusion activates the same brain areas as physical pain (Eisenberger, Lieberman & Williams, 2003), and baseline sensitivity to physical pain has been shown to predict sensitivity to social rejection and exclusion (Eisenberger et al, 2006).

Cruwys and colleagues (2013), as part of a growing body of social research work, have identified that, in depression, social connectedness (ie. membership of social groups) has both a protective *and* a curative quality. They found depressed participants with no group memberships reduced their risk of relapse by 24% by joining one group, and their risk of relapse reduced to 63% if they were members of three groups. Crucially, this is not solely about the potential beneficial opportunities for physical interaction but also relates to the ability of social group membership to develop a sense of shared identity with others. As Arendt puts it, we lose ourselves and our identities if we have no sense of the past, and, moreover, who we are is revealed in the stories we tell of ourselves and of our world shared with others (Arendt, 1998).

Rising to this ringing proclamation, having told my story of struggling with the role of leadership, I will now hand over to my author-colleague to tell his story of being a student in the Recovery College project.

Part 2: Steven Prosser's 'student' experience of attending the Recovery College

Four thousand words, FOUR THOUSAND WORDS! You idiot (that's me). After all, what do I know about the Recovery College? I don't know how it works or how the idea came about; all I know is what I experienced.

Let me take you back 12 months. I had lost my job as a civil servant through gross misconduct due to my mental health condition. I had attempted suicide by ligation and was taking assorted medications to ease the pain and turmoil going on in my mind. Help didn't exist as far as I was concerned. For three months I shook with fear and jumped at loud noises. My depression felt as if I had an actual weight on my body, I understood what the term 'being pressed' meant. At times, just getting out of bed was a major effort and all the doctors could offer me was a so-called fit note, but no other help unless you count increasing the dosage of my medication. That's right – offer an addictive personality stronger drugs.

Counselling was mentioned briefly and I was promised that my name would be added to the waiting list. I made some tentative enquiries and found out that the list was 18 weeks before an initial assessment and a further wait after that to actually get some counselling. Therefore, I didn't hold out much hope of assistance from the NHS, bless them; there's only so much money and physical health has always had a greater priority. Actually, I didn't have much hope in the NHS as a way of getting better. I was aware that mental health was talked about at a high level and its importance stressed. It's great to hear a health minister talk about how much money is being spent and how much in real terms the money for mental health has increased but I was also aware that, at the grass roots, nothing much was being done to alleviate the queues and suffering this caused. Actually, I didn't have any expectations of recovery; all I was looking forward to was mental illness and the idea that I would probably deteriorate further into what I referred to as The Beast.

The Beast presented itself to me in many forms and guises. My temper was one form that I had had issues with most of my life. So I had anger issues; didn't everyone? Apparently not. Once, when working in an ex-offender hostel, I had been ordered to attend counselling about my anger issues. That was just after I broke a man's fingers. He was remonstrating with me about something and to make his point clearer he was poking me in the chest, rather painfully. It seemed reasonable to me that I should defend myself.

The Beast manifested itself in depression: that terrible blackness, like a velvet net covering one's soul. So many people suffer in silence and so many take their own lives. Robin Williams said: 'The saddest people always try their hardest to make people happy because they know what it is like to feel absolutely worthless and they don't want anyone else to feel like that.' Many speak about it but only those few who suffer can really understand what it's like when, as Churchill called it, 'the Black Dog' comes. I had been given a diagnosis of bipolar – as it was called back in the early 1980s: I was a manic depressive. Then, in 2015, I was told that I wasn't bipolar but probably had personality disorder traits that caused me never to be on an even keel – I was either high or low, never level. The Beast again.

Alcohol had played a large part in my life for many years and so had my dependence on it. From my early 20s I had sought help. I had tried many ways to control my thirst over more than 30 years but the only thing that continued to work was the complete abstinence of the 12-Step Alcoholics Anonymous programme. I'd been on that for nine years, 'one day at a time', fighting The Beast.

I decided to attend a Mind group. I don't know why or from whom I got the idea but I gave them a call and found out about their opening times. Mind in Bradford allows a group called Moving Forward to meet on its premises on Wednesdays. Moving Forward is a men-only group run by facilitators who have 'come up through the ranks': in other words, they use their own mental health experience to help others. I have always believed that, in order to tackle and ultimately beat The Beast, I have to know The Beast and fight it head on. Before too long, I was helping out with facilitating, coming up with ideas and fully joining in the discussions; I was learning. A book called *The Curse of the Strong* by Tim Cantopher was highly recommended. It's written in language that I can understand and the author shows an insight that I believed, at that time, to be almost unique (Cantopher, 2012).

I do enjoy taking an active part in things and like to lead; I do not enjoy following, especially when I believe I can contribute. In fact, my ideas on what I can contribute have led me to voice my opinions to my detriment on many occasions. I am renowned for putting my foot in it. I just need to make the final statement, have the last word and make that unnecessary wisecrack. Too many years watching Humphrey Bogart films is my excuse, if I ever get the chance to apologise, but usually it's been too late for apologies.

One Thursday, at a Moving Forward meeting in a different location, I was told that someone was coming to do Mindfulness with us. Mindfulness? What was Mindfulness? This rather softly spoken, young (well, to me) man gave me my first taste of mindfulness. I felt relaxed, at ease, the tension and stiffness in the back of my neck was less than normal; in fact, I was at peace. This bloke was onto something; I didn't know what but he had something. He spoke of his own life experiences in mental health and I found out that he worked at the university. An academic no less.

Stephen Williams (as he turned out to be) then mentioned something that has had a profound effect on my life from that point on – the Recovery College at

Bradford University. University! My ears pricked up, like Spock's in Star Trek. A chance to attend Bradford University; to be able to say that I was at 'Uni'. I needed to know more: how, when, how much, where, what? We were given details of some courses and a website. I didn't take the website address in, as I was still hearing the word 'university'.

Within a short time, I knew I had to attend. My brain was already dreaming of a degree, maybe a doctorate, who knows how high I could go? Doctor Steven sounded good. My runaway brain was yet again dreaming of the future through a rose-coloured lens, never really ready to put in the hard work, just looking for the plaudits.

Just a note – my father didn't really encourage education or approve of 'further education', not when you should be out earning money. As a child, I hated school. I was bullied quite a lot and grew a mask of humour to hide my true feelings. Hence my distress at losing Robin Williams, who I felt expressed my feelings. Why have so many comedy greats been depressed? Why do people like Robin, Tony Hancock and others feel so down?

Because I failed to make a note of the website, I couldn't find the curriculum. Luckily, some kind person provided me with Stephen Williams' phone number. During a spluttering, by me, phone call I got the correct web address and I also got an invite to a meeting at the university to discuss the Recovery College. My ego knew no bounds; he wanted me to help! My confidence was boosted and I felt that there was a chance that life hadn't discarded me after all. The doctorate was back on the cards again. Maybe I was of some use to my family and society after all.

I met people at the meeting who had this plan to help people with mental health problems outside the normal (ie. NHS) settings. They were doing it because they believed they could make a change for the better. I didn't understand much of what was said; as we know, most people use acronyms for anything they deal with on a regular basis, so the room was full of 'mental-health speak', but what I did understand was that I was being treated as an equal and that I was being listened to by people with real qualifications, who cared so much that they wanted to do things to alleviate the problems people like me with mental health difficulties were finding.

I had to help. I volunteered to do anything that was needed and made up a few jobs that were not. About this time, I discovered that there were no formal qualifications on offer, but I didn't mind not getting the professorship this year. By now I had learnt that something positive was happening and some of my treatment was within my own control. For the first time, I could make some choices as to what therapy I was going to get. WRAP was mentioned. I googled it, discovered Wellness Recovery Action Planning and read of how its originator, Mary Ellen Copeland, had reacted to her mother's treatment and her own. Wellness Recovery Action Planning – the clue for me was in recovery. It's said, where there's life there's hope, and now I was getting hope.

Mindfulness was planned; once more I turned to Google and the name Jon Kabat-Zinn came up. YouTube furnished me with some rather long lectures by Mr Kabat-Zinn. I think that I will always refer to him as Mister even if I ever have the privilege of meeting him and he asks me to call him Jon. He is someone to whom I owe such a great deal. I bought some books by him and proceeded to read and pursue a state of Mindfulness. Even if I didn't understand what was happening, I knew that something was happening for my recovery.

Induction sessions were planned over a number of days and I volunteered to attend them all, so that my fellow students would have someone they could recognise who wasn't a tutor or from the faculty. It also made me feel important. I volunteered to act as liaison for my fellow students with their problems and difficulties. I do like to stand out from the crowd.

There is an art to listening. Most of us can hear but listening takes concentration. I wanted to understand. I needed a reason for why I am me. At the first session, I found a reason: people looked to me for guidance; my opinion was important. Yes, I was just a student; yes, we were all just students, but we were there because we wanted. No doctor, no health visitor, no psychiatrist had told us we had to attend. No court order, no judgment, not even a strong suggestion. We were there because we chose; because we wanted to understand; because we wanted some control of our own treatment.

Control of our treatment is something that so many people with mental health problems long for. Decisions are made for us; at best they are explained, at the worst we're told, 'It's for your own good.' At the Recovery College, there was a group of people who not only understood but could provide answers. I don't mean the facilitators; I mean my fellow students. We had been prodded, poked, drugged, sometimes unwillingly, sectioned, released into the community but rarely listened to. We knew all about treatments, all about new drugs and new ideas. Some of us had been around that long that the new ideas were old ideas coming back into fashion.

Here at the Recovery College, people listened to us. The facilitators were interested in our opinions and some delighted in our opinions of some of their colleagues. They learnt from us that we were aware of our problems and wanted to help in our treatments. WRAP was being done by some for the second time and at least one had completed it three times, not just as something to pass away the time but because it was important, because it could work. We need things that work; even if we have to sit through them three times or 23 times, as long as it's *our* choice.

I'm not the fastest at taking things in; I listen but I have a short attention span, so gazing out the window or observing what others are doing is more interesting after a while, but I found myself interested. The various subjects had to be listened to or I would miss something important. Homework, yes homework was handed out, with the expectation that it was going to be done and it was, willingly, because we wanted to do it.

I found a number of jobs to do – for instance, meeting one person by the main entrance and walking with them to their lecture room. They just wanted a friendly face among the crowds of 'real' students. Another had a wait between morning and afternoon sessions. We lunched together every week before going to our separate afternoon classes, or so they thought. I actually then went home because I didn't have an afternoon session, but for me it was nice to be needed, to be of some use. I had stopped feeling cast aside and was feeling a definite improvement in my health.

Quite early on, we started asking for ideas for the next year, or indeed if a next year was wanted. At meetings over coffee, we discussed what we would like to see. Yes, was the resounding answer to another Recovery College, and more of the same courses with a few added extras like a WRAP facilitators course and possibly a Mindfulness facilitators course, something about addictions, fitness or outdoor activities and gardening – the list was long and, in some cases, impractical. Driving lessons was one that I recall with fondness – try explaining to someone that the costs would be prohibitive when their argument was that, if they could drive, they could then find employment.

Now the not-so-good stuff. Whenever people meet, there is a likelihood of clashes of personality. The Recovery College was no different. Some were used to being in the front, of feeling important, but now they were one of a group and could not dominate the rest. 'My opinion is right as it's my opinion.' A few egos were popped, including my own, and some people chose to leave the group, either distancing themselves while still attending or, in a very few cases, not coming back.

I think that because I had attended the initial meet-and-greet sessions, most of my fellows trusted me and quickly pointed out disagreements and fallings out. I attempted to pour oil on troubled waters if I could, but in the case of those who left, all I could do was inform Stephen, and he would endeavour to contact them. I only know of one who continues to refuse to speak or communicate with me, despite all my attempts.

Room bookings sometimes went wrong. The Brexit referendum was a challenge as the local council took over to use as polling offices the lecture rooms we had booked and no one told us until that morning. Apparently they didn't ask before ordering the polling cards and literature; they assumed it would be okay. Luckily it wasn't raining, as I had to walk around the campus gathering up my strays like a shepherd finding his lost flock.

What did I gain from the Recovery College? Confidence? Most certainly. I got my mojo back – whatever the heck it is. I didn't know I'd lost it until I got it back and I'm still not sure but I know I can joke about it now without making depreciating remarks about myself. Yes, my humour is different: it's a more thoughtful type of humour. My wisecracks and jokes don't target individuals who can't fend for themselves. Less Frankie Boyle, more Billy Connolly. Certainly my temper is much better; ask my wife. (I did).

I am in more control of me, my inner me. I know what to do to relax. Yes, I isolate myself still but only because I want to do things that others don't enjoy as much - that certain TV programme I want to watch or the book I want to read in peace. I have become an enthusiastic gardener and have an allotment where I find peace with what I call 'mindfulness gardening'. What I greatly enjoy is how the simple concentration on what I'm doing helps me block out the negativity that tries to take me prisoner.

I have started work, in the civil service, and I have a fantastic manager who cares about me and my condition. The managers are brilliant and actually want to help rather than hinder; they want me to be happy. I practise Mindfulness meditation at my desk. The first couple of times, some colleagues made jokes about it; they didn't realise that I could hear and understand them while meditating until I gave suitable answers to their quips after I had finished. Now no one takes any notice; it's accepted as the norm for me and I have heard colleagues proudly defending me: 'No, he's not sleeping, Steve's meditating,' and, 'I wish I could do that, just blot out the surroundings and find some peace.'

If I were asked what was the most important aspect of the whole Recovery College, it would not be any course or individual; it would be the choices. We first chose to attend; then we chose which course to attend; next we chose to actually turn up, and finally we chose to participate. As I have written above, so many times people with mental health difficulties lose the power of choice. The Recovery College, for its duration, empowered the participants and this empowerment gave us strength to take more of an active part in the decisions that are being taken about us. No one among us is ready to take over all the decisions; I am still unable to look after money – if I have it, I spend it. But we can now express ourselves in a more confident way, a way that deserves being listened to and deferred to, rather than just a nodding way. If you don't know what I mean, watch someone who has no interest in your opinion and notice how good they are at pretending that your opinions matter by nodding their head while the rest of their body language tells you they don't care.

I have a plan now: thanks to WRAP, I know roughly what I will be doing on a daily basis and how to cope. For the most part, I am at peace and, if I do get agitated, angry or sad, I know what to do: meditate, take myself away from the problem, listen to the sound of my own breathing for a while, get some sleep, eat – any or all of these can offer help, it just depends on the circumstances and my location. For the most part, I now know when things are wrong and that means I can attempt to rectify the situation, or at least remove myself from it.

If it wasn't for the Recovery College, I don't know where I would be now but certainly Iwouldn't be writing about it.

Part 3: the Atrium meeting

Having written our accounts separately, we met, having read them for the first time, to discuss each other's experiences.

Steve W: To get the ball rolling, can I say something about how I found it reading your account as a student?

Steve P: Certainly.

Steve W: I was really moved by what you wrote. I found it a really powerful story. It told me a lot more about how difficult it was for you before you even got through the doors of the Recovery College. Early on, you talked about the very first telephone conversation we had. It strikes me how different you are now a couple of years on from that moment. You mentioned how nervous you felt. I remember listening to you on that day and thinking to myself, 'This is a guy who could really do with someone showing a bit of faith and confidence in him.' That's what was stirred up for me when I read that bit of your account.

Steve P: My biggest gain from reading yours was the insight into your own mental health and the wonderful bit about you writing down who you were in felt-tip pen when you were sectioned. It really humanised the piece. Reading your section as well as getting used to using the dictionary made me appreciate I haven't used words in the way I could have done and should have done, from a lack of needing to. In some of my work now, I am now expressing myself for the first time. As to my opinion of the Recovery College, I don't think I would be alive without it because I learned so much.

Steve W: That became so apparent to me when I read your account, because you wrote very elegantly and succinctly about the difficulties you had with depression and the events at work that led up to it. I'm wondering how much the relationship we developed through being leader and student in the Recovery College might have changed if I had known more about your earlier personal circumstances.

Steve P: I remember, when I was at sixth-form college as a young man, my wife told me that all the girls were afraid of me. I wondered why that was. But apparently they were afraid.

Steve W: I guess that speaks to how people judge one another by how we appear to each other – both visually and how we talk to and with each other, what we know about each other and what we tell each other.

Steve P: I remember my old college principal saying to me that the angry young man had gone and been replaced by a gentler person. I think, with the Recovery College, I came to it with a lot of anger and a lot of fear. I approached it with, 'Well, I've got to give it a try even though it's not going to work.' Once I'd started the WRAP course, I learned you've got to plan your life. Once I'd started doing that, I gained a lot more confidence.

Steve W: What I take away from that is you wanted to go to the Recovery College wanting to go to it – knowing that you needed to make a change but not really sure that the College was going to be able to do anything for you. The very first thing I wrote about running the Recovery College was feeling really uncertain about whether it was going to pan out, whether we were doing the right thing and whether anyone was going to turn up at all. I really didn't want it to be like services when I was younger, where you didn't get any choice and no one really cared about what you said. These things could be used against you – for example, you might not be allowed to leave the unit if you said something other people didn't like or felt was 'inappropriate'. These were some of the things I was striving to stay away from.

Steve P: Yeah, people were there because they wanted to be there and make choices that they hadn't had with mainstream rehabilitation. With my alcoholism, the only thing that worked for me was AA, and there are no professionals in AA.

Steve W: So, are you telling me that being among peers – with people with experiences – was significant in helping you recover at the College?

Steve P: Yes definitely – peer mentoring works. I think of that research – if you are depressed and join a group, you are 26% less likely to relapse, and if you join three or more social groups, that gets you to 66%. I've got three groups that interest me now and things that occupy and relax me. Mindfulness gardening, for instance, helps me now – it's a wonderful way of relaxing because I can devote my thoughts to exactly what I'm doing, which is sometimes really creating life.

Steve W: I wonder if there is a relationship between creating a life for yourself, or the possibility of creating a life for yourself, and what has come out of going through the Recovery College?

Steve P: Possibly, yes.

Steve W: So, some of the things you are talking about are getting into groups, being with other people and regaining a sense of community. But I also get the sense that you also have regained a sense of purpose?

Steve P: The whole thing is I gained confidence in myself. As I wrote, my first dream was to be an academic. What I wanted was hope for the future. When we students discussed things, I found so many people knew a lot about each other's treatments. Lots of suggestions were made – there was an interchange of ideas between us. This was so important – to have the freedom to discuss these things, and also that people had the freedom to opt out and say no.

Steve W: I was always disappointed when people didn't get out of the course what they wanted and left, but content about them being able to exercise that choice.

Steve P: I'm still in contact with people from the College – we've formed friendships – and they have got so much out of it too. One is playing football in a team, another is learning to drive after years of being terrified. We celebrate each other's achievements.

Steve W: So, people have been able to gain confidence – they've got some hope going and gained a sense of community from the experience. They've started to believe they can transform themselves and be more than someone stuck in a traumatised or distressed past. Not everybody, but many.

Steve P: You learn to stand up straighter. You don't feel as tired. There's a purpose. Even after a couple of sessions, you knew there was a purpose. There was a light at the end of the tunnel for everybody who could reach for it.

Steve W: And what drove me to form the community at the university were memories of being controlled, being coerced, being told what to do and how I needed to behave. All the very opposite to how I wanted things to be for people when they attended the College.

Steve P: To be listened to by academics and professionals and realise that you valued my opinions on things was a great uplift for me.

Steve W: I was really struck by the impact learning about mindfulness had for you – that you had a sense that something was happening for your recovery even if you didn't know what that was.

Steve P: I had three minutes of mindfulness at work today, waiting for my call to be put through. I've woven it into my everyday now. It just expands your mind.

Steve W: It seems like you've taken away some tools and that, on top of this, the camaraderie of being with others and growing friendships and being heard seriously have been important to you.

Steve P: Yes, we laughed with each other as we told our stories and we enjoyed each other's stories as a fellowship.

Steve W: Do you think there is a better way of talking about the Recovery College?

Steve P: In a lot of ways, we know what it means – and just the word 'college' is a problem. Maybe this is confusing.

Steve W: At the moment we are calling it a Wellness Academy.

Steve P: I still like Recovery, because that means hope. We have to keep moving and keep learning, reading and talking and trying to understand. When I learned about WRAP I had to go and find out why Mary Ellen developed it after her experiences with other kinds of treatment, to try and understand more about it for myself.

Steve W: What we tried to do was invite people to come together in nice spaces without spending too much time going through their personal history and becoming overly fixated on risk assessment. We wanted to give people space to find their own way through, accessing the College for what they needed.

Steve P: By not asking us what our 'problem' was all the time, we probably made a lot more progress. Instead, we were allowed to choose what we wanted to work on and what courses we thought might be helpful to us. We had an exchange of opinions, views and solutions. It's so important that people listen to us without then telling us what's wrong with us or what we need to do about it.

Further reading

McAdams DP, McLean KC (2013). Narrative identity. *Current Directions in Psychological Science 22*(3): 233–238.

Sherman DK, Cohen GL (2006). The psychology of self-defense: self-affirmation theory. In: Zanna MP (ed). *Advances in Experimental Social Psychology* vol 38. San Diego, CA: Academic Press (pp183–242).

References

Arendt H (1998). *Human condition* (2nd ed). Chicago: University of Chicago Press.

Arendt H (1963). *Eichmann in Jerusalem: a report on the banality of evil*. New York, NY: Viking Press.

Bahktin M (1929/1985). *Problems of Dostoyevsky's Poetics* (C Emerson trans). Minneapolis MN: University of Minnesota Press.

Burns JK, Tomita A, Kapadia AS (2014). Income inequality and schizophrenia incidence in countries with high levels of income inequality. *International Journal of Social Psychiatry 60*(2): 185–196.

Butler J (1990). *Gender Trouble: feminism and the subversion of identity*. New York, NY: Routledge.

Cantopher T (2012). *Depressive Illness: the curse of the strong* (3rd ed). London: SPCK Publishing.

Clark DM, Wells A (1995). A cognitive model of social phobia. In: Heimberg RG, Liebowitz MR, Hope DA, Schneier FR (eds). *Social Phobia: diagnosis, assessment, and treatment*. New York, NY: Guilford Press (pp69–93).

Cooke A (2017). *Understanding Psychosis and Schizophrenia: why people sometimes hear voices, believe things that others find strange, or appear out of touch with reality, and what can help*. Leicester: British Psychological Society.

Cruwys T, Dingle GA, Haslam C, Haslam SA, Jetten J, Morton TA (2013). Social group memberships protect against future depression, alleviate depression symptoms and prevent depression relapse. *Social Science and Medicine 98*: 179–186.

Dennett DC (1991). *Consciousness Explained*. Boston, MA: Little, Brown & Company.

Dickerson SS, Kemeny ME (2004). Acute stressors and cortisol responses: a theoretical integration and synthesis of laboratory research. *Psychological Bulletin 130*(3): 355–391.

Eisenberger NI, Jarcho JM, Lieberman MD, Naliboff BD (2006). An experimental study of shared sensitivity to physical pain and social rejection. *Pain 126*(1-3): 132–138.

Eisenberger NI, Lieberman MD, Williams KD (2003). Does rejection hurt? An FMRI study of social exclusion. *Science 302*(5643): 290–292.

Grant A (2016). Storying the world: a posthumanist critique of phenomenological-humanist representational practices in mental health nurse qualitative inquiry. *Nursing Philosophy 17*(4): 290–297.

Harper D, Speed E (2014). Uncovering recovery: the resistible rise of recovery and resilience. In: Speed E, Moncrieff J, Rapley M (eds). *De-Medicalizing Misery II*. Basingstoke: Palgrave Macmillan (pp40–57).

Lysaker PH, Lysaker JT (2001). Psychosis and the disintegration of dialogical self-structure: problems posed by schizophrenia for the maintenance of dialogue. *British Journal of Medical Psychology 74*(1): 23–33.

Messias E, Eaton WW, Grooms AN (2011). Economic grand rounds: income inequality and depression prevalence across the United States: an ecological study. *Psychiatric Services 62*(7): 710–712.

Perkins R, Slade M (2012). Recovery in England: transforming statutory services? *International Review of Psychiatry 24*(1): 29–39.

Pickett KE, James OW, Wilkinson RG (2006). Income inequality and the prevalence of mental illness: a preliminary international analysis. *Journal of Epidemiological Community Health 60*(7): 646–647.

Pickett KE, Wilkinson RG (2010). Inequality: an underacknowledged source of mental illness and distress. *British Journal of Psychiatry 197*(6): 426–428.

Rhodes E (2015). Something's burning. [Online.] *The Psychologist*, 16 June. https://thepsychologist.bps.org.uk/somethings-burning (accessed 15 May 2018).

Rosenhan DL (1973). On being sane in insane places. *Science 179*(4070): 250–258.

Sapolsky R (2005). Sick of poverty. *Scientific American 293*(6): 92–99.

Short NP, Turner L, Grant A (eds) (2013). *Contemporary British Autoethnography*. Rotterdam: Sense Publishers.

Singh SP, Burns T, Amin S, Jones PB, Harrison G (2004). Acute and transient psychotic disorders: precursors, epidemiology, course and outcome. *British Journal of Psychiatry 185*(December): 452–459.

Williams S (2016). *Recovering from Psychosis: empirical evidence and lived experience*. Abingdon: Routledge.

Zelazo PD, Astington JW, Olson DR (1999). *Developing Theories of Intention: social understanding and self-control*. Mahwah, NJ: Lawrence Erlbaum Associates.

4 | A balancing act?[1]

Darren Mills

It normally begins with a phone call. A heartbeat thumps to acknowledge the first ring. Like Pavlov's dog, a number of physiological changes kick in, heightening my senses, speeding my thoughts and accentuating my being. Here I am. About to be. A being as a voice on the end of the phone.

How will the caller perceive me? Empathic, sympathetic, a validator, a challenger, a realist, a supporter, a rejecter, inspirational, helpful, dogmatic, pragmatic, a bastard, a connection, a fellow being, a human being? I hope that the caller perceives my humanity. Within the next three to four rings, several thoughts invade my mind, swiftly followed by a number of standard replies:

What if the caller is too distressed to speak to me clearly?

That is okay; I can give them time, reassure, thank them for calling, and wait. I can validate their distress and support the caller with breathing exercises. Then talk. (Empathic, a connection, hopeful.)

What if the caller is rude or abusive?

I can ask them to stop swearing, let them know I am here to support but I will not tolerate abuse. I hope that I can de-escalate their anger or, if they continue to be abusive, I can inform the caller I will terminate the call. If I need to, I can hang up. (Pragmatic, dogmatic, no doubt a bastard if I hang up.)

---

1. None of the incidents or people mentioned in this ethnography are real, although the occurrences are authentic and based on events that frequently occur in a mental health crisis assessment. Although a fictional piece, the components of the narrative depict the reality often faced by people involved in mental health crisis situations. The themes it raises are supported by cuttings and briefings from news agencies and national and international organisations and institutions.

What if the caller is in imminent danger?

Easy –explain clearly that they need to call the police for personal safety if they are at risk from someone else. If they persist in wanting immediate attendance from the crisis team, I can briefly explain our resources and times of response – that is, we have four mental health clinicians covering an area the size of a small African country and we can be there within six hours. I can also call the police if they give me an address.

If they are calling with an imminent suicide plan, I can thank the caller for making contact and get them to talk, which will include finding out where they are, who they are with and why they want to end their life. If they are calling, then it is likely some part of them does not want to die and they are seeking help. However, with suicide rates being so high in New Zealand, I am not taking anything for granted.

The highest rate of teen suicide in the developed world[2]

New Zealand has the highest rate of teen suicide in the developed world, an OECD report reiterates.

Despite the alarming information, the report revealed nothing new.

New Zealand continuously ranked among the worst in the world for our levels of teen suicide.

In a normal week two teenagers or two children kill themselves, Youthline director Stephen Bell says. About 20 young people will be hospitalised for self-harm each week, he estimated.

This was New Zealand's shame, he said. If suicide was a contagious disease, Bell said, the country would have demanded action. (McConnell, 2017)

Small talk can help to get to know the person a little better, build basic rapport and trust while I direct a colleague to call the police, if I am not alone, without the caller's knowledge, potentially with their knowledge. (Pragmatic, empathic, supportive, hopeful.)

What if I cannot hear the caller properly, or I have difficulty getting their demographics and clarifying their address, contact details and the nature of the mental health crisis? (Silence. Hello? Anxiety.)

Louder heart thump. I pick up the phone.

---

2. All quotes in boxes are quoted verbatim from contemporary media sources.

'Hello, Crisis Mental Health Line, you are speaking with Darren.' I put the emphasis on 'Darren', as in, 'I am a person, you have not got through to a computerised answer phone service'… yet.

'How can I help?' I say in a measured tone.

'Hello, I was hoping you could give me some advice.' The caller sounds elderly; she is quietly spoken and cautious.

'Certainly, how can I help you today?' The next heartbeat is slower and quieter.

'I am calling about my grandson,' she says.

'Tell me about your grandson… how old is he and what are you worried about?' I ask.

'He has been getting so… angry recently. Oh, he is 19 years and living with me and his *tatao* (siblings). He's been getting mad for the last few months now, shouting and punching the walls. He won't tell us what is bothering him.' Her hesitancy is less now, but I cannot discern any anxiety or concern in her voice.

> *This has been going on for a while. What is the mental health component besides anger? Maybe I need to direct this conversation a little more. She sounds very calm about it all, though.*

'Sorry, I didn't ask for your name or the name of your grandson,' I say, taking control at this point.

'I'm Mia and my grandson is called Jono.'

'Nice to talk to you, Mia. Is Jono his full name or nickname?' (I am now focused on his demographics). 'It would be helpful for me to have his full first and last name so that I can look your grandson up on our system here to see if we have had previous contact with him. Do you know if he has had contact with mental health services before?'

'I don't think he has. His name is Jonathon W___ and he lives with me here in F___. He's been living with me since he was nine… or… 10 years of age. After his parents split, his mum couldn't manage all the kids so I agreed to take a few.'

'Okay. Thanks Mia. I am just going to start looking up Jono on the computer while I ask a few questions, if that's okay?' I start to type his name into the computer. There are two different possibilities, the first showing a date of birth from the 1960s. The other entry matches the age. I click and confirm the village mentioned by Mia.

'Of course,' says Mia, after a long pause. 'I'm not sure if I can answer everything though.'

'No worries,' I say, injecting some energy into the conversation through heightening my tone. 'So, Jono has been living with you for a number of years. Has he had problems with anger in the past or has this been a more recent thing?'

'No, he has always been a very good boy.' I can hear the pride in her voice, the word good is drawn out and slightly musical. 'Of course, sometimes he has had his moments, like his brothers, but he's never been directly angry towards me… or threatened me before.'

'He threatened you? What did he say and when was this?' I ask, putting emphasis on the word 'threatened'.

'Oh, he told me that he would,' she pauses, possibly reaching for the right word, then says, 'Thump me. Often when I ask him not to be so noisy or try and get him to eat.'

'He's not eating? What about sleep?'

'Oh no, he hasn't been sleeping well for weeks now, I think. I mean, mmm, it's hard for me to know exactly, but I sometimes wake at three or four in the morning with him shouting and arguing and banging in his room. When I've asked him to be quiet… because he's disturbing my *moko* (grandchildren)… he tells me to fuck off otherwise he'll...' she trails off. 'Came running at me once, screaming and shouting and waving his arms about.' The tone of her voice changes. I can detect fear. 'Other times, he just sits there and won't talk to anyone, staring at nothing. He's a bit like that at the moment,' she says, flatly.

'Who is he arguing with?' I ask, sure that the answer will be 'no one' but not wanting to assume.

'No one that's been coming round… his friends,' she says defensively. 'He's often been talking with people lately, all alone,' she goes on, more softly. 'Laughs,' she laughs, 'to himself as well sometimes. He seems a bit worse when he's been drinking with his cousins.'

This is not looking good.

'Okay, I'm sorry to hear that,' I say sincerely. 'Must be upsetting for you and your *moko*. How old is the youngest child in the house? Has he ever threatened to harm them or anyone else?'

'Yes, he did threaten to bash Whiri' she says, omitting his age. 'Whiri just avoids his big brother whenever he can now. Such a… shame… as Jono has always gotten on well with his brother… often acted like a father. Their father doesn't have any contact. With one of the gangs, in and out of prison. His mum has her own demons to deal with,' she says, indicating potential mental health, drug or alcohol issues, and with a note of intolerance in her voice – a suggestion of patience long gone. 'My husband died a long time ago,' she notes wistfully. 'Rawiri was quite well known,' she said. 'Played rugby.'

She is on her own, I think. Yet another grandparent responsible for bringing up the grandchildren, struggling to get financial support while the parents are struggling with addictions. I check my emotive reflections and biases, though it's not uncommon to hear through the media about the growing struggles of grandparents and their difficulties with the state benefit system.

Grandparents' struggles to bring up their *mokopuna*

Grandparents bringing up babies for the second time around say that navigating their way through the welfare system is one of the toughest parts of the job...

Many of these grandparents or *kaumatua* are stepping in because they don't want to see their grandchildren or *mokopuna* go into care.

Social agencies like the Manukau Urban Māori Authority (MUMA) say that they've seen an increase in grandparents or kaumatua seeking their help. Many want help dealing with Work and Income, Housing New Zealand and Oranga Tamariki...

Often these children come into their grandparents' lives under difficult or tragic circumstances involving family violence, drugs or alcohol. (Perera, 2017)

'Have you tried to get him help before? Like see his GP, general practitioner or...?' I trail off, not sure what to add.

'No, I did try once to take him to see the family doctor. However, Jono said there was nothing wrong with him and wouldn't go. He accused me of putting things in his food.' (Pause.) 'Maybe that's why he isn't eating,' she says, with sudden recognition.

'What do you think he would do if we turned up there, Mia, and asked him if he wanted some support?'

'I don't think he will want to speak with you, but you can ask him. I'll get him.' She suddenly disappears and there is a clunk as she puts the phone down. I can hear mumbled speaking, mainly her, no raised voices. It sounds like she is pleading. After about a minute, I hear steps coming back in my direction.

'Hello,' says a soft voice without emotion.

'Hi Jono, my name is Darren and I am calling from the mental health services. Your Nan is a bit worried about you at the moment and I wondered what you think?'

(Silence… 10 seconds.)

'Do you think you would like to see someone to talk about how you are feeling at the moment?'

(Silence… 10 seconds.)

> *Where can I go with this? Do I push that we would like to come out and see him or might he take off? Why did he come to the phone but not talk? He sounds unwell. There are clearly risks. I wonder why Mia phoned today and not yesterday, and when did he last threaten her? Is he scared of me? What is he thinking? Is he at risk from suicide?*

Chief Coroner releases provisional annual suicide figures

Chief Coroner Judge Deborah Marshall today released the annual provisional suicide statistics, which show 606 people died by suicide in the 2016/17 year – the third year in a row that the number has increased.

This is the highest number of suicide deaths since the provisional statistics were first recorded for the 2007/08 year, and follows last year's total of 579 (2015/16), and 564 in the year before that (2014/15)… This year's figures show:

The 20–24 year-old age cohort recorded the highest number of suicide deaths (79), followed by 64 each in both the 25–29 and 40–44 year-old cohorts. Last year, the 25–29-year-old age cohort recorded the highest number of suicide deaths (66), followed by the 20–24-year-old cohort (60) and 45-49 age group (57).

Māori suicide death numbers are up by one from last year with 130, which was the same as two years earlier. Māori continue to have the highest suicide rate of all ethnic groups at 21.73. (Office of the Chief Coroner New Zealand, 2017)

'Jono, I would like to come out and meet with your Nan if that is okay and talk about why she is worried about you. It would be good if you would talk to me as well. Would that be okay?'

(Silence.) 'No.'

There is the sound of the phone being put down, picked up again.

'Hi, it's Mia. He handed the phone back to me. Looks like he is going over to Tamati's house… Tamati is a decent boy, his cous [meaning his cousin]. What can he do? What can I do?' she asks, with desperation in her voice now.

'Well Mia, I'm really worried about your grandson. It sounds like he could be very unwell at the moment and I am worried about his and your safety with his outbursts. We do need to see him and see him this evening. Do you think he needs to go into hospital?' I cringe at my awkward questions and jumbled response to her request.

'I suppose so. I don't really know about that. That's why I'm calling,' she says.

Of course she is, you idiot [I am addressing myself].

'Sure. I wanted to know your thoughts, as it sounds to me that we will need Jono to see one of our doctors, and I'm afraid that we may need to ask the police for some help to do that, as Jono has refused to meet up with me.'

Bringing in the police at this point is inevitable, once he's said 'No'. It could have meant anything. He may not have understood my question, but my clinical reasoning suggests a lack of insight. A lack of reasoning. Madness. A state of being that allows me to take control. And I have the authority to act according the Mental Health (Compulsory Assessment and Treatment) Act, 1992.

'Okay,' says Mia in an even tone. 'I suppose it's for the best. When will you get here?'

'It may be a few hours. I need to have a chat with my colleagues here about how we best do this without causing your grandson too much distress. But I do think we will need to have police support as we are not able to restrain him or stop him if he takes off. I'm worried that he might hurt himself if he took off. It can take quite a while for the police sometimes, as this is not an emergency. However, if he becomes threatening to you or others or tries to hurt himself, please phone 111. You can tell the police that you have had contact with us, but tell them you are worried for yourself and the children in the house, or his safety, if things escalate. Would you do that?'

'Yes, I suppose so,' she says. I confirm her address, telephone number, and ask her whether she has any questions. 'No, I don't think so' she says. 'Thank you for helping my boy.'

'I will call you with a time as soon as I know we can come out. Thanks for the call, Mia, and see you soon.' I hang on for any last questions, then hang up the phone after a period of silence and a click.

I look around the room. It is a messy office, with empty mugs, empty crisp bags and a half-eaten salad scattered over the desks, next to antiquated computers, monitors, mobile phones, scraps of paper and a few files. The heater is humming noisily. The windows are grimy and the carpets soiled with trampled-in food stains from over the years. My colleague, who is coordinating this evening's shift, is on another call. I am not sure where the other two nurses are now. I glance at the time.

It's the start of another shift.

One of my colleagues comes into the room with a cup of coffee and bowl of salad. She is a petite lady in her early 50s with an eccentric taste in mismatched second-hand clothing and a shock of silver hair, styled by a connection to the national grid. Tonight she is wearing a green outfit that resembles a jungle of seaweed bleached by a nuclear blast.

Jean has been a nurse with the crisis team for at least 10 years; she is highly experienced, very professional and a great reflector, from my point of view.

'Jean,' I say, 'we have a job.' We both look at Bob, who is coordinating our shift tonight. The crisis team 'after-hours' coordinator is a rotating role among all of us and based on our roster patterns. This means that one of the four shifts is taking the phone calls in the office, triaging them and then directing the work to the others. For the other three shifts, you are mainly out, seeing people in police stations or emergency departments, occasionally in their own homes. Bob appears deeply involved in supporting someone to manage their distress through validation and mindfulness techniques.

'Tell me about the assessment,' says Jean, munching on her salad.

'The caller was his grandmother,' I reply. 'Male, 19 years old, no previous history with us or anyone else, from what I can see. Lived with his Nan for about half his life. Mia, his Nan, called about his anger problems, I don't think she knows what is wrong apart from something being wrong, but she clearly described someone who is presenting with a psychotic episode, likely been going on for weeks… if not months.'

'What are the symptoms?' she asks, her interest validating my concerns.

'Arguing with himself and responding to voices, verbally aggressive at times, poor sleep for weeks, reduced eating because he thinks he is being poisoned. Has threatened Mia and his little brother. Major change from his normal self. I tried to speak with him but he didn't respond apart from saying "No", when I asked to come over and meet him.'

'What about drugs,' she asks.

'Sorry, didn't ask.' I silently kick myself. 'However, using alcohol at times, which makes his behaviours worse. Mia did not seem to be distressed. She was phoning for some advice. I am worried. I think we need to see him this evening, and I think we need to use police.'

'Why police?'

'He's not interested in meeting up. My feeling is that he is psychotic and will need an admission. I cannot see him coming with us. He's unknown and there's been an escalation in threats. Who knows how he will react to us turning up? Perhaps the police can wait in the wings to begin with.'

'Makes sense. We need to run it by Bob. I'm not sure what else is on this evening, but if we do go out it will take up most of the night. Do you want to phone through to the police for assistance, see how busy they are?' she asks.

I look at Bob. He appears to be ending the conversation, thanking the person for the call, summarising the plan. I wait. He puts down the phone. He looks angry.

'That wouldn't have happened, *if* her bloody team had made contact today liked we asked from last night's contact.'

'Who's the key worker?' I ask.

'Sally M_____. Useless!'

'Well, that's because she has a caseload of 45, and probably covering for others,' responds Jean.

Nine in 10 healthcare workers feel understaffed and under-resourced

Understaffing and fears of burnout among health workers could be jeopardising patient safety, and reducing access to care, unions have warned.

A survey of almost 6000 paramedics, nurses, mental health workers and support staff has found 90 per cent felt the healthcare system was understaffed and under-resourced.

The same proportion said funding was affecting access to healthcare, and 72 per cent said their workload and work pressures were not reasonable. (Canin, 2017).

'Anyway, what do we have on? Darren has a potential assessment,' Jean adds.

Bob looks down at the sprawl of scribbled notes on his desk. 'Two in the emergency department. Both overdoses. I can't imagine how the woman who took five sleeping tablets and half a bottle of whisky three hours ago is going to be ready for interview, though the nurse has already called. Needing the bed probably.'

'Well it's not the first time that ED has been at full capacity, if that's the case,' retorts Jean. 'People can't afford to see their GP, if they are lucky to have one in their area, so turn up at ED with chipped toenails and a bit of fluff in their eye. No wonder the emergency staff are as stressed as we are.'

All Auckland hospitals at capacity, all non-urgent patients asked to stay away

More and more hospitals are feeling the pressure of winter illnesses, with patients being told to stay away unless they are seriously sick.

Both North Shore Hospital and Waitakere Hospital in Auckland were experiencing high demand and occupancy levels, Waitemata District Health Board said on Thursday.

The DHB's acting chief medical officer Dr. Jonathan Christiansen asked people to 'think twice' before going to the emergency department at either hospital... 'Emergency departments are for seriously unwell patients in need of emergency care, and patients with less serious health concerns could delay treatment for patients in serious emergency situations,' he said. (Stuff, 2017)

I explain the phone call and the plan to Bob, as soon as Jean takes a breath. 'Why tonight?' asks Bob. 'That will take up most of the night, and this has been going on for weeks!'

'Because she called us and now he knows we know. Who knows how he will react. He might take off. Nan's on her own and there are kids there,' I say, emphasising risks. Then I add: 'The ED jobs can wait, they are in a safe place, even though we're supposed to assess them within six hours.'

'Okay,' says Bob, clearly not looking for an argument tonight, which makes a pleasant change, and probably due to his phone ringing again at that point.

I dial the number for police communications and speak to a person in the call centre.

'You're speaking with Matt from police communications, how can I help?' says a muffled voice with a few clicks in between words.

'Hi, my name's Darren, I'm a duly authorised officer calling from B_____ crisis mental health services. I would like police assistance to support a mental health assessment, under the Mental Health Act.' I explain the situation briefly, emphasising that the young man has been verbally aggressive, is declining assessment, lives with his elderly Nan and that there are children in the house. I confirm that I have not seen him yet. When asked, however, I put forward my concerns regarding potential risks. Matt requests I go the property and wait for police to show up. He is unable to give a timeframe but gives a police job number for me to call once I'm there, for updates.

My next call is to the psychiatric registrar on duty. I am happy to hear it's Frances, who is helpful and agreeable to the plan. She asks me to keep her 'in the loop' as things progress, after asking about how I am. She says: 'Take some prn (*pro re nata*, meaning 'take as needed') out and call me if you need to use any.' She's referring to a one-off dose of medication that can reduce agitation, which we can take from a small box of medications held in the office.

I next call the coordinator of the S_____ in-patient unit. Jolene is in charge tonight. 'Well, I don't know where we are going to put him. I don't have any beds,' she says, as soon as I indicate that there is a potential admission. 'Why tonight?' she asks, meaning on her shift. 'I know,' I say, likely echoing her thoughts: the S_____ unit has been at full capacity for months now. One of the issues is people who 'block' beds – that is, people who cannot be discharged from the wards when well enough, as they do not have a suitable place to go. Some of them are homeless, a growing number. A few people have been stuck on an acute inpatient ward for months, as there are no facilities in the community appropriate to support their complex needs. It has not been uncommon for new patients to sleep on a mattress in an interview room.

Opinion: Mental health service in crisis – still

This week we are once more reminded that the mental health system is in crisis, with the update by Kirsty Johnson in the *Herald* on autistic man, Ashley Peacock, who has been locked in an isolated mental health unit for five years; a place so isolated his long-suffering parents have never been inside.

This is a heart-breaking story, and certainly not an isolated case.

The care of psychotic patients is, of course, extremely complicated. But the key part of the story is identified by psychologists working in the system themselves: Ashley, and people like him with 'complex needs', do not have services – or not enough services – in enough places around the country that will allow them and their families decent quality of life. (DeBoni, 2016).

'Right, ready to go?' I ask Jean after hanging up the phone to the coordinator.

I park the car about five houses down from number 14B_____ Street. A faint drizzle mists up the windows, making it difficult to see out. It is a muggy evening and the outside temperature is on the warm side for winter. Dusk is settling in. Jean is attempting to force chocolate and crisps into me, her mothering tendencies to the fore.

'So, how is the thesis going?' she asks.

I had started a master's research thesis on the emergence of recovery philosophy in New Zealand's mental health service provision how it first appeared, who key players were, its use in policy and practice. I was trying to put a Foucauldian spin on it by looking at power relationships – that is, how different groups could access power through the discourse of recovery. I was also interested in enduring knowledge, the kinds of beliefs that may have been around 200 years ago and are still prevalent as knowledge in today's society. I was interested in the possible tensions created through the discourse of recovery, through the creation of subjects, the circulation of truth as socio-political comment and Panoptic power as a form of self-governance.

'Great,' I say.

> I am a fraud and Jean will figure that out as I inarticulately babble some nonsense and try to make sense of what I have read and attempt to demonstrate that I know what I am talking about. My 'intellectual ambitions amount to little more than an elaborate hoax' (Fleming, 2006: 30).

'I've been writing about resiliency at the moment, the new buzzword in recovery discourse,' I tell her. 'The promotion of health literacy and personal responsibility in current health policy has shifted attention away from the providers of mental health services, to those that use them.'

'Explain!' says Jean.

'At the beginning of this century, policy emphasis was on providers of services, clinicians, to adopt recovery philosophy in their practice. It was used to tackle the stigma and discrimination coming from the mental health workforce, which was acting as a barrier to social inclusion, among other things. That whole shift from institutional to community-based care required a change in clinical attitudes. It appears that *we* have adopted recovery as now the attention is on the service user.'

'Well, nothing wrong with that, if it's about treating people with dignity, helping people to achieve their goals and focusing on strengths,' responds Jean.

'That's all well and good, Jean,' I say, 'but what about the expectations that come with resiliency?'

'I'm not sure what you mean.'

'Resiliency rightly suggests that the solutions that support recovery come from the person experiencing mental illness. As long as their solutions match the values of our society and psychiatric discourse, we see the person as engaging with recovery. However, resiliency not only situates the solutions but also the problem within the individual. It is their fault for not being resilient enough in the first place and becoming unwell.'

'That's a bit of a generalisation, but I can go with that.'

'My concern with the concept of resiliency is that it could be used by groups – for example, our policy makers – to further draw attention away from the socio-political and environmental factors that can cause illness in the first place. How can we expect people to be resilient when they are living in poverty and dealing with the detrimental factors attached to poverty? Look how many kids are living in poverty currently; how can they develop resiliency while living in volatile situations without the basics, like food?'

Child poverty is a reality in New Zealand

Right now, 28% of New Zealand children – about 295,000 – currently live in income poverty.*

When a child grows up in poverty they miss out on things most New Zealanders take for granted. They are living in cold, damp, over-crowded houses, they do not have warm or rain-proof clothing, their shoes are worn, and many days they go hungry. It can mean doing badly at school, not getting a good job, having poor health and falling into a life of crime. (UNICEF, 2017)

*According to the *2016 Technical Report* from the Child Poverty Monitor

---

'I agree, as a concept, resiliency may be meaningless to those people caught up in a cycle of poverty and abuse,' she responds.

'It may be more than meaningless,' I say. 'With a new focus on resiliency, recovery as a discourse endorses people who are able to regain autonomy, productivity and a sense of self, but it can be exclusionary for persons who struggle or fail to engage in the recovery journey. Recovery as a discourse could be used to label these types of people as problematic.'

'So you are not saying recovery is problematic; rather, that groups can use recovery to label people problematic if they don't follow all the rules and advice of mental health services?' Jean asks.

'Right,' I say. 'Recovery, as a discourse, has shifted from being a power for service users in previous decades to critique psychiatry and the lack of basic human rights experienced by service users, towards a measurement tool that can represent people as recovery focused or problematic. It's not recovery's fault,' I add, 'but if we use recovery to measure and judge a person's resiliency and their engagement with recovery discourse, we potentially constrain those people who live in low socio-economic environments. How do you recover from depression when you wake up each morning to a damp, mouldy house, lack of food, an abusive partner or parent and limited opportunities?'

'That's just for some people, though,' says Jean. 'It's possible that Jono was brought up in a neglectful or abusive environment, but it sounds like Mia has been there for him since he started living with her.'

'True,' I respond. 'But what we don't know is whether any abuse Jono may have experienced as a child may increase susceptibility to psychosis. And Mia may be loving, but the house is possibly cold and damp. Unemployment is high in this town and methamphetamine is cheaper and more accessible than cannabis. For those who like to escape, the gangs create easy access.'

'Well, we may get an answer or two now,' says Jean, noting the headlights of a car with a small blue light box on the roof.

The police car pulls up alongside and I can see a young male officer named Rei with a keen look in his eyes and a stylish comb-over, and a slightly older, very helpful female officer called Jenny, whom I've met a couple of times at the central station when assessing 'potential clients'. After exchanging introductions and some pleasantries, Jean looks to me pointedly to initiate conversation about the current situation.

We have parked outside a small row of houses that are foreground to some stunning hills and bush. Overall, gardens are overgrown or sparse, with children's toys dotted around the gardens. A group of pre-teen kids are kicking a ball on the road, under the street lamps. We can see Jono's house at the end of the cul-de-sac, next to a field that slopes down to the river. Paint is peeling from the window frames and the roof looks like it has seen better days – all in all, a rather gloomy aspect in the growing darkness and drizzle, until I see a flower bed bursting with vibrant winter plants on the front lawn.

I give the police a brief overview of the phone call with Mia. I request that they stay back initially while we talk to Jono, so we can explain our visit and concerns and 'request' for him to come and see one of our doctors.

It's already a foregone conclusion. However he presents, whatever he says, we have to act on the concerns of his grandmother, start the Mental Health Act process and put him in front of a doctor.

'Can I ask you to chip in if we are getting nowhere?' I ask the police, as I know from experience they can be a calming and reassuring element (sometimes) in the dynamics of these situations. They both nod their heads.

I hate this type of job; it creates too much tension in me. Dragging someone off to hospital with the help of the police. I feel a sense of anxiety and doom; a conflict with my values regarding client-centred practice. Conceptual models and frameworks of occupational therapy seem meaningless.

To counteract this gloom, I think of the struggles of Jono's grandmother and his siblings and his likely downward spiral into psychotic madness and the impact of his mental state on his relationships, functioning and overall wellbeing. To counteract this optimism, I think about the uncertainty of his future relationship with mental health services, the luck of the draw concerning the personality and competency of his psychiatrist and keyworker.

I walk up the path with Jean, skirting a child's tricycle, and up to the front door, while the police hang back on the pavement. Hoping that Jean cannot hear my heartbeat, I knock on the door.

I am about to radically change someone's life and impose a knowledge of madness that was first produced in the 18th century as truth, a knowledge that clings onto the 21st century through the rhetoric of psychiatry.

My hand connects with my face. I feel the flaky thickened skin on my left cheek, a symptom of psoriasis, and I feel ugly – a reflection of my impending actions. The glass particles in the front door show a shadow approaching and there's a brief fumble with the lock. Then the door swings inwards and I get to meet Mia.

My first thought is that she reminds me of my deceased grandmother: small in stature, wearing pink slippers and navy blue polyester trousers that would give off an electric shock if you touched them, a white blouse and brown woolly cardigan. She has short, curly hair, growing grey in places, and a warm smile. Unlike my grandmother, uncertainty and fear look at me through her eyes.

'Kia ora,' she says gently through her smile. Her face is lined. She emanates warmth in her welcome. Her acceptance of me before I even speak increases my confidence and reduces my anxiety.

'Good to meet you, Mia,' I say, 'though sorry to have to meet you in these circumstances.'

'Kia ora, kia ora,' she says, looking at Jean and then me.

Jean smiles and nods slightly and then looks at me.

I look at Mia and smile.

All good. Everything seems to be going okay.

I am standing outside in the rain, my trainers sinking into the wet grass and mud. I can feel the water soaking up my trouser legs while a continuous downpour drenches me from above, plastering my hair onto my forehead. The rain obscures my vision. Jono had made it up to his waist in the river before Rei managed to grab him and pull him back onto the bank. Jono is screaming and crying. I can hear the fear in his cries as he struggles to break free. Jenny supports Rei to overturn Jono onto his stomach and place his hands into the handcuffs, securing them behind him. It takes several seconds to do this, seeming more like minutes. I attempt to calm Jono, with clumsy apologies and statements that I am concerned about his health and that we do not want to hurt him.

This is so wrong. I hate this job. I feel useless.

I turn around and see Jean attempting to console Mia with a hug. Mia appears to be in a state of shock.

Sometimes events can race away, just as Jono did when he must have heard me talking to Mia about taking him up to hospital with the police if he was uncooperative, among other things. He had crashed out of a side door and headed for the fields and the river. Several seconds of inaction grounded me to the floor while my brain caught up with what had happened. Luckily, the police had taken off after Jono while my brain was still processing the situation. Jono had turned around once to stare at us, a face full of panic and fear.

This is my fault, talking about the outcome before we have even spoken to him. It makes things easy though. Jono running into the river for whatever reason has sealed his fate – no doctor would consider not holding him in hospital under the Act for a period of observation.

Rei and Jenny help Jono into the back seat of the police car and his crying subsides. Mia returns with towels for her grandson and Rei, who are both pooling water. Jean sticks close to her, letting her know what will be happening. I can see Mia is torn, wanting to come but needing to stay home to look after her other grandchildren. Jenny sits in the back of the car with Jono and I climb into the front seat next to Rei, in front of Jono. My position makes it difficult to converse with him appropriately and I let Jenny continue to lead the conversation, thanking him for the sudden exercise – 'I've been eating too much chocolate recently' – and checking how he is doing – 'Sorry about the handcuffs, but we all need to remain safe while we drive to the hospital.' Jono asks where we are taking him, in a slow, monotonous voice. I tell him that he is going to the hospital to meet with one of our doctors. I again feel the need to apologise but refrain from doing so as Jenny makes a joke with Jono about how frizzled her hair is with all the rain. We drive through the darkness to the hospital, the police radio emitting snatches of conversation that break the silence.

Somehow, Jean manages to get the hospital before us, even though she left after us, and I see that Mia is with her. She must have asked a neighbour to look after her little ones. Once we are in the confines of a small room in a locked ward, the police remove the handcuffs and Jenny manages to get a smile from Jono while she reassures him. The police depart with our thanks and a nurse and nursing assistant come over with some towels and direct Jono to another room where he can change into the dry clothes Mia has brought. Offering drinks, as if in a café, the nurse departs with the orders and the assistant stays. Jean goes off to start writing our assessment and hand over the events to the psychiatric registrar. I sit next to Mia and Jono joins us when he returns. Jono sits and stares into space. I try asking him a few questions but he ignores me. I make some small talk with Mia instead and explain that Jono will be seen first by one doctor but that they will be likely to confirm the need for a consultant to carry out an assessment.

About 30 minutes later, Frances, the psychiatric registrar, bustles in clutching a notebook, handbag, phone and pager with one hand and a plastic cup filled with water in her other hand. She smiles warmly at Mia and Jono and takes a seat in the now crowded room, introducing herself and her role. Frances begins by telling Jono and Mia that Jean has told her about the events leading up to their being here, and asks a few brief questions to confirm some of the concerns that Mia had told me over the phone. Jono remains silent through much of the interview, his slow monotone and brief responses reflecting his flat affect. He doesn't move. Frances has apparently seen and heard enough after 10 minutes to continue with the sectioning process. She thanks Mia and Jono and leaves the room. I also depart with Frances and the nurse, who has returned with drinks, leaving the nursing assistant with Jono and Mia. I fill out the paperwork (Section 9 of the Mental Health Act, 1992) that will inform Jono of his pending appointment with the consultant psychiatrist and his rights in relation to the Act.

Felix, another nurse with the crisis team, and Fay, one of the psychiatric assistants working in the crisis team, are sitting in the nursing office, along with one of the ward nurses, when I enter. Screaming, shouting and profanities come from a locked door opposite the office.

'Did you upset someone again?' I ask Felix.

Felix gives a wry smile. 'Not guilty. All was going fine until she heard that she was being admitted to hospital under the Mental Health Act.'

My questioning look is enough for Felix to continue. 'Overdose. Background of domestic abuse, boyfriend been using her as a punching bag for the last few months.

Likely raped her recently, which resulted in a pregnancy and then a miscarriage. Took a handful of sleeping pills with half a bottle of whisky. Not the first time, poor thing. We thought we could get her home with an auntie who was there supporting her but she continued to voice suicidality so we put her in front of the registrar. They agreed for a voluntary admission into hospital.'

Family violence: 525,000 New Zealanders harmed every year

New Zealand has the worst rate of family and intimate-partner violence in the world. A shocking 80 per cent of incidents go unreported — so what we know of family violence in our community is barely the tip of the iceberg....

Just under 115,000 people live in Tauranga. Imagine if every one of those people was the victim of family violence. Imagine that every person who lived in Tauranga had been physically, sexually, emotionally or psychologically abused by a member of their immediate family. A husband, an ex-partner, a parent. Imagine if, every five minutes, the police were called in Tauranga because someone was beaten, tormented, bullied, tortured, abused or savaged in their home by someone who was supposed to love and care for them. While this scenario is imaginary, the statistics are real. In 2015, police around New Zealand attended about 105,000 family violence callouts. If each of those incidents was represented by a person, that's getting close to the population of Tauranga. (Leask, 2017)

'So how come she is in seclusion under the Mental Health Act?' I ask.

'Well, that's what you get with a risk-averse consultant,' says Felix. 'He was worried that she would want to leave the ward for a cigarette, and told Frances to start the Act – she had asked him for an informal admission. Frances did try to tell him that Sue had been through enough abuse recently, but he wouldn't listen. Frances was quite upset by it all. Poor old Sue went crazy when she was told the Act was being initiated and that she would be detained in hospital. It probably didn't help that she told the consultant where he could stick his nicotine patches.'

'That's great!' I say (meaning the opposite).

> As soon as she is discharged and taken off the Act, it's unlikely she will have anything to do with community mental health follow-up.

With Sue's screams in the background, I fill out the section paperwork and return to Jono and Mia. It's possibly the last time I will see them.

Jono stares into space when I read him his rights and inform him that he will be meeting a consultant psychiatrist for further assessment. I tell him the possible outcomes from assessment and the likely one. I am supposed to ask Mia to sign his formal section papers as a witness to ensure that I have gone through the rights process appropriately. I rarely do ask relatives to sign and instead record their name for them, with a brief explanation: 'Not wanting potential future relationship issues.' Some family members have told me that signing the papers has damaged their relationship with their son, daughter, mother, father, brother, sister, grandchild, grandparent, cousin, friend, as their loved one had believed that it was their signature that had committed them to hospital. I shake Mia's hand. She thanks me, wishes me well. Jono ignores me when I say good-bye. *I wish you luck,* I think.

By the time I get back to the nurses station, Felix and Fay have left and Jean is putting on her coat. 'We've got someone in C_____ police station needing assessment. Police picked him up for beating his girlfriend. Tried to strangle himself with his T-shirt. Likely high on methamphetamine, according to the police. Let's go.'

References

Canin G (2017). Nine in 10 healthcare workers feel understaffed and under-resourced. [Online.] *Stuff*; 1 March. www.stuff.co.nz/national/health/89932971/nine-in-10-healthcare-workers-feel-understaffed-and-underresourced (accessed 10 September 2017).

DeBoni D (2016). Opinion: Mental health service in crisis – still. [Online.] *1 News Now*; 8 June. www.tvnz.co.nz/one-news/new-zealand/opinion-mental-health-service-in-crisis-still (accessed 8 September 2017).

Fleming C (2006). Diseases of the thesis. *Australian Universities Review 48*(2): 30–31.

Leask A (2017). Family violence: 525,000 New Zealanders harmed every year. [Online.] *New Zealand Herald*; 26 March. www.nzherald.co.nz/family-violence/news/article.cfm?c_id=178&objectid=11634543 (accessed 15 October 2017).

McConnell G (2017). The highest rate of teen suicide in the developed world. [Online.] *Stuff*; 16 October. www.stuff.co.nz/national/health/94948665/all-auckland-hospitals-at-capacity-all-nonurgent-patients-asked-to-stay-away (accessed 22 October 2017).

Office of the Chief Coroner New Zealand (2017). *Chief Coroner releases provisional annual suicide figures.* [Online.] Wellington: Office of the Chief Coroner, 28 August. https://coronialservices.justice.govt.nz/assets/Documents/Publications/suicide-statistics-media-release-20170828.pdf (accessed 10 September 2017).

Perera R (2017). Grandparents' struggles to bring up their mokopuna. [Online.] *Newshub*; 23 July. www.newshub.co.nz/home/shows/2017/07/grandparents-struggles-to-bring-up-their-mokopuna.html (accessed 18 October 2017).

Stuff (2017). All Auckland hospitals at capacity, all non-urgent patients asked to stay away. [Online.] *Stuff*; 20 July. www.stuff.co.nz/national/health/94948665/all-auckland-hospitals-at-capacity-all-nonurgent-patients-asked-to-stay-away (accessed 15 October 2017).

The Mental Health (Compulsory Assessment and Treatment) Act 1992. New Zealand: Parliamentary Counsel Office. www.legislation.govt.nz/act/public/1992/0046/latest/whole.html (accessed 22 October 2017).

UNICEF New Zealand (2017). *Child poverty in NZ*. [Online.] Wellington: UNICEF New Zealand. www.unicef.org.nz/learn/in-new-zealand/child-poverty (accessed 3 September 2017).

5 | Power at play: the Doctor-Nurse Game in acute mental health care

Anne Felton and Gemma Stacey

The internal beliefs and morals that we hold represent our perceptions of the world and what is important. These are the characteristics of values. Values-based practice (VBP), advocated by Bill Fulford and Kim Woodbridge (2004), recognises that the decisions made by mental health professionals, including nurses, are significantly influenced by values. Mental health practice is therefore not only guided by research, evidence and policy but also by our own values.

According to this definition of VBP, conflict of values would be inevitable. However, by recognising, discussing and understanding each other's positions, a more democratic outcome could be achieved. This appears to present the potential to encourage decision-making structures that recognise the voice of the person receiving mental health services as equal to that of those delivering them. Although all parties may not agree with the outcome, if all stakeholders have inclusion within the decision-making process, this would be more empowering for all involved.

This chapter takes values-based practice as a springboard for a critique of decision-making in acute mental health care, drawing on research data gathered in focus groups with doctors and nurses working in this setting.

Both the authors are mental health nurses who have worked in the higher education sector for a number of years, predominantly in pre-registration nurse education. The principles of VBP seemed to us to offer a useful framework to disseminate to pre-registration mental health nursing students. Encouraging students to develop an awareness of their own values and motivations and engaging them in critical dialogue to uncover the attitudinal, structural and cultural barriers to valuing the voice of the person using services made for a challenging and reflective teaching session. Moreover, this ethos underpins our teaching philosophy and the emphasis we are able to bring to our mental health nursing programmes. How this would translate into nursing practice, however, was less apparent to us – and, indeed, less observable among our students and newly qualified nurses, particularly those working in areas where compulsory care was part of day-to-day practice.

The research study

The Critical Values-Based Practice Network[1] (CVBPN), of which the authors are members, developed as a group of practitioners and people with lived experience interested in this area of practice. The network was established more than 10 years ago as a local interest group to explore how the VBP approach could be supported within the local mental health trust. Learning from this work, the network evolved to recognise that organisational culture created a barrier to the VBP democratic approach in decision-making. Consequently, the CVBPN endeavoured to conduct a research study that explicitly explored the issues of power, positioning, performance and hierarchy in decision-making forums, such as acute mental health admissions unit ward rounds. It was our view that these factors presented real structural and cultural barriers to VBP becoming a reality in this setting. We conducted focus groups with people who had recently used or were working in acute mental health care, and with family members from a range of personal and professional backgrounds. The data were analysed collaboratively, using the conventions of critical narrative discourse analysis. A full overview and discussion of this study is reported in Stacey et al (2016).

This chapter will focus on the findings of a secondary analysis of the data collected from the focus groups. This aimed to explore the extent to which decisions are shared in acute inpatient settings. We draw specifically on two focus groups: one with nurses (n=7) and the other with consultant psychiatrists (n=7). The data were re-analysed using the rules of the Doctor-Nurse Game (Stein, 1967). This provides a critical deductive framework for the discussion of these professional relationships in the context of mental health nursing work. The chapter explores the implications of the power relationships between these disciplinary groups, which are themselves embedded within an organisational and social context that supports them.

A significant finding of the main study was the way in which groups positioned themselves as outsiders to the decision-making process and viewed the psychiatrist as the professional with overriding influence and accountability. While the other professional groups were often dissatisfied with this position, they also used it to absolve themselves of responsibility for making the unpopular decisions, such as depriving people of their liberty. The nurses, in particular, perceived themselves to be reluctant enforcers of the decisions of the psychiatrists, with which they went along in an apparently passive manner.

As nurse educators, we have observed a national shift in the content of pre-registration mental health nursing programmes to a more social and psychological

---

1. www.criticalvaluesbasedpracticenetwork.co.uk

understanding of mental distress. This aims to enable nurses to challenge traditional practice and offer critical perspectives. This was arguably influenced by the Chief Nursing Officer's review of mental health nursing, *From Values to Action* (Department of Health, 2006), which had an explicit focus on the nurse's role in promoting the recovery of people with mental health problems and challenging discrimination. In addition, the Nursing and Midwifery Council's standards for pre-registration education (2018) emphasise the competences required of mental health nurses in terms of engagement, emotional intelligence and prioritising the relational aspects of care.

It was demoralising therefore to learn of this passivity among the nurses in the focus group, which implied these political shifts remained aspirational, as opposed to a practice reality. On reflection, our own personal reaction to the nurses' accounts was to feel disheartened, because in many respects they undermined the defence we had created as our reason for moving from practice into the higher education setting. We had become comfortable with the stance that this was motivated by our belief that working with a critical mass of mental health nurses presented more opportunity to influence practice than would be possible as lone voices working in mental health services. The focus group data presented us with a stark picture of the limited influence education could have on a culture where the professional hierarchy and power structures are so ingrained.

It became apparent that the nurses and doctors were describing current decision-making processes in a manner reminiscent of the original rules outlined by Leonard Stein in his 1967 paper 'The Doctor-Nurse Game'. Stein (1967) identified that the doctor-nurse relationship is hierarchical and that doctors are always superior. Nurses are able to make recommendations based on their experience and this is an important part of the game, but the nurses' recommendations had to appear to be initiated by the doctor. In contrast to the premise of VBP, which encourages the airing of diverse perspectives, Stein observed that open disagreement had to be avoided and when doctors wanted to know what the nurses would recommend, they needed to appear not to be asking for their views. If a doctor failed to acknowledge and act on the nurses' recommendations, or did not agree with their advice, there was potential for a breakdown in the accepted relational dynamics. Doctors who contravened this unwritten code by not acting on the nurse's advice were treated as 'rule breakers'. Nurses who were outspoken when making recommendations or who overtly made a worthwhile contribution risked being ostracised and excluded from the decision-making forum.

It is acknowledged that the medical profession is accomplished in engaging in practice that supports its professional project by defining and controlling specialist or expert knowledge. This knowledge then enables the profession to construct an identity that separates it from the other occupational groups in healthcare. This is often achieved through control over access to education, formalisation of knowledge through accreditation and delineation of available career paths (Freidson, 2001). Nursing, however, demonstrates an enduring difficulty in articulating a distinctive, privileged system of knowledge that can be clearly distinguished as unique to nursing. McNamara notes:

> ...the justification of higher education for nurses, in terms of improved status and professional advancement, exposes nursing to the accusation that its educational aspirations are related to a desire for recognition, status and improved pay, rather than a need to enhance the teaching or learning of knowledge and skills in the interests of improved standards of patient care. (2005: 57)

Opponents of the move to shift nurse training into higher education were quick to highlight the apparent self-interest in this, constructing nurses as self-serving and lacking the distinct epistemological base to become learned professionals who could legitimately contribute to clinical decision-making in a way that would be viewed as valid or useful by the medical profession (Fealy & McNamara, 2007).

These arguments reinforce the notion of nursing as an oppressed profession articulated by Roberts and colleagues (2009). Roberts explains the nursing profession's defensiveness about its status as a reaction against a culture that defines its role as inferior. He maintains that the anti-intellectualism discourse that has emerged from within the profession is a form of rebellion against the prevailing view held by society and reproduced in the media (Meerabeau, 2004). This is achieved by defending practical activity and belittling the relevance and value of abstract thought.

A similar criticism could be levelled at the role of VBP in healthcare. VBP allows evidence-based practice to maintain the illusion of objectivity as it situates the influence of values, and therefore subjectivity, in the decision-making process and in individual practice. Critique of the influence of subjectivity in the construction and consumption of research is therefore avoided, allowing evidence-based practice to continue to appear value free. VBP's focus on the democratic, without acknowledging the power and knowledge structures within which mental health practice is nested, continues to perpetuate this lack of critique.

Freire (1971) identifies that defensive reactions within an oppressed profession allows society to further label the oppressed as unintelligent. He sees dialogue as essential to free both parties from accepted cultural norms. However, the gendered perception of nursing, the hierarchy engrained in organisational structures and the nature of the profession's association with medicine often inhibits such dialogue. We recognise that this discussion of power and the oppression of professional groups is insignificant in the context of the lived experience of coercion, forced treatment and disempowerment experienced by people diagnosed with mental health problems in services and wider society. However, as nurses who have always adopted a questioning and critical perspective and have hope that different ways of practising are possible, we find ourselves frequently in forums where criticisms are rightly levelled at the work of mental health professionals. Yet responses to these criticisms are often tokenistic, such as better training or better understanding of co-production or recovery, and lack a critical examination of the power and organisational relationships impacting on the actions of practitioners. Examining the professional and organisational culture in which mental health nursing operates exposes the challenges to creating change.

Findings of the secondary analysis

This next part of the chapter will focus on the data emerging from the secondary analysis of the two focus groups, using the rules of Stein's (1967) Doctor-Nurse Game. Two rules were identified as frequently being reinforced:

- doctors are superior in decision-making
- when nurses make recommendations, these should appear to be initiated by the doctor.

However, some patterns of rule-breaking were also recognised, such as:

- when doctors fail to acknowledge and act on nurses' recommendations.

In 1990 Stein argued that the rules of the game had changed in light of a shift to multidisciplinary models of practice, which encouraged a flatter hierarchy (Stein, Watts & Howell, 1990). It could be argued that mental health care has a long history of multidisciplinary practice, due to the bio/psycho/social influences on mental wellbeing. This analysis will consider to what extent this has influenced the games that are played today between doctors and nurses.

Doctors are superior in the decision-making hierarchy

Within the nurses' accounts, there was a clear consensus that the doctor controlled the decision-making process:

> I do feel that, personally, that there's a lot of emphasis on the power behind the consultant's decision, just because they're a consultant. (Nurse)

> There's a lot of skill, a lot of experience, and a lot of documented evidence that a nurse will have prior to any discussion of that kind and still that doesn't necessarily drive the decision making. (Nurse)

If forums such as ward rounds were called 'nurse-led', this was at the consultant's discretion and the nurse was required to read from a pre-written summary sheet prepared by another member of the team, even when they had not recently had contact with the person using the service. Therefore, the nurse-led aspect appeared purely administrative and the quality of the information was doubted by the doctors.

> We tried different ways of getting information, like having a special document that the nurses fill out with all the details in, but then they wouldn't even bother with that, and, you know, I think we tried lots of different things but... [it] just seems to sort of go back to the same old ways. (Doctor)

Where the person was considered a 'complex case' or requiring in-depth initial assessment, this was viewed as the role of the doctor, due to the perceived advanced nature of this work.

> Where we have more complex cases and therefore, you tend to find the consultant takes a bit more of the lead with that, or if someone's brought into hospital and it's a first introduction, the consultant will introduce himself and they'll do a very thorough interview and discussion around that individual, how they are, what their mental state is like and the symptoms they're experiencing. Because I'm a nurse, we then take a more sort of back seat in that situation. (Nurse)

Despite this perceived superiority, the nurses identified that the communication of decisions to the person and their family and their implementation were often their responsibility. The nurses perceived themselves as mediating between the powerful decision-maker (the doctor) and the person on the receiving end of the decision, which often meant they were the recipients of the service user's and carers' frustrations and discontent.

> It sometimes can be difficult trying to please everyone, because obviously as a nurse, we try and be a support to the carers, be the main support to the patient because they're there on the ward, they're sharing things with us. I find that quite challenging in ward rounds if the decision isn't going their way. (Nurse)

> Sometimes, decisions are made that are not as popular. And then we have dynamics with the family, if they're not happy with the decisions, or we get consent and confidentiality issues where family are really worried but their relative is not happy for us to share certain information and everybody has that right to have the confidentiality, but the family are looking towards us, to support them. They're worried, they're anxious, they don't feel we're making good decisions so that applies a lot of pressure, and beyond that ward round process, you've still got to try and work one-to-one to maintain a therapeutic relationship. (Nurse)

> In terms of enforced treatment, keeping somebody behind a door, stopping leave, removing leave and that's – we're seen as the enforcer of certain decisions. And that doesn't always sit comfortably. These people are not in

prison, but, you know, we keep people in, if the consultant says they have no leave, they have no leave, we're the one who are left enforcing that decision. I think, you have to do it and be around to see it to appreciate the magnitude of that, you know – [there are] very few times consultants are aware or actually physically see the impact of that. I think the patients tend to remember what we do rather than what the consultants do… Like when they sometimes, if they come back into hospital… 'I remember you, you held me down, and did this to me.' They don't say that to the consultant. (Nurse)

A lot of the negative experiences that they have… they remember the faces and the people that were involved and it tends to be us. And you have to try and reinforce to them, at the time, it's as disturbing to you as it is for them. I've been in situations before where I've been accused of enjoying and getting a thrill out of restraining somebody, and that is the worst feeling because you know for a fact, of course you're not enjoying it. It's uncomfortable for a start; it's disturbing mentally and draining mentally and physically. But unfortunately, sometimes, the patient misinterprets that into some sort of power trip over them. I've really tried to reinforce the fact that I am not enjoying this, it is uncomfortable, it's disturbing… I'm as upset about this as you are, and really try and get that through to them. Because I think we are seen as the nasty one – 'You're the evil one, you've injected me, you've held me down', and it's us that's seen as the bad guys in that, in those situations. (Nurse)

Nurses' recommendations should appear to be initiated by the doctor

Examples were given where nurses felt that their views were actively considered in the decision-making process. The accountability of the decision itself, however, clearly remained with the doctor.

We've actually got two consultants, both of which do listen and take our views on board and I think that makes a massive difference. I think it makes somebody feel more at ease in general because we can phone our consultants, you know; we just pick the phone up and, wherever they are, we'll ring them if we need the advice or we need something doing, and both of them are happy for that to happen. (Nurse)

The nurses could identify their unique clinical knowledge, which arose from the 24-hour nature of their interactions with the people using the service. They perceived this as a more credible source of information to underpin decisions but maintained this was often undervalued or overlooked in the factors contributing to the ultimate outcome, which was decided by the doctor.

> A lot of what goes off in a multidisciplinary team meeting depends on your consultant and the relationship you have with your consultant to a certain degree. But certainly, as nurses, sometimes we feel that, you know, consultants come to the ward, they see a very brief snapshot of a patient based on a 20-minute interview and then they, obviously, make decisions based on that interview. However, they've not been around on the ward when you've seen that patient, you know, and the behaviours that are associated with certain conditions. They've not seen that. So they're basing their evidence on what they see, and sometime it doesn't always marry and we try and put forward our clinical view on how that patient has presented but sometimes it doesn't work out. (Nurse)

The psychiatrists acknowledged the potential for the nurses' understanding of the person to contribute to decision-making but were sceptical about their willingness to both share and take responsibility for the outcome.

> ... because you're not there a lot of the time... when thing happen... suddenly everything comes back to you to... sort it, when in actual fact, it should be somebody else that should be held responsible and accountable rather than you. It's also default to the consultant. (Doctor)

The perceived lack of value placed on their knowledge was a source of discontent and frustration among nurses. They went so far as to say it negatively influenced the quality of care offered to the person and, in some cases, led to increased risk due to the lack of responsiveness. This was viewed to have consequences for the person's level of distress and increased the potential for the need to use enforced treatment.

> It's the same with medication. Sometimes we feel, because obviously we get a lot of people who are quite poorly, psychotic and very, very unwell, emotionally unwell, and we would like to see our doctors be more proactive in terms of reviewing medication, in providing therapeutic medication reviews. But we feel there's like a lagging because they're lagging behind, and when you expect or anticipate a decision to be made, it's not made. Which means that the poor patient is then left for another week. I don't think we always do the best for our patients. So that's the conflict I've experienced. (Nurse)

> I think it's the potential for risk being increased on the ward, for the nursing staff and the patient as well, because every time you have to go hands-on, they're in danger, we're in danger, other patients are in danger, and the ward's unsettled. And I think that the actual impact of their decision-making, they should consider that more, and actually take what we're saying into consideration, rather than almost them being dismissive. (Nurse)

Doctors fail to acknowledge and act on nurses' recommendations

Risk appeared to be the main motivation when anyone departed from the rules of the Doctor-Nurse Game. There was a sense that the doctor was not directly involved in the challenges of caring for a person who might be violent as a result of their distress, and therefore did not make decisions with the safety of the staff and other patients in mind. An example of this challenge was articulated by an experienced nurse (their description) who had been unhappy with a junior doctor's decision-making capabilities and failure to acknowledge the nurses' recommendations. Here the rules were contravened when the nurse engaged in open disagreement with the doctor. In this situation, it could be argued that the hierarchy is less well defined and therefore the rules are less concrete.

> I guess, because I'm quite experienced nurse, I will challenge situations in the review. Not with the patient involved because it would increase the stress, but say in case of the risks, I have had instances where I've escalated that... either with my direct manager or a matron to see what they feel about the risk decisions that are being taken at that time, and documented, as is reasonable to do. We don't have as many career psychiatrists of late seeming to be coming through the rotation so the other clinicians that are around that aren't psychiatrists, their level of knowledge is very limited. It's not so easy to kind of manage that situation so you're very dependent on that consultant. I telephone consultants out of hours. I've even bothered them at home at the weekend if I've been uncomfortable with somebody. I've even said as much in that review – 'I'll be coming back to you even out of hours if I'm concerned'. And I've actually had acceptance of that. But that is probably not what you should have as a standard for managing multidisciplinary decisions and risks. (Nurse)

Further examples were given of nurses using the organisational hierarchy to challenge doctors who were not taking their views into account and were justified as being in the best interests of good patient care. This threw into further relief the consequences for working relationships where the rules of the game were not followed.

> ... in the past, we've had some really terrible experiences that we've had to actually take it to the management level and they've actually had to report on one consultant because they just weren't doing what we thought was best, and it turned out that they really were[n't] doing what was best. So, I think it really does matter. The problem is, you do kind of think, 'Oh well, they're the consultant, maybe they do know best'. Why? Why do they know best? They don't always know best and I think, if you can challenge them, do challenge them. And then, if you get a bad response, at least you've made your point and at least you've done the best you can for your patient. (Nurse)

The desire to influence decision-making and willingness to challenge decisions does not however indicate a desire to take responsibility for the outcome. Despite expressing clearly the unique and well-informed expertise that they held, when decisions about risk were passed to the nurse, there was categorical reluctance to accept this responsibility.

> We have had decisions where we want leave or we don't want leave for a service user around risk, and you think you're going to get one decision based on this and the consultant completely out of the blue makes another decision, but, ultimately, then the nurse is left with another dilemma of, 'Well, the consultant has said yes.' However, if the nurse feels that that leave is not safe, then that leave shouldn't happen. And then, you're left, again, with the pressure and fall-out of that decision when you do decide to allow leave, with good clinical reason, even if the consultant has agreed, if something untoward happens. The nurse saw that patient, and, sadly, if it ended in something really untoward, then it's the nurses that are subject to the root cause analysis, at the initial point. It almost feels like the buck stops [with the nurse]… especially where they state 'at nursing staff's discretion…' (Nurse)

> Some decisions are seen as the responsibility of the consultant who is obviously getting paid a lot more money to make those decisions, and the consultant has normally, you know, been working for many more years in psychiatry and taken those risks based on the analysing those risks. (Nurse)

Furthermore, psychiatrists viewed the quality and detail of the information given by nurses as limited and that they lacked the confidence or tools to articulate their views within a ward round setting.

> … they'd be having informal discussion about what they thought about a patient, there'd be tons of information, they did this and they did that and they did this, and then they'd come to the ward round and they'd say nothing, really; not much to feed back, and I wondered whether it was a difficulty with them framing it in a language which they felt would be appropriate to the setting of a ward [round]… it would have been great… hearing it in a ward round setting but I think… they feel that there's a particular language that needs to be spoken on the ward round and then it all disappears. (Doctor)

The issue of disparity of knowledge and social positioning reflected in salaries was also acknowledged by the psychiatrists who were resigned to maintaining their responsibility as a justification for their position as the superior profession.

> With regard to the hierarchy in respect of how much the [pay] gap has been breached… whether people think that people have different levels of

knowledge or people have different pay scales... 'You get more money so you should be the one taking responsibility here, you know, rather than me.' So I think those sort of things will remain and will continue to remain, I guess. (Doctor)

With regard to improving decision-making practices, the nurses suggested that consultants should spend more time with patients to inform their decisions; they did not propose that they should have a more active role or that the person using services should be able to contribute in a more meaningful way.

Discussion

Despite Stein's assertions, over 25 years ago, that the rules of the original Doctor-Nurse Game have been superseded, analysis of very recent focus group data from psychiatrists and mental health nurses working in acute mental health care suggests the game is still being played. The long-standing relative positions and power of each professional group are consistently reinforced. However, the vignettes from the participants suggest some interesting subtleties in the details of the game and justification for the rules that reflect some key concerns for critical perspectives on mental health care. These particularly relate to coercion, risk and blame.

Coercion and 'dirty work'

The nurses identified that they were the enforcers of unpopular and coercive actions that were distressing for service users and for the nurses themselves. These decisions related particularly to restrictive practices such as restraint. The nurses position themselves as having to implement the decisions made by more powerful others that expose them to emotional pain of carrying out practices that they can see are difficult for service users. Psychiatrists are identified by the nurses as distanced from these painful experiences as they are often not physically present when these practices take place. Mental health nurses' responsibilities for enacting coercion have led to a well-documented critique of their role as enforcers of the moral and social order in accordance with the ideals of a neoliberal society (Szmukler & Rose, 2013).

Mental health professionals have been recognised as participating in what Hughes (1958) defines as 'dirty work' through their association with people diagnosed as mentally ill (Godin, 2000). 'Dirty work' is conceptualised in physical, social and moral terms (Ashforth & Kreiner, 1999). The mental health profession engages in all three dimensions of dirty work, but the social and the moral are primarily reflected here. Mental health nurses are tainted by their links with a group seen to transgress social norms and excluded as 'other' (social), and also by their practices, which involve coercion for the maintenance of control (moral) (Godin, 2000). The concept of dirty work, therefore, links with ideological beliefs about maintaining order (Dick, 2005). Workers undertake practices or work that is perceived as dirty by society because it threatens the sense of boundaries and stability (Douglas & Kalender, 1966). The work is stigmatised by the social world that creates and defines this work in the first place. Although critique of the role and function of mental health nursing exists and is, indeed, a core theme of this book, the profession does not define itself in terms of performing tainted work. This was also reflected in the findings of the research study on shared decision-making, in which nurses positioned themselves as the experts in decision-making, justified by their proximal relationship to service users. This tension about the nature of mental health nursing, therefore, leads to an important question: how do mental health nurses create a positive professional identity when performing such morally difficult work?

Occupations can adopt ideological mechanisms to manage their identity, reframing aspects of their role that incorporate dirty work (Ashforth & Kreiner, 1999; Dick, 2005). The extracts from the nurses' focus group in our research clearly highlight the difficulties they experienced when performing practices that place restrictions on service users. By locating with psychiatrists the responsibility for the necessity of these actions, the nurses are also distancing themselves from these emotionally and morally complex practices. By positioning doctors as superior in the decision-making hierarchy, in accordance with the rules of the Doctor-Nurse Game, the nurses are engaging in a mechanism that allows these actions to be reframed and protects their identity against association with the 'dirtiness' of this work.

Douglas and Kalender (1966) highlight that dirt and being associated with it are to be avoided. Its avoidance in this case relates to the coercive aspects of the mental health professional's role and their proximity to the stigmatised group. Distancing from these aspects of the role reflects assumptions about social order, including the relative social positions of different groups and their relationships to each other, where people with mental health problems are seen as marginalised, stigmatised and excluded. The relational rules acted out in the Doctor-Nurse Game may thus serve to reinforce the social position of each group. Higher status professions, such as medicine, are recognised as delegating tasks deemed to be dirty – in this example, implementing restrictive practices such as restraint or refusing leave to groups that are still lower in the hierarchy (Dick, 2005). In the focus groups, the doctors describe their power to do this as part of the responsibility for decision-making they have to undertake because of their higher pay and status, but also voice their lack of confidence in nurses' ability to take on this responsibility. The nurses recognise the costs of this delegation in terms of the emotional impact of undertaking the work. However, while the apparent cost to mental health nursing is its lower status, its identity is protected as it is able to disassociate itself from the accountability for doing the 'dirty work', such as coercive practices, by locating responsibility for it with the doctors, a higher authority. However, unlike the implication of Stein's original work that the nursing profession lacked autonomy, this response may also actively serve the interests of mental health nursing as it creates and protects a positive professional identity.

Risk and blame

The notion of mental health nurses being involved in dirty work has been recognised as part of the association with a tainted group treated as 'other' and perceived as threatening to social order. The increasing dominance of risk in the practice of mental health professionals and mental health services further taints people using those services. People diagnosed with mental health problems are seen to pose a risk to others and to be dangerous, rendering other aspects of their identity or experience of distress invisible and so further perpetuating an emphasis on risk (Felton, 2015).

Managing risk becomes part of the dirty work of mental health nurses, associated with their practice and close proximity to this 'dangerous' group (in line with the social conceptualisation of dirty work). However, in the focus groups, nurses deferred accountability for decision-making to doctors, in particular when these decisions related to risk. This may represent a further strategy to maintain a positive professional identity in relation to this type of work. Here nurses are reinforcing the rules of the Doctor-Nurse Game hierarchy by avoiding the responsibility for decisions related to risk management. In this way, they distance themselves not only from dealing with the risk but also from an anticipated consequence of failed risk management. In the nurses' accounts there is an implicit and, in some cases, explicit reference to fears of being blamed for 'something untoward' taking place. Interestingly, this fear takes precedence over any recognition of the consequences of unnecessary restrictions being placed on service users. Instead, the nurses' chief concern is that they may be seen as responsible for failures in risk management, and therefore, to avoid this responsibility and any blame if things do go wrong, they evade decision-making about risk.

Blame has been explained as evaluation of an individual based on the belief that they have acted in a way or displayed an aspect of character that is considered bad, wrong or impermissible and for which they have no valid excuse (Sher, 2006), and have thus violated a moral code. Blame is often associated with anger, hostility and reproach (Williams, 2003; Sher, 2006). Blame is linked with the values and beliefs of contemporary Western society and as such is perpetuated by modernist mentality (Lau, 2009) in that the attribution of blame is part of modernist thinking that defines tragic events as preventable and therefore predictable, and holds individuals to blame when they occur (Douglas, 1992; Lau, 2009). In this way, a culture of blame can develop as individuals are seen as responsible for failing to act properly (Locke, 2009). In this respect, blame is inextricably linked with risk and perceived failures of risk management by professionals who are seen to have failed to foresee and prevent tragic events. According to Douglas (1992), this forms part of a new blaming system linked with risk reduction in modern society. A fear of being blamed is a common experience for healthcare professionals and has been described as being part of an organisational culture (Kendall & Wiles, 2010). A culture of blame has been widely recognised in health services and is largely seen as a negative force that undermines safe and effective care (Freeman, 2009; Woodward, Lemer & Wu, 2009).

Being blamed exposes professionals to loss of status and social or moral standing and even to loss of employment. This emphasises the affective experience of being blamed, judged as acting badly or having a bad character, and so contravening a moral code. The feared consequences of failures in risk management may therefore also form part of the dirty work of mental health nursing, associated with the moral taint of shame. Blame, according to Woodward and colleagues (2009), provides the mechanism whereby shame is assigned and it is this experience of shame that is damaging to both professionals and safety within healthcare systems. It is an experience that individuals would seek to avoid. Blame and responsibility are deeply frightening, in part due to the associated implication that we exist in a social and physical environment that is difficult to predict and impossible to control (O'Connor, Kotze & Wright, 2011; Lau, 2009). This reinforces the position that blame should be avoided and control promoted through accurate predictions and careful management, notably as inaccurate judgments of risk are seen to expose mental health professionals to blame and shame (Undrill, 2007). Arguably, the deferring of complex decisions to those with authority, in this study from nurses to doctors, may be a strategy to avoid blame should something bad happen. Traditionally, nurses have lacked power and status to collectively resist increases in management and governance in the NHS – medicine has been much more successful in doing so (Traynor et al, 2013). This may provide insight into the tendency for nurses to perceive psychiatrists as responsible for complex decisions that may pose a risk of being blamed, particularly as, according to Kendra (2007), the more power that is possessed by the person, the less the likelihood of them being blamed for a negative event.

A desire for more responsibility and voice in decision-making is part of the discourse of today's university-educated nursing profession. This perspective was echoed in the voices of the nurses in this study who were frustrated by the lack of influence their expertise and relationship with service users played in decision-making on acute wards. However, this existed in parallel to practices that sought to avoid the authority and responsibility for such decisions or, perhaps more significantly, any evidence of challenge to the hierarchy to facilitate the participation of service users in the decision-making process. This may create an inverse rule for the contemporary version of the Doctor-Nurse Game: rather than maintaining hierarchical relationships by nurses making suggestions without appearing to, in this rule nurses appear to desire empowerment and an end to the game, while actually acting to reinforce it.

Conclusion

VBP has been presented as a framework that would facilitate collaborative decision-making in which the voices of service users and professionals are equally valued. The research undertaken by the CVBPN highlighted that this approach lacks a critique of power relationships and overlooks the ingrained structural and cultural barriers to shared democratic decision-making. Although not a key focus of the research, the focus groups undertaken with psychiatrists and nurses revealed interesting relational dynamics between these two professional groups. In this chapter, we have re-analysed these data to propose that Stein's (1967) Doctor-Nurse Game provides a critical framework through which to examine the reproduction of traditional professional power relationships. The examination has provided insight into the maintenance of status quo within mental health care that protects hierarchical structures and perpetuates the exclusion of people who have experienced mental distress from participating in decision-making in inpatient care. It is important to recognise that these power relationships are embedded within an organisational and social context that supports them.

Although our role as outsiders has made the critique possible in many respects, it is also limited by this outsider status: as nursing academics, we share a professional identity but are no longer tainted by 'dirty work'. Offering a framework to explain the maintenance of power relationships in mental health practice also provides us with a justification for our perceived limited impact in tackling them through education. However, we also acknowledge that this study hasn't explored the experiences of those nurses who actively rebel and subvert the rules in other ways in order to become more empowered.

While nursing remains largely associated with medicine and the web of traditional hierarchy, social positioning and valuing of medical expertise, nurses will remain oppressed and therefore limited in their attempts to promote social and psychological ways of understanding and dealing with distress.

Acknowledgements

With thanks to the Critical Values-Based Practice Network.

References

Ashforth BE, Kreiner GE (1999). 'How can you do it?': dirty work and the challenge of constructing a positive identity. *Academy of Management Review 24*(3): 413–434.

Department of Health (2006). *From Values to Action: the Chief Nursing Officer's Review of Mental Health Nursing*. London: the Stationery Office.

Dick P (2005). Dirty work designations: now police officers account for their use of coercive force. *Human Relations 58*(11): 1363–1390.

Douglas M (1992). *Risk and Blame: essays in cultural theory*. London: Routledge.

Douglas M, Kalender M (1966). *Purity and Danger: an analysis of concepts of pollution and taboo*. London: Routledge & Kegan Paul.

Fealy GM, McNamara MS (2007). A discourse analysis of debates surrounding the entry of nursing into higher education in Ireland. *International Journal of Nursing Studies 44*(7): 1187–1195.

Felton A (2015). *'Psychiatry is a Risk Business': the construction of mental health service users as objects of risk: a multiple case study inquiry.* Doctoral dissertation. Nottingham: University of Nottingham.

Freeman G (2009). Rogue nurse highlights dilemma over blame vs root cause. *Healthcare Risk Management 31*(12): 133–144.

Freidson E (2001). *Professionalism: the third logic.* Cambridge: Polity Press.

Freire P (1971). *Pedagogy of the Oppressed.* New York, NY: Herder & Herder.

Fulford KWM, Woodbridge K (2004). *Whose Values? A workbook for values-based practice in mental health care.* London: Sainsbury Centre for Mental Health.

Godin P (2000). A dirty business: caring for people who are a nuisance or a danger. *Journal of Advanced Nursing 32*(6): 1396–1402.

Hughes EC (1958.) *Men and their Work.* Glencoe, IL: Free Press.

Kendall K, Wiles R (2010). Resisting blame and managing emotion in general practice: the case of patient suicide. *Social Science and Medicine 70*(11): 1714–1720.

Kendra J (2007). The reconstitution of risk objects. *Journal of Risk Research 10*(1): 29–48.

Lau R (2009). The contemporary culture of blame and the fetishization of the modernist mentality. *Current Sociology 57*(5): 661–683.

Locke S (2009). Conspiracy culture, blame culture and rationalisation. *The Sociological Review 57*(4): 568–585.

McNamara M (2005). 'Dr Nightingale, I presume?': Irish nursing education enters the academy. In: Fealy GM (ed). *Care to Remember: nursing and midwifery in Ireland.* Cork: Mercier Press (pp54–68).

Meerabeau E (2004). Be good, sweet maid, and let who can be clever: a counter reformation in English nursing education? *International Journal of Nursing Studies 41*(3): 285–292.

Nursing & Midwifery Council (2018). *Future Nurse: standards of proficiency for registered nurses.* London: Nursing & Midwifery Council.

O'Connor N, Kotze B, Wright M (2011). Blame and accountability 1: understanding blame and blame pathologies. *Australasian Psychiatry 19*(2): 113–118.

Roberts SJ, Demarco R, Griffin M (2009). The effect of oppressed group behaviours on the culture of the nursing workplace: a review of the evidence and interventions for change. *Journal of Nursing Management 17*(3): 288–293.

Sher G (2006). *In Praise of Blame.* Oxford: Oxford University Press.

Stacey G, Felton A, Morgan A, Stickley T, Willis M, Diamond B, Houghton P, Johnson B, Dumanya J (2016). A critical narrative analysis of shared decision-making in acute inpatient mental health care. *Journal of Interprofessional Care 30*(1): 35–41.

Stein LI (1967). The Doctor-Nurse Game. *Archives of General Psychiatry 16*(6): 699–703.

Stein LI, Watts DT, Howell T (1990). The Doctor-Nurse Game revisited. *New England Journal of Medicine 322*(8): 546–549.

Szmukler G, Rose N (2013). Risk assessment in mental health care: values and costs. *Behavioral Sciences & the Law 31*(1): 125–140.

Traynor M, Stone K, Cook H, Gould D, Maben J (2013). Disciplinary processes and the management of poor performance among UK nurses: bad apple or systemic failure? A scoping study. *Nursing Inquiry* *21*(1): 51–58.

Undrill G (2007). The risks of risk assessment. *Advances in Psychiatric Treatment 13*(4): 290–297.

Williams G (2003). Blame and responsibility. *Ethical Theory and Moral Practice 6*(4): 427–445.

Woodward H, Lemer C, Wu A (2009). An end to the witch hunts: responding to the defenders of blame and shame. A commentary on Collins, Block, Arnold and Christakis. *Social Science and Medicine 69*(9): 1291–1293.

6 Colluding with prejudice? Mental health nurses and the Mental Health Act

Gary Sidley

The prominent mental-health activist Jacqui Dillon has claimed that, 'Fighting for the rights of people deemed mad, many of whom have already suffered enough, is the last great civil rights movement' (Dillon, 2011). Given the habitual acts of discrimination and human-rights violations endured by people labelled as 'mentally ill', her assertion is valid. Could mental health nurses be instrumental in determining how long this widespread injustice continues against those already suffering anguish and emotional overwhelm?

In this chapter, I will suggest that the engine room for these modern-day discriminatory practices is the Mental Health Act (1983, 2007) – a framework that not only constitutes a form of legalised discrimination but also sponsors mental health professionals to guarantee its implementation. Such an argument raises the disturbing spectre that mental health nurses – and all psychiatric professionals – are routinely colluding with discriminatory practices, the prejudicial nature of which is akin to the starkest examples of racism and sexism witnessed throughout the world.

I will highlight the key elements of the current mental health legislation to support my argument that it constitutes a form of legalised discrimination by infringing basic human rights. In particular, I will question the prominence given within the present legal framework to the dubious activities of identifying 'mental disorder' and the estimation of risk and will discuss preferable alternatives, focusing on decision-making capacity and 'best interests'. I will also explore the possible reasons why nurses collude with the prevailing legal framework and its associated prejudicial practices and discuss actions health professionals might consider to bring about its radical revision.

The legislation discussed in this chapter refers chiefly to the Mental Health Act (MHA) operating in England and Wales at the time of writing (July 2018). However, while there may be differences in detail, the mental health laws in other Western countries tend to adhere to similar principles.

Evolution of the Mental Health Act

Up until the second half of the 18th century, the care of those deemed insane typically defaulted to the family and religious organisations. The enduring alliance between the state and the medical profession in taking collective responsibility for this group of people began with the Madhouse Act of 1774, when, for the first time, a physician was installed as arbiter of the insane. A requirement of this legislation was that all private asylums must be licensed and inspected annually, with doctors in the role of overseers. From this point onwards, a letter from a medical practitioner was necessary to legitimise confinement (although paupers were exempt from this requirement).

Further piecemeal legislation followed through the 19th and early 20th centuries, much of it delegating additional powers to the medical profession in the management of those identified as displaying 'mental disorders'. The landmark Mental Health Act 1959 allowed the state effectively to surrender its role in determining who should be incarcerated in psychiatric institutions, leaving the way clear for psychiatrists to gatekeep this process (Szmukler & Holloway, 2000; Moncrieff, 2003).

The next major piece of mental health law – the Mental Health Act 1983 – appropriately addressed rising concerns about patients' human rights, placing some restrictions on non-consensual treatments and establishing the Mental Health Act Commission to scrutinise the implementation process and thereby protect the interests of service users. As will be shown, by the beginning of the 21st century, the British government was demonstrating an irrational preoccupation with the risk posed by people with mental health problems and strove to be credited with the role of noble protectors of the general public (Morgan & Felton, 2013; Pilgrim & Tomasini, 2013). Thus, in the prelude to the 2007 revisions to the Mental Health Act, the authorities sought to use mental health legislation as a way of controlling people deemed to be challenging and difficult, even inventing another fictitious diagnostic category – 'dangerous and severe personality disorder' – to allow the detention of these troublesome individuals without any requirement to demonstrate that a crime had been committed (Freshwater & Westwood, 2006).

The result of these changes was that, following the 2007 revisions, England and Wales operated under a draconian mental health legislation that explicitly sanctioned human rights violations.

The Mental Health Act as legalised discrimination

Citizens of a civilised society expect certain freedoms and safeguards. Two of these basic human rights are relevant here: first, the assurance that, if you abide by the law, you will be immune from incarceration; second, you have the opportunity to make an informed decision as to whether or not to accept a medical treatment.

The existing MHA rides roughshod over these cherished cornerstones of a free, democratic nation.

Under the current legislation, people deemed to be displaying a 'mental disorder' who have committed no crime can be forcibly confined in a psychiatric hospital – 'sectioned' – against their will and without recourse to a court hearing. This vulnerability to detention without trial, without having committed a demonstrable criminal act, accords psychiatric patients the same status as suspected terrorists (Vassilev & Pilgrim, 2007). Once incarcerated, invasive medical procedures, typically involving the intramuscular injection of psychotropic drugs, can be repeatedly administered without the person's consent.

By legitimising the detention of people who are suffering anguish and emotional overwhelm, the MHA also infringes Article 14 of the United Nations Convention on the Rights of Persons with Disabilities (United Nations, 2006), which states that 'the existence of a disability shall in no case justify a deprivation of liberty'.

Arguably, two of the most glaring injustices associated with the MHA are evident in relation to community treatment orders (CTOs) and advance decisions.

Community treatment orders

One of the most contentious elements of the 2007 revisions to the MHA was the concept of supervised community treatment, a legal instrument that enables psychiatry's coercive tentacles to stretch beyond the walls of a hospital. Patients incarcerated under particular sections of the MHA can be placed on a CTO following discharge, which imposes specified conditions and restrictions on their freedoms in their own homes. Their ongoing liberty is made contingent on their continuing to comply with a prescribed treatment regime, typically a nurse-administered depot injection. They can also be required to attend (or avoid) certain places and to take part in specified activities. Failure to comply can result in a compulsory return to the psychiatric hospital (Care Quality Commission, 2017).

The central repercussion of a CTO – and one that blatantly trespasses over basic human rights – is that law-abiding citizens with the wherewithal to make their own informed decisions can be compelled to take toxic drugs and face incarceration if they refuse. Such a violation of a person's freedoms is rendered even more appalling when one considers the physical health consequences, and relative ineffectiveness, of the mainstream psychiatric medications (Jakobsen et al, 2013; Moncrieff, 2013; Whitaker, 2015). Furthermore, since CTOs were introduced in 2008, black people have been consistently over-represented in those placed under their restrictions (Care Quality Commission, 2016), raising the likelihood of a racist element to their implementation.

The human rights violations inherent to CTOs could, arguably, be a price worth paying if these coercive measures achieved significant clinical benefits. Although advocates of CTOs occasionally claim some positive outcomes – see Light (2014) for a review – two wide-ranging studies have reported a lack of evidence for any meaningful gains for the service users snared within them. In an appraisal of studies conducted abroad, Churchill and colleagues (2007) found no indication of any positive effects in relation to patient satisfaction, hospital readmission rates or length of hospital stays. Similarly, a more recent evaluation of over 300 UK people with psychotic experiences concluded of CTOs: '... there is strong evidence that liberty is being substantially curtailed without any obvious clinical benefit to justify it' (Burns & Molodynski, 2014).

The combination of lack of effectiveness and human-rights violations makes it hard to disagree with the conclusion of Morgan and Felton (2013) that the implementation of CTOs was a politically motivated act, intended to appease the general public's irrational fears about risk rather than benefit those suffering with mental health problems.

Advance decisions

Originally called advance directives, the 'advance decision' emerged as part of a different piece of legislation, the Mental Capacity Act 2005 (MCA). This, unlike the MHA, emphasises the central importance of a person's decision-making capacity in determining future planning and the appropriateness of any potential coercion. An advance decision is a legal instrument that allows people with mental capacity the option of stating which medical treatments they do not wish to receive should they, in the future, lose the wherewithal to make their own informed choices.

In essence, the advance decision empowers users of healthcare services with the opportunity to influence service responses should a health problem subsequently render them incapable of autonomous decision-making. It is legally binding; any professional who ignores its stipulations risks prosecution, as they would if they proceeded with a clinical treatment without a patient's informed consent.

Unsurprisingly, people who require recurrent contact with psychiatric services seem to value the opportunity afforded by advance decisions; they appreciate being treated as responsible, capacitated adults and actively participating in shaping their future care (Sidley, 2012). Advance decisions are also formally recognised as an important part of a high-quality psychiatric service, warranting a specific reference in best-practice guidance for the management of 'schizophrenia' (National Institute for Health & Care Excellence, 2009).

Regrettably, the experience of completing an advance decision with the confidence that the requirements enshrined therein will be respected is yet another right denied the 'mentally disordered' as a direct result of the MHA. If a person is formally detained under the auspices of the MHA, their expressed wishes detailed in an advance decision can be over-ridden by the 'responsible clinician' (a psychiatrist, in almost all cases).

This potential corruption of advance decisions leads to a curious anomaly. Any citizen can construct an advance decision to refuse life-saving treatment for a future physical illness and, if it is drawn up correctly, health professionals are required to respect the decision, even if it leads directly to the person's premature death. In stark contrast, the legalised discrimination that is the MHA means that a person recurrently struggling with emotional distress and overwhelm cannot even refuse a specific medication with any confidence that their wishes will be respected.

Following their 2015/16 inspection, the Care Quality Commission (CQC), the formal regulatory body for the NHS, acknowledged – albeit in understated language – that the MHA had 'failings that may disempower patients, prevent people exercising legal rights, and ultimately impede recovery or even amount to unlawful and unethical practice' (Care Quality Commission, 2016).

How did a democratic society end up with discriminatory mental health laws?

It is informative to consider the process whereby the UK, a Western democracy, developed a comprehensive law that explicitly discriminates against a section of its citizens who are already suffering emotional pain and overwhelm. As persuasively argued by Szmukler (Szmukler, Daw & Dawson, 2010a, 2010b, 2010c), a crucial factor in the evolution of this prejudicial MHA is that it emerged independently of capacity-based law (as represented in the UK by the MCA). Whereas the latter piece of legislation demands the demonstration of a loss of decision-making capacity before a person may be treated without their consent for physical health problems – any compulsion being deemed to be in the 'best interests' of the individual – the MHA merely requires the presence of a 'mental disorder' and an assessment suggesting a risk to self or others as justification for coercive treatment of people with mental health problems. And, importantly, the requirements of the MHA override those of the MCA.

The implicit assumption within the MHA is that the existence of a 'mental disorder' is synonymous with a loss of capacity: that all people so labelled will not possess the mental ability to make their own decisions. Biological psychiatry's enduring insistence that brain abnormalities are the primary cause of the range of human suffering with which people present in their clinics has reinforced this misconception by colluding with the premise that a psychiatric diagnosis usually indicates a less than fully autonomous person. Similarly, mental health nurses who resort to the 'illness like any other' mantra when describing the distress of their patients will also be perpetuating this spurious notion.

Contrary to this implicit assumption in the MHA, most psychiatric service users do retain the ability to make informed choices. Even when they are enduring the peak of distress and overwhelm, research suggests many retain this ability: for example, in one study, between 40 and 60 per cent of patients admitted to an acute psychiatric ward displayed decision-making capacity (Owen et al, 2008).

While failure to consider whether patients are capable of making their own decisions is a major flaw in the MHA, the fundamental problems with the legislation derive from the fact that the judgment as to whether coercive treatment is deemed appropriate depends on two dubious and unreliable constructs: the identification of a 'mental disorder' and an assessment of risk.

Dubious construct 1: 'mental disorder'

The spurious notion that there is a clear dividing line between those with and without 'mental illnesses' continues to underpin biological psychiatry. Diagnostic classification systems – the *Diagnostic and Statistical Manual of Mental Disorders* (*DSM-5*) published by the American Psychiatric Association (2013) and the *International Statistical Classification of Diseases and Related Health Problems* (*ICD-10*, shortly to be reissued as *ICD-11*) produced by the World Health Organization (WHO, 2011) – are routinely relied upon in professional communications about mental health problems. Thus, when the MHA refers to the presence of a 'mental disorder', this is assumed to indicate that a person's symptoms match one or more of the diagnoses listed in these manuals.

The question of which symptoms should be included under each diagnostic label is defined by groups of self-appointed psychiatrists voting in committee (Davies, 2013). In the absence of physiological 'markers' for almost all mental disorders, this is a far from scientific process. As such, it is a subjective exercise that can be grossly influenced by the political and cultural context of the time. This is illustrated by the range of 'illnesses' identified in various past editions of the *DSM*: 'masturbatory insanity' (requiring genital mutilation as a form of treatment); homosexuality (considered a medical illness up until 1987); 'drapetomania' (created to explain why slaves attempted to escape from their owners); and 'sluggish schizophrenia' (a term used in Russia to discredit the political views of dissidents). As argued above, more recently, the UK government invented the diagnosis 'dangerous and severe personality disorder' for political purposes (Freshwater & Westwood, 2006), in order to enable the indefinite incarceration of people deemed to pose a major risk to society.

The presence of a 'mental disorder' – a fundamental requirement of the MHA sectioning process – relies on these flawed diagnostic classification systems (for a review, see Bentall, 2009: 89–109). Diagnostic labels such as 'schizophrenia' and 'bipolar disorder' are subjective, unreliable, poor predictors of response to interventions and not underpinned by science. Yet a person's liberty and the legitimacy of forced treatment often hinge on their identification.

Dubious construct 2: estimation of risk

The underlying assumption that people struggling with mental health problems are inherently risky is often used by the psychiatric profession to defend human-rights violations. Furthermore, the assessment of the level of danger (to self and/or others) posed by the individual patient is central to the operation of coercive intervention under the auspices of the MHA. However, the combination of inflated expectations of threat and the inaccuracy of the measures to assess it render risk estimation a woefully inadequate construct for justifying incarceration and forced treatment.

It is true that people in contact with psychiatric services constitute a higher risk of self-harm and suicide when compared with the general population – a predictable finding, given that many risk factors for developing mental health problems also predispose a person to suicidality (for example, social deprivation, disempowerment, previous traumatisation) and that risk to self is often a key factor in people's entry into psychiatric services. Nonetheless, between two-thirds and three-quarters of people who take their own life do not have a recognised psychiatric problem and have had no previous contact with mental health services (Luoma, Martin & Pearson, 2002; Lee et al, 2008; Appleby et al, 2013). Thus, the potential impact of current psychiatric practice on the suicide rate in our communities is limited.

By contrast, the evidence that people with mental health problems pose a greater risk of harm to others than the general population is weak and contradictory. While a few studies focusing on specific groups have suggested an association between 'mental disorder' and violent behaviour (for example, Bentall & Taylor, 2006; Silver, Felson & Vaneseltine, 2008), other research in this area has failed to highlight any substantial link. A Dutch study (Vinkers et al, 2012) calculated that only 0.07 per cent of all crime could be directly attributable to mental health problems. Even when the focus is exclusively on people with psychotic experiences, there is no convincing support for the assertion that delusions and hallucinations significantly predict violence (Appelbaum, Robbins & Monahan, 2000; Douglas, Guy & Hart, 2009). People diagnosed with 'schizophrenia' account for only five per cent of all murders, and alcohol and drug misuse are contributory factors in more than 60 per cent of such cases (Shaw et al, 2006; Swinson et al, 2007).

A couple of further statistics illustrate the irrationality of the notion that specific legislation (the MHA) is required to protect the general public from people with mental health problems. Szmukler (2000) calculated that the probability of a member of the general public being murdered by someone with a 'schizophrenia' diagnosis is one in 10 million – a risk on a par with dying from a lightning strike. Furthermore, psychiatric patients are 14 times more likely to be the victims of violent crime than they are to be the assailants (Brekke et al, 2001).

Even if those suffering emotional anguish did represent a substantial threat to others, the MHA constraints would only be justifiable if the risk level could be accurately estimated. This is not the case. Risk assessments – a substantial component of a mental health nurse's role – are so riddled with inaccuracies that they are unlikely to reduce the frequency of high-profile incidents of violence that grab media attention (Witteman, 2004; Morgan, 2007). In particular, formal risk assessments are fundamentally flawed by their low specificity, in that they identify many people as 'high-risk' who do not subsequently engage in violent or suicidal behaviour. One important consequence of these 'false positives' is that, for every homicide correctly predicted, there would be at least 2,000 people wrongly identified as posing such a risk (Szmukler, 2000). Risk predictions by psychiatric professionals may be only marginally more accurate than those generated by chance (Doyle & Dolan, 2002).

Furthermore, there is no evidence that risk assessment is any more precise with 'mentally disordered' groups than with potentially dangerous people outside of the psychiatric system. Nor is there any evidence that psychiatric 'treatments' are any more effective in reducing risk in people with mental health problems than they are with people who pose risk but are outside the psychiatric system. On the contrary, community-wide interventions like anger management (McGuire, 2008) and controlled drinking programmes (Raistrick, Heather & Godfrey, 2006), accessible to all on a voluntary basis, may be more likely to reduce the number of violent incidents in society than forced consumption of psychotropic drugs.

Preventative detention and the increasing use of coercion

The vast majority of people who constitute a threat to the safety of others are not part of the psychiatric population. Yet risk in the context of mental health problems is interpreted and managed in a completely different way to risks inherent in society as a whole (Pilgrim & Tomasini, 2013). This difference of approach is most evident in preventative detention, where sectioning under the MHA is typically based on the *potential* risk to others.

Psychiatric patients are susceptible to a form of preventative detention, legitimised by the MHA, that, if applied to any other sections of the community, would be emphatically rejected. As Pilgrim and Tomasini (2013) persuasively argue, a fair approach demands that we use preventative detention for all or for none, as opposed to singling out the 'mentally disordered'. There is no plausible justification for these double standards. If the fundamental driver of legislation were risk reduction, it would be much more effective to impose night-time restrictions on all teenagers and young adults – an intervention that would, of course, be construed as an unacceptable infringement of personal freedom.

A degree of reassurance might be drawn if it could be shown that these MHA-inspired human rights violations are a rare and diminishing occurrence. The official statistics suggest otherwise. In 2015/16 there were 63,622 detentions, a 47 per cent increase on the 2005/06 figure (NHS Digital, 2016). Recently, the use of sectioning has escalated at a rate of around 10 per cent a year. At the end of March 2016, 25,577 patients remained under detention; the comparable figure for this snapshot at the end of 2005/06 was 14,625. Almost one in three of these detainees are now housed in independent hospitals.

With regards to CTOs, their implementation in Australia and the US prior to their arrival in the UK seemed to find favour with psychiatrists: some three-quarters reported that they found them useful (Churchill et al, 2007). This affinity with CTOs has continued, Australia in particular reporting high rates of application (Light, Kerridge & Ryan, 2012). In England and Wales, the Royal

College of Psychiatrists initially opposed their introduction, but here too they now appear to be an accepted part of service provision: some 4,500 CTOs are imposed each year (NHS Digital, 2016).

Alternatives to the MHA

In light of the fundamental flaws and injustices intrinsic to the MHA, it is appropriate to explore whether there are alternative legal frameworks that could be more helpful. It is generally recognised that some form of non-consensual intervention may be necessary at times when a person is suffering extreme emotional overwhelm, displaying troubled or troubling behaviour and presenting an imminent risk to self or others. However, any legal framework that regulates the use of coercion in these circumstances must apply equally to all citizens if it is to be judged to be fair and non-discriminatory. Are there other, more egalitarian forms of legislation that would avoid the human rights violations associated with the MHA while still retaining sufficient power to safeguard both the individual and the general public?

One option might be to extend the use of the MCA into routine psychiatric practice. As previously mentioned, the MCA is a broad, non-discriminatory framework applicable across the health spectrum (physical and mental) for people who lack the capacity to make their own decisions. It operates on the assumption that a person has capacity unless proven otherwise. As described in the Mental Capacity Act 2005 Code of Practice, to be deemed to have capacity, a person must be able to understand why a decision needs to be made; understand the likely consequences of not making a decision; understand the information relevant to making a decision; retain the relevant information in memory long enough to be able to choose between the options, and communicate the decision, via whatever means. It is up to others to demonstrate that a person has lost capacity; the default assumption is that the person can make his/her own decisions.

Under such circumstances, deprivation of liberty safeguards may be legally applied in the 'best interests' of the patient and if offering the least restrictive option. This would mean only those who genuinely lack capacity to consent to treatment could be treated without their consent.

Psychiatric professionals, with their focus on 'mental disorder' and level of risk, often fail to consider the appropriateness of the MCA when detaining people with mental health problems, automatically relying on the MHA to manage patients in acute crisis. In addition to its fairness, the MCA does not discriminate against those labelled with 'mental disorders'. Its use is supported by research suggesting that professionals usually agree on whether a person retains decision-making capacity, even when the assessments are conducted independently (Cairns et al, 2005). However, an important weakness of the MCA when used in a mental health context is that it provides very little guidance on the use of force in non-consensual treatment and detention when a patient has lost decision-making capacity.

Szmukler and colleagues have proposed a 'Fusion Law' that strives to build on the strengths of the MHA and MCA (Dawson & Szmukler, 2006; Szmukler, Daw & Dawson, 2010a, 2010b, 2010c). This would provide one legislative framework governing non-consensual treatment that would be applicable across the spectrum of physical and mental health problems. Under this proposal, the central justification for all non-consensual detentions and treatments would be incapacity to make decisions, thereby reducing legal discrimination against the 'mentally disordered'.

Although the details of this 'Fusion Law' continue to be debated, particularly around how to create practical safeguards to protect vulnerable people without capacity from unnecessary interventions, there is a growing consensus that inclusive legislation of this kind is both imperative and achievable.

Both these alternatives – Fusion Law and the expansion of the MCA into psychiatric settings – recognise that psychiatric interventions do not need to be the subject of special legislation. Furthermore, each also recognises that 'mental disorder' is often not synonymous with loss of capacity to make decisions. These normalising messages would help counter the common, spurious assumption that those tagged with a psychiatric diagnosis are inherently defective and that their emotional suffering is the direct consequence of a brain abnormality. By not colluding with this myth, these proposed legal frameworks would reduce the stigma and other significant disadvantages of assuming an illness-like-any-other understanding of human distress (Sidley, 2015a).

Why no collective protest from nurses?

Given its inherent destructive prejudices, why do nurses – along with other mental health professionals – continue to collude with the use of the MHA?

Mental health nurses constitute the largest professional group working within the current psychiatric system. As such, their attitudes towards, and degree of collusion with, the MHA are a major factor in prolonging the lifespan of the existing discriminatory framework. Although only a few hold the formal role of 'Approved Mental Health Professional', which accords them a recognised role in the sectioning process (Coffey & Hannigan, 2013), mental health nurses are centrally involved in implementing the requirements of the MHA around statutory detention and forced treatment. As such, they are typically the human barrier that prevents involuntary patients from leaving psychiatric units; they are also the clinicians who administer drugs against the wishes of the recipients.

Considering their numerical superiority in the psychiatric system, along with their direct involvement in pervasive coercive practices, it is reasonable to suggest that any collective dissent by nurses to the MHA would necessitate an immediate government review of the mental health legislation. So what level of clamour for change can be heard from this group of psychiatric professionals?

Extensive searches of Google and publication databases – inputting terms such as 'Mental Health Act' and 'mental health nurses' – failed to identify any nurse-informed critiques of the current legal framework. Informal discussions with nursing educators involved in the Critical Mental Health Nurses' Network (CMHNN), together with the responses to an article I submitted about the Mental Health Act on the same site (Sidley, 2015b), clearly indicate that some nurse academics and educators are giving this considerable thought. However, this critical thinking has yet to reach the legions of mental health nurses who staff our inpatient units and community teams and silently collude with the discriminatory practices and human-rights violations inherent to the MHA.

What could be the reasons for this blanket conformity? Why is there no collective scream of disapproval from professional nurses? Given the absence of published debate about this issue, any attempts to answer these questions are purely personal speculation. Four possible reasons suggest themselves to me.

Explanation 1: lack of awareness

It may be that nurses do not recognise the relevance of the broader political and legal context in which they operate. Perhaps the laws of the land are assumed to be fixed background factors and therefore it rarely occurs to nurses to question them in the course of their demanding roles. So, despite the grotesque injustices within it, the MHA is accepted as 'the way it is'; something we all must accept.

With this explanation, the MHA is considered to be outside of the clinical domain and, therefore, the concern of others – politicians and law-makers – rather than a legitimate focus for nursing discussion. Hence, there is a dearth of writings in the mental health nursing literature about the topic, and comments about its appropriateness and implications are rarely heard in the everyday chatter of multi-disciplinary teams.

Explanation 2: power and status

Szasz (1973) coined the term 'institutional psychiatry' and argued that mental health legislation inevitably results in psychiatrists acting as agents of the state, in cahoots with the government of the day. In line with this, the psychiatric profession is empowered to confine and control troublesome and unwanted members of the community (Summerfield, 2001). Although such a process raises serious ethical issues, it results in the role of a psychiatrist being formalised and instilled with enhanced power and status. Perhaps the mental health nursing profession also benefits from this MHA-inspired increase in authority, and so overlooks or tolerates the inherent discriminatory practices.

Under section 5(4) of the MHA, mental health nurses are granted an exclusive, profession-specific power to detain a voluntary patient in hospital for up to six hours if the nurse believes that, by not doing so, there will be an immediate risk to the individual or to the general public. Although this particular legal responsibility may confer some degree of status, the power associated with this 'holding' function is dwarfed by that accredited to the 'responsible clinician', a role almost always fulfilled by a psychiatrist. Given the enduring, symbiotic relationship between medical psychiatrists and mental health nurses, it is reasonable to suggest that the latter benefit much more from their longstanding association with their ideological allies (the former) than from any specified role within the MHA.

Explanation 3: acceptance of 'the inherently defective' model

A third potential explanation for nursing collusion with the MHA may relate to their dominant explanatory model of mental health problems. In keeping with their strong alliance and historical ties with the medical profession, it is plausible to suggest that a large majority of mental health nurses concur with the 'illness-like-any-other' understanding of the suffering and anguish of their patients. Therefore, they may accept as valid the implicit assumptions that form the foundation of a discriminatory MHA.

A belief that a primary cause of human suffering is a biological deficit or brain abnormality could logically lead to the acceptance that all patients with a 'mental disorder' are inherently defective and lack the capacity to make their own decisions. Following on from this reasoning, there is likely to be acceptance of the need for special legislation to manage and control psychiatric patients. Human rights violations may then be construed as a price worth paying for public protection and the safety of the people in their care. If this explanation is valid, collusion with the MHA by mental health nurses derives from a belief that the existing legal framework is reasonable and fit for purpose.

Explanation 4: low self-esteem and high burnout among psychiatric nurses

The role of a psychiatric nurse in our underfunded mental health system is often a very stressful one. Frontline work with people experiencing extremes of emotional distress can inevitably lead to high levels of burnout and low self-esteem among practitioners (Carson et al, 1997; Edwards et al, 2000; Nolan & Smojkis, 2003). High bureaucratic demands and relatively low remuneration may add to this psychological burden.

It may be that many nurses exposed to these day-to-day realities feel undervalued and demotivated – a state of mind that would not be conducive to collective efforts to change the wider world in which they operate. Negotiating the daily demands of their micro-environment might leave many with insufficient energy and confidence to scream disapproval about something as relatively remote as the MHA.

Potential acts of resistance by nurses

Considering the potential explanations for why mental health nurses generally remain silent about the MHA, it is unclear whether there is a desire within the profession to agitate for change. Nonetheless, it is pertinent to explore the options open to mental health nurses should they wish to highlight the fundamental injustices associated with the MHA.

The most obvious and accessible act of resistance – and one that many nurses will already deploy – is to advocate on behalf of their patients when issues such as sectioning, community treatment orders and advance decisions are raised during multi-disciplinary team discussions. Questioning the appropriateness of MHA-informed decisions in this context can require courage, particularly if the nurse's view is at odds with that of the psychiatrist and given the risk-averse milieu of psychiatric services. Yet discussions of this type – although important – are likely to be limited to the particular set of conditions surrounding the individual patient; the broader question of the legitimacy of the MHA itself will rarely arise.

Perhaps a more productive way to achieve a radical revision of the MHA would involve political activism in all its various forms. Individual actions might include lobbying local Members of Parliament to raise the issue of the discriminatory mental health legislation in the House of Commons. Collective action would, potentially, be more influential, involving campaigns by the relevant professional bodies and trade unions. These formal organisations representing the interests of nursing practitioners should be deeply concerned that their paying members are routinely required to engage in discriminatory actions against vulnerable, suffering people in our society.

While advocacy and political campaigning by nurses could helpfully raise awareness of the injustices of the MHA, direct action in the form of 'conscientious objection' to implementing some of its specific requirements would powerfully demonstrate disapproval and the urgent need for reform. Indeed, a collective lack of cooperation with some of the more blatant discriminatory practices – such as non-consensual treatments for patients retaining the capacity to make their own decisions – would impede the workings of the MHA to such an extent that an urgent review would be unavoidable.

There are precedents for conscientious objection in healthcare provision. In the UK, it currently is lawful for nurses and midwives to opt out of involvement in abortions and technological procedures to achieve conception if these medical interventions violate the practitioner's moral or ethical values (Nursing & Midwifery Council, 2015). The conscientious objection concept is also valid in other parts of the world, with reproductive activities and end-of-life care typically amenable to such opt-outs.

The detailed guidance from professional bodies regarding conscientious objection rightly emphasises that patients should not be disadvantaged as a result of a nurse's moral convictions. In particular, tensions may arise where the rights of patients to undergo a legal procedure – such as a termination of pregnancy – clash with nurses' rights to conscientiously object (Lachman, 2014). However, in the field of mental health nursing, these patient-professional tensions are unlikely to arise as it is hard to imagine service users with decision-making capacity taking legal action against staff members who, for example, refuse to force psychotropic drugs on them.

Barriers to implementing conscientious objections in mental health services would most probably originate not from patients but from service managers and fellow professionals. A minority voice in the orthodox psychiatric machine typically attracts hostility and censorship. To reasonably expect mental health nurses to engage in non-cooperation with aspects of the MHA would require robust safeguards that these brave individuals are not disadvantaged, whether it be through harassment, social exclusion, threats to career development or even loss of jobs or professional conduct sanctions.

Reasons for optimism?

In February 2016, the Independent Mental Health Taskforce published *The Five Year Forward View for Mental Health* (Mental Health Taskforce, 2016). Although, regrettably, much of the document calls for more-of-the-same traditional services, one of the recommendations is that the Department of Health should work with a broad range of stakeholders to review the MHA. Consistent with this stated aim, the Mental Health Alliance – a coalition of more than 65 organisations – has, since 2000, been highlighting its concerns about the MHA and, more recently, campaigning for radical revision.

In June 2017, this alliance published a document titled *A Mental Health Act Fit for Tomorrow: an agenda for reform* (Mental Health Alliance, 2017). The document, based on a survey of more than 8,000 stakeholders (service users, carers and professionals), reported a wide range of concerns, including human rights violations, lack of dignity, the disregarding of advance decisions and the overuse of CTOs. The overarching conclusion was that the MHA was 'not fit for purpose', leading to a demand that the Government 'deliver a fundamental review'.

There are signs too of a growing political momentum for radical revision of the MHA. The 2017 Conservative Party pre-election manifesto contained a commitment to reform the mental health legislation, and the Prime Minister, Theresa May, referred to 'burning injustices' caused by 'discriminatory use of a law passed more than three decades ago' (Savage, 2017). Despite a reduced majority following the election – and a subsequent contraction of the policy programme of the minority administration – Theresa May's government retained its intention to reform mental health legislation (Queen's Speech, 2017) and an 'independent review' of the Mental Health Act was announced in May 2018, led by one of the UK's foremost psychiatrists, Professor Sir Simon Wessely. It was due to report as this book went to print but early indications are that its main focus will be how the MHA is implemented, not a revision of the legislation itself.

A significant and welcome addition to the debate is the recently published report *The Power, Threat, Meaning Framework* (Johnstone & Boyle, 2018), which offers a radical, psychological alternative to the biomedical, 'illness-like-any-other' approach and a comprehensive and normalising way of making sense of human suffering. If widely adopted, this framework could remove the need for dedicated 'mental health' legislation. A primary aim is to offer a 'fundamentally different perspective on the origins, experience and expression of emotional distress and troubled or troubling behaviour' (p8). This new paradigm attributes the misery and anguish of any person – psychiatric patient or otherwise – to the negative experience of power, past and present, in their life and the subsequent meanings they attach to these experiences. In shifting the focus away from the identification of individual deficits ('mental disorders') as a means of explaining human suffering, the framework raises fundamental questions about the relevance and validity of distinctive 'mental health' laws.

In light of these encouraging developments, it is reasonable to believe that the current political context is receptive to the idea of a radical rewrite of the MHA. Given that this piece of mental health legislation, as well as infringing basic human rights, also drives much that is awry with current health and social care provision for people suffering anguish and overwhelm, there could be no better time for mental health nurses to add their own distinctive – and potentially decisive – contribution to the campaign for change.

References

American Psychiatric Association (2013). *Diagnostic and Statistical Manual of Mental Disorders* (5th ed). Washington, DC: American Psychiatric Association.

Appelbaum P, Robbins P, Monahan J (2000). Violence and delusions: data from the MacArthur Violence Risk Assessment Study. *American Journal of Psychiatry 157*(4): 566–572.

Appleby L, Kapur N, Shaw J, Hunt IM, While D, Flynn S et al (2013). *The National Confidential Inquiry into Suicide and Homicide by People with Mental Illness. Annual report: England, Northern Ireland, Scotland and Wales*. Manchester: Centre for Mental Health and Risk, University of Manchester.

Bentall RP (2009). *Doctoring the Mind: why psychiatric treatments fail*. London: Penguin Books.

Bentall R, Taylor J (2006). Psychological processes and paranoia: implications for forensic behavioural science. *Behavioural Sciences and the Law 24*(3): 277–294.

Brekke JS, Prindle C, Bae W, Long JD (2001). Risks for individuals with schizophrenia who are living in the community. *Psychiatric Services 52*(10): 1358–1366.

Burns T, Molodynski A (2014). Community treatment orders: background and implications of OCTET trial. *Psychiatric Bulletin 38*(1): 3–5.

Cairns R, Maddock C, Buchanan A, David AS, Hayward P, Richardson G et al (2005). Reliability of mental capacity assessments in psychiatric in-patients. *British Journal of Psychiatry 187*: 372–378.

Care Quality Commission (2017). *Information for people subject to community treatment orders (CTOs)*. London: Care Quality Commission.

Care Quality Commission (2016). *Monitoring the Mental Health Act in 2016/17*. London: Care Quality Commission.

Carson J, Fagin L, Bromn, D, Leary J, Bartlett H (1997). Self-esteem in mental health nurses: its relationship to stress, coping and burnout. *Journal of Research in Nursing 2*(5): 361–369.

Churchill R, Owen G, Singh S, Hotopf M (2007). *International Experience of Using Community Treatment Orders*. London: Institute of Psychiatry.

Coffey M, Hannigan B (2013). New roles for nurses as approved mental health professionals in England and Wales. *International Journal of Nursing Studies 50*(10): 1423–1430.

Davies J (2013). *Cracked: why psychiatry is doing more harm than good*. London: Icon Press.

Dawson J, Szmukler G (2006). Fusion of mental health and incapacity legislation. *British Journal of Psychiatry 188*: 504–509.

Dillon J (2011). The personal is the political. In: Rapley M, Moncrieff J, Dillon J (eds). *De-Medicalising Misery: psychiatry, psychology and the human condition*. Basingstoke: Palgrave Macmillan (pp141–157).

Douglas K, Guy L, Hart S (2009). Psychosis as a risk factor for violence to others: a meta-analysis. *Psychological Bulletin 135* (5): 679–706.

Doyle M, Dolan M (2002). Violence risk assessment: combining actuarial and clinical information to structure clinical judgements for the formulation and management of risk. *Journal of Psychiatric and Mental Health Nursing 9*(6): 649–657.

Edwards D, Burnard P, Coyle D, Fothergill A, Hannigan B (2000). Stressors, moderators and stress outcomes: findings from the All-Wales Community Mental Health Nurse Study. *Journal of Psychiatric and Mental Health Nursing 7*(6): 529–537.

Freshwater D, Westwood T (2006). Risk, detention and evidence: humanizing mental health reform. *Journal of Psychiatric and Mental Health Nursing 13*(3): 257–259.

Jakobsen JC, Katakam KK, Schou A, Hellmuth SG, Stallknecht SE, Leth-Moller K et al (2013). Selective serotonin reuptake inhibitors versus placebo in patients with major depressive disorder: a systematic review with meta-analysis and Trial Sequential Analysis. *BMC Psychiatry 17*: 58. https://doi.org/10.1186/s12888-016-1173-2

Johnstone L, Boyle M with Cromby J, Dillon J, Harper D, Kinderman P, Longden E, Pilgrim D, Read J (2018). *The Power Threat Meaning Framework: overview*. Leicester: British Psychological Society.

Lachman VD (2014). Conscientious objection in nursing: definition and criteria for acceptance. *MEDSURG Nursing 23*(3): 196–198.

Lee HC, Lin HC, Liu TC, Lin SY (2008). Contact of mental and non-mental health care providers prior to suicide in Taiwan: a population-based study. *Canadian Journal of Psychiatry 53*(6): 377–383.

Light E (2014). The epistemic challenges of CTOs: commentary on community treatment orders. *Psychiatric Bulletin 38*(1): 6–8.

Light E, Kerridge I, Ryan C (2012). Community Treatment Orders in Australia: rates and patterns of use. *Australasian Psychiatry 20*(6): 478–482.

Luoma JB, Martin CE, Pearson JL (2002). Contact with mental health and primary care providers before suicide: a review of the evidence. *American Journal of Psychiatry 159*(6): 909–916.

McGuire J (2008). A review of effective interventions for reducing aggression and violence. *Philosophical Transactions B 363*(1503): 2577–2597.

Mental Health Alliance (2017). *A Mental Health Act fit for tomorrow: an agenda for reform*. London: Rethink.

Mental Health Taskforce (2016). *The Five-Year Forward View for Mental Health: a report from the Independent Mental Health Taskforce to the NHS in England.* London: NHS England.

Moncrieff J (2013). *The Bitterest Pills: the troubling story of antipsychotic drugs.* Basingstoke: Palgrave Macmillan.

Moncrieff J (2003). The politics of a new Mental Health Act. *British Journal of Psychiatry 183*(1): 8–9.

Morgan J (2007). *'Giving Up the Culture of Blame': risk assessment and risk management in psychiatric practice.* London: Royal College of Psychiatrists.

Morgan A, Felton A (2013). From constructive engagement to coerced recovery. In: Coles S, Keenan S, Diamond B (eds). *Madness Contested: power and practice.* Ross-on-Wye: PCCS Books (pp56–73).

National Institute for Health and Care Excellence (2009). *Schizophrenia: core interventions in the treatment and management of schizophrenia in adults in primary and secondary care.* London: National Institute for Health and Care Excellence.

NHS Digital (2016). *Inpatients formally detained in hospitals under the Mental Health Act 1983 and patients subject to Supervised Community Treatment: 2015/16. Annual figures.* [Online.] www.content.digital.nhs.uk/catalogue/PUB22571 (accessed 12th June 2017).

Nolan P, Smojkis M (2003). The mental health of nurses in the UK. *Advances in Psychiatric Treatment 9*(5): 374–379.

Nursing & Midwifery Council (2015). *The Code: professional standards of practice and behaviour of nurses and midwives.* London: NMC.

Owen GS, Richardson G, David AS, Szmukler G, Hayward, P, Hotopf M (2008). Mental capacity to make decisions on treatment in people admitted to psychiatric hospitals: cross sectional study. *British Medical Journal 337*(7660): 40–42.

Pilgrim D, Tomasini F (2013). Mental disorder and the socio-ethical challenge of reasonableness. In: Coles S, Keenan S, Diamond B (eds). *Madness Contested: power and practice.* Ross-on-Wye: PCCS Books (pp74–89).

Queen's Speech (2017). *Her Majesty's most gracious speech to both Houses of Parliament.* [Online.] www.gov.uk/government/speeches/queens-speech-2017 (accessed 30 June 2017).

Raistrick D, Heather N, Godfrey C (2006). *Review of the Effectiveness of Treatment for Alcohol Problems.* London: National Treatment Agency for Substance Misuse.

Savage M (2017). Theresa May pledges mental health revolution will reduce detentions. [Online.] *The Observer;* 7 May. www.theguardian.com/politics/2017/may/07/theresa-may-pledges-mental-health-revolution-will-reduce-detentions (accessed 1 July 2018).

Shaw J, Hunt IM, Flynn S, Meehan J, Robinson J, Bickley H et al (2006). Rates of mental disorder in people convicted of homicide: national clinical survey. *British Journal of Psychiatry 188*: 143–147.

Sidley G (2015a). *Tales from the Madhouse: an insider critique of psychiatric services.* Ross-on-Wye: PCCS Books.

Sidley GL (2015b). The Mental Health Act: legalised discrimination. [Online.] *Critical Mental Health Nurses' Network.* https://criticalmhnursing.org/2015/05/29/the-mental-health-act-legalised-discrimination (accessed 20 June 2017).

Sidley GL (2012). Advance decisions in secondary mental health services. *Nursing Standard 26*(21): 44–48.

Silver E, Felson RB, Vaneseltine M (2008). The relationship between mental health problems and violence among criminal offenders. *Criminal Justice and Behavior 35*(4): 405–426.

Summerfield D (2001). Does psychiatry stigmatize? *Journal of the Royal Society of Medicine, 94*(3): 148–49.

Swinson NA, Ashim B, Windfuhr KL, Kapur NN, Appleby L, Shaw J (2007). National Confidential Inquiry into Suicide and Homicide by People with Mental Illness: new directions. *Psychiatric Bulletin 31*: 161–63.

Szasz TS (1973). *The Manufacture of Madness: a comparative study of the inquisition and the mental health movement.* London: Routledge & Kegan Paul.

Szmukler G (2000). Homicide inquiries: what sense do they make? *Psychiatric Bulletin 24*(1): 6–10.

Szmukler G, Holloway F (2000). Reform of the Mental Health Act: health or safety? *British Journal of Psychiatry 177*: 196–200.

Szmukler G, Daw R, Dawson J (2010a). 1. A model law fusing incapacity and mental health legislation. *International Journal of Mental Health Law 20*: 9–22.

Szmukler G, Daw R, Dawson J (2010b). Response to the commentaries. *International Journal of Mental Health Law 20*: 89–98.

Szmukler G, Daw R, Dawson J (2010c). Outline of the model law. *International Journal of Mental Health Law 20*: 99–122.

United Nations (2006). *United Nations Convention on the Rights of Persons with Disabilities and Optional Protocol.* New York, NY: United Nations.

Vassilev I, Pilgrim D (2007). Risk, trust and the myth of mental health services. *Journal of Mental Health 16*(3): 347–357.

Vinkers DJ, De Beurs E, Barendregt M, Rinne T, Hoeck HW (2012). Proportion of crimes attributable to mental disorders in the Netherlands. *World Psychiatry 11*(2): 134.

Whitaker R (2015). *Antipsychotics/schizophrenia.* [Blogpost.] Mad in America. www.madinamerica.com/mia-manual/antipsychoticsschizophrenia (accessed 29 May 2017).

Witteman C (2004). Violent figures; risky stories: invited commentary on... psychodynamic methods in risk assessment and management. *Advances in Psychiatric Treatment 10*: 275–276.

World Health Organization (2011). *The ICD-10 Classification of Mental and Behavioural Disorders.* Geneva: World Health Organization.

7

The development of a critically orientated mental health nursing practice: Michel Foucault's 'history of the present'

Marc Roberts

Contemporary mental health care is a complex, challenging and contested field of professional practice. What were once considered acceptable and productive ways of understanding and responding to mental distress are increasingly being challenged by those who work in and those who use mental health services (Rapley, Moncrieff & Dillon, 2011; Cromby, Harper & Reavey, 2013; Roberts, 2018). The authority of mental health professionals and the legitimacy of their interventions are subject to ongoing critical examination, and people who use mental health services are increasingly calling for greater involvement in how their experiences are understood and addressed (Beresford, 2010; Campbell, 2013).

To provide informed, effective and responsive mental health care in this challenging and changing context, and in response to the requirement to practise in an evidence-based, collaborative and recovery-focused way, there is a recognition of the need for mental health nurses to possess sophisticated critical thinking and reflective capabilities (McKie & Naysmith, 2014; McKeown & White, 2015; Roberts, 2015). The ability to think and reflect critically not only enables practitioners to identify, examine and evaluate the range of theory, research and evidence that informs contemporary mental health care; it is also necessary for the development of a critical awareness of how the assumptions, values and beliefs of mental health professionals may affect their practice in both productive and non-productive ways. Indeed, such critical capabilities are essential for preventing the provision of potentially ineffective, dogmatic and paternalistic mental health care by questioning, challenging and seeking to change that which does not withstand critical examination, especially in response to contemporary research and evidence, the emergence of new theoretical perspectives and because of the innovative work of those who use mental health services.

Beyond asserting the importance of these capabilities, however, the character of such a critically orientated mental health nursing practice and the manner in which practitioners might engage in such activity have been infrequently articulated. Therefore, while recognising that many mental health nurses already possess sophisticated critical thinking and reflective capabilities – and also acknowledging the variety of means by which these can be acquired (Brookfield, 2001) – this chapter will suggest that those capabilities can be productively situated within the context of the work of the 20th century French philosopher Michel Foucault. One of the most challenging, innovative and influential thinkers of the 20th century, Foucault produced a prodigious body of work that dealt philosophically with a variety of interdependent themes such as knowledge, power and subjectivity. In doing so, he typically examined these themes in the context of various historical studies, such as the transformation in the understanding and treatment of those designated 'mad' or 'mentally ill'; the development of practices of punishment and the emergence of the penal system, and analyses of the forms of sexual conduct and ethics that characterised classical antiquity, Christianity and the modern era (Foucault 1990a, 1991a, 1998a, 1998b, 2001).

Rather than focusing exclusively on the content of Foucault's work, however, this chapter will propose that it is possible to discern a general methodological approach across that work, which Foucault refers to as the 'history of the present' (Foucault 1991a: 31). An accessible account of that approach in relation to contemporary mental health care will be presented in order to propose that the history of the present provides a framework in which to situate the critical capabilities of mental health nurses and thereby contribute to the development of a critically orientated mental health nursing practice.

Self-evidence

To begin to understand how the critical capabilities of mental health nurses can be situated within the context of Foucault's work, it is first productive to clarify the character of those capabilities. However, it can be a particular challenge to encapsulate in a succinct manner the features that comprise an activity as complex as critical, reflective thinking. For example, Foucault suggests that such activity – which he variously refers to as 'criticism', 'critique' or simply 'thought' – ranges from 'unearthing' and examining the assumptions that underlie our various practices to a form of personal transformation that can involve a change in our thinking and even a transformation of our identity or 'self' (Foucault 1990b, 1990c). Of course, various definitions of this critical activity have been proposed but the attempt to do so in a concise manner often means that one definition will minimise or omit features that another emphasises (see, for example, Boyd & Fales, 1983; Boud, Keogh & Walker, 1985; Dewey, 2012). However, while acknowledging the challenge in providing such a concise definition – as well as those conceptual considerations surrounding the possible distinction between critical thinking and reflection (Fook, White & Gardner, 2006) – this critically reflective activity can broadly be understood as a multifaceted cognitive and affective capability that requires a variety of intellectual skills and emotional attributes (Paul & Elder, 2014). In particular, these intellectual skills and emotional attributes are employed in a purposeful, disciplined and often creative manner to meet various critical and clinical objectives. This can include the analysis and clarification of issues and areas of concern; the gathering and appraisal of evidence, research and theory; the questioning and challenging of assumptions, values and beliefs, and the synthesis and application of information to produce alternative and innovative ways of thinking and behaving.

In addition to this challenge of definition, a variety of obstacles can impede, oppose and even negate the attempt to facilitate critical thinking and reflection in mental health care and the healthcare professions in general. These can manifest at personal, social and institutional levels, and can include misunderstandings about the purpose and character of this critical activity; an under-appreciation of its value and significance for clinical practice, and an 'anti-intellectualism' that can be expressed as an implicit or even explicit hostility towards those who think and reflect critically (Thompson & Thompson, 2008; Taylor, 2010; Roberts, 2015).

For Foucault (2002a), however, one of the most pervasive and persistent impediments to the development of such critical capabilities is what he refers to simply as the 'self-evident' (p226). In its broadest sense, the self-evident can be understood as the way in which an individual, a group or entire organisation can maintain that something is obvious, universal and even natural. In what can be understood as a concise formulation of the character of the self-evident, and the way in which it can obstruct an engagement in critical thinking and reflection, Foucault's philosophical contemporary, Gilles Deleuze (2001), proposed that it characteristically takes the form of 'Everybody knows; no one can deny...' (p130). Indeed, in considering the manner in which the self-evident can impede the employment of critically reflective thinking, it is instructive to note that the use of such a capability to question something that has been presented as obvious and that, supposedly, 'everybody knows' can not only come to be seen as unnecessary and unproductive but can also be dismissed as disruptive, unreasonable and even irrational.

In mental health care, the self-evident can become manifest in a multiplicity of forms. At the individual, organisational and societal levels, any theoretical and therapeutic approach to mental distress can come to be held as obvious, universal or natural. Indeed, Foucault's *Madness and Civilization* (2001) and *History of Madness* (2006) – the former being a significantly abridged version of the latter work – can be understood, among other things, as detailing the way in which a variety of approaches to mental distress have been held as self-evident at various stages throughout the history of the West. Similarly, in the context of contemporary mental health care, it has been suggested that there exists a model, framework or paradigm that has become the dominant approach to mental distress and that, while it is the focus of critique in some quarters, is often uncritically maintained by many as being self-evident (Boyle, 2011; Bracken et al, 2012; Middleton, 2015). This dominant approach, or what has been referred to as the 'technological model of mental distress', is said to be largely individualistic and acontextual in so far as it conceptualises mental distress as primarily having its origin 'within' the individual, a consequence of some form of biological or psychological 'dysfunction'. In doing so, it proposes that the most appropriate way to respond to that distress is through the expert application of various technical interventions, such as psychiatric medication or cognitive behavioural therapy. In articulating the main features of this dominant framework, Coles and colleagues (2015) make it clear that, while it is:

> not entirely homogenous, the current paradigm centres on the technical scientific expert, who utilises the tools of biological treatments and cognitive therapies. It is predicated on an individualistic conceptualisation of madness, where people are diagnosed with disorders of assumed biological origin or as having psychological deficits or distortions. (pvii)

To suggest that contemporary mental health care is characterised by a dominant model or framework, a framework whose particular manner of understanding and responding to mental distress is maintained by many as self-evident, is not to propose that it should simply be disregarded in order to facilitate critical, reflective thinking. Such frameworks – or what have been referred to as 'frames of reference' (Mezirow, 1991) – can be profoundly productive in so far as they provide practitioners with a particular perspective or point of reference by which to frame, organise and comprehend what can occur in the clinical setting. Moreover, to the extent that they provide a common vocabulary that comes to be shared by many, those frames of reference also enable mental health professionals to coherently communicate their clinical understandings with others and to discuss and determine their interventions on the basis of those shared understandings.

However, it is important to recognise that, once any one of those frameworks comes to be held by an individual practitioner, a professional group or even an entire organisation as self-evident, then the ability to develop alternative and potentially more productive ways to understand and respond to mental distress can become significantly impaired. That is, to the extent that any frame of reference comes to be understood as obvious, universal or natural, then the need to critically engage with the particular perspective or 'way of seeing' that it instantiates can come to be seen as unnecessary, unproductive and even unreasonable. As Morgan (2006) suggests, when this occurs:

> Ways of seeing become ways of not seeing. All the forces that help people and their organizations create the shared systems of meaning that allow them to negotiate their world in an orderly way, can become constraints that prevent them from acting in other ways. (p209)

History

It is in the context of the self-evident that we can begin to understand the significance of Foucault's work and the methodological approach that he refers to as the history of the present for the development of a critically orientated mental health nursing practice. However, while many of Foucault's works are explicitly concerned with the analysis of particular historical periods and events, they challenge various assumptions that have traditionally been associated with the methods and objectives of historical study. In distancing himself from these assumptions, he suggests that many of the works that he has produced 'are studies of "history" by reason of the domain they deal with and the references they appeal to; but they are not the work of a "historian"' (Foucault 1998a: 9). In the context of contemporary mental health care, for example, his work should not simply be understood as an attempt to detail how different historical periods have approached what has variously been referred to as 'mental illness', 'disorder' or 'distress'. Moreover, in contrast to what have been described as conventional and comforting 'Whig histories' of psychiatry (Bentall, 2010: xvii–xviii; Newnes, 2012: 20), Foucault (2001) is not concerned with characterising the present as a 'happy age' in which the current approach to mental distress is the culmination of a period of enlightened scientific and medical progress (p229). In explicitly positioning his work against such an understanding of history, and the way in which it seeks to unify disparate, contingent and singular historical events into an overarching, necessary and teleological progression, Foucault (1991b) asserts that '[t]he traditional devices for constructing a comprehensive view of history and for retracing the past as a patient and continuous development must be systematically dismantled' (p88).

To distance himself from the assumptions that he presents as being associated with the methods and objectives of historical study, and in seeking to explain his own methodological employment of history, Foucault (1991a) suggests that he is concerned with writing the 'history of the present' (p31). While it may seem somewhat paradoxical, Foucault's description of his work as a history of the present can be understood as a concise expression of the characteristic way in which he begins with something – an idea, a practice or an institution, say – in the present that, while he discerns within it potential 'cracks', 'fault lines' and 'malfunctionings' (Foucault 1990b: 156, 2000a: 263), is often regarded as obvious, universal and even natural. He then engages in historical research to show that, far from being self-evident, this supposedly natural feature of the present has actually emerged as a result of myriad complex processes. As noted above, however, Foucault is not seeking to reveal how what is currently regarded as self-evident is a result of a necessary, inevitable and unproblematic historical progression. Rather, he is attempting to show how a seemingly self-evident feature of the present is a consequence of a plurality of previous accidents, forgotten events and haphazard conflicts. His point is that what is now seen as obvious, given different conditions, could have been otherwise. In a concise statement of his particular purpose and methodological manner of using history across his work, Foucault (1990d) therefore suggests that it is meaningful:

> ... to the extent that history serves to show how that-which-is has not always been; i.e., that the things which seem most evident to us are always formed in the confluence of encounters and chances, during the course of a precarious and fragile history. (p37)

In *Madness and Civilization*, for example, Foucault employs history in this way to problematise a conceptual distinction that is fundamental to the theoretical perspectives and therapeutic practices of mental health care: the seemingly obvious, universal and natural distinction between reason and madness or, in terms characteristic of contemporary psychiatric discourse, the distinction between mental health and mental disorder. In doing so, however, it is important to remember that Foucault is not simply seeking to detail the way in which different historical periods have understood and responded to those experiences that are associated with mental distress. Indeed, in outlining his objectives in *Madness and Civilization*, he proposes that 'rather than asking *what*, in a given period, is regarded as sanity or insanity, as mental illness or normal behavior, I wanted to ask *how* these divisions are effected' (Foucault 2002a: 224). That is, in accordance with his aim of investigating the history of the present, Foucault takes a seemingly self-evident distinction that is characteristic of mental health care and engages in extensive historical research to suggest that, rather than being obvious, the distinction between reason and madness (and the subsequent reconceptualisation of madness as mental illness) emerged during 'the classical age' – a period that lasted from the middle of the 17th century until the end of the 18th century (Foucault 2001: xi–viv). Foucault is therefore not examining the history of madness with recourse to the seemingly self-evident conceptual categories of contemporary mental health care, and thereby writing a history of the past in terms of the present. Rather, he is concerned with revealing how our current conceptual distinctions emerged at a particular period during the history of the West, and using history to detail, disrupt and displace the conceptual self-evidences of the present with recourse to the past.

To the extent that contemporary mental health professionals are required to possess the knowledge, skills and experience to be able to practise effectively in the context of increasingly complex and technologically advanced healthcare settings, the significance of history for those practitioners has commonly been considered unnecessary, irrelevant and dispensable (Madsen, 2008; Alpers, Jarrell & Wotring, 2011). In contrast with such assessments, it has been suggested that history possesses a contemporary relevance for healthcare professionals in so far as it can contribute to a more comprehensive understanding of current healthcare issues, enable a more complete sense of professional identity and, through a knowledge of past mistakes, promote a vision of how things ought to be done differently in the future (Ion & Beer, 2003; Lewenson, 2004; Holme, 2015). However, Foucault's work can be understood as proposing that history continues to possess both a critical and clinical significance for contemporary mental health care through its ability to orientate the purpose and process of critical, reflective thinking for mental health nurses. In particular, the methodological approach that he refers to as the history of the present can be understood as an invitation for practitioners to develop a historical awareness of the theoretical and therapeutic approaches that characterise contemporary mental health care and, by doing so, guard against the way in which a critical engagement with those approaches can be obstructed by the potential for them to become understood as obvious, universal and natural. As Foucault (2002a) makes clear:

> It's a matter of shaking this false self-evidence, of demonstrating its precariousness, of making visible not its arbitrariness but its complex interaction with a multiplicity of historical processes, many of them of recent date. (p225)

Interests

In considering the significance of Foucault's history of the present for the development of a critically orientated mental health nursing practice, it is important to recognise that this approach is not simply concerned with disclosing the way in which those seemingly self-evident features of the present are the result of a multiplicity of historical processes. Rather, in an attempt to destabilise the ostensible self-evidence that can impede the employment of critically reflective thinking, the history of the present can also be understood as attempting to discern the interests that were implicated in the emergence of those supposedly self-evident features of the present and the interests that continue to be implicated in the maintenance of those features as self-evident. For example, in addition to disrupting that which is uncritically accepted as obvious, Foucault (2002a) suggests that his work is also concerned with 'rediscovering the connections, encounters, supports, blockages, plays of forces, strategies, and so on, that at a given moment establish what subsequently counts as being self-evident, universal, and necessary' (pp227–228).

Therefore, in considering how Foucault's history of the present can provide a productive framework in which to situate the critical capabilities of mental health nurses, it is important to recognise that his work does not simply suggest the need to 'historicise' the theoretical perspectives and therapeutic practices of contemporary mental health care by placing them in a historical context. Rather, it also suggests the need to 'politicise' those perspectives and practices by considering the variety of interests that have established, and that continue to sustain, those supposedly self-evident ways of understanding and responding to mental distress (Roberts, 2005).

In *Madness and Civilization*, for example, Foucault does not only seek to historicise the seemingly self-evident conceptual distinction between reason and madness by disclosing the way in which it emerged at a particular period during the history of the West. Rather, he also politicises that distinction by proposing that a multiplicity of social, economic and ethical interests was implicated in its establishment and maintenance during the classical age. In particular, Foucault (2001) suggests:

> The new meanings assigned to poverty, the importance given to the obligation to work, and all the ethical values that are linked to labor, ultimately determined the experience of madness and inflected its course. (p59)

In elaborating this thesis, Foucault engages in extensive historical research to clarify how these various interests were implicated in the emergence of the conceptual distinction between reason and madness. In broad terms, he can be understood as proposing that there was a shift in the social and ethical sensibilities of the developing industrial societies of the classical age such that to be unable or unwilling to work was no longer tolerated, and this intolerance found its concrete expression in the establishment of the houses of confinement across Europe (Foucault 2000b: 337, 2001: 52–53). In the context of this new sensibility, those who were designated as 'idle' (a category that incorporated those who were perceived as 'mad') progressively came to be conceptually and physically excluded from the emerging industrial and what was considered 'rational' socio-economic order. As Foucault (2001) makes clear:

> In the classical age, for the first time, madness was perceived through a condemnation of idleness and in a social immanence guaranteed by the community of labor. This community acquired an ethical power of segregation, which permitted it to eject, as into another world, all forms of social uselessness. (p54)

Similarly, it has been suggested that a multiplicity of complex interests is implicated in the establishment and maintenance of the individualistic, technical model of mental distress that has come to dominate contemporary mental health care. That is, rather than this dominance being attributable to this model's supposed theoretical and therapeutic superiority over alternative ways of understanding and responding to mental distress, a variety of concerns and motives are implicated in how mental distress has come to be framed as a manifestation of some form of individual dysfunction that can be addressed through the expert application of various technical interventions.

For example, it has been argued that an understanding of mental distress as an individual and, in particular, biological dysfunction that can be addressed through psychiatric medication serves the commercial interests of the pharmaceutical industry, who use their corporate influence to perpetuate the ostensible self-evidence of that way of understanding and responding to mental distress (Bentall,

2010; Busfield, 2015; Whitaker & Cosgrove, 2015). In addition, it has been proposed that this technical approach to mental distress legitimises the role of the mental health 'expert' or 'professional' who possesses a body of specialist knowledge and the associated therapeutic interventions to treat such distress, which, in turn, ensures the professional recognition, continued employment and financial rewards of those who are positioned in such a role (Bostock, Noble & Winter, 2012; Moloney, 2013). Moreover, it has been suggested that the dominance of this technical and largely acontextual model of mental distress is politically expedient in so far as it diverts attention away from the need to address the social context and material conditions that can contribute to mental distress and the need to improve people's environments so that they are more conducive to psychological wellbeing (Boyle, 2011; Shim et al, 2014; Smail, 2014).

The suggestion that a variety of often implicit, obscured or hidden interests are implicated in the establishment and maintenance of the dominance and supposed self-evidence of the individualistic, technical approach to mental distress may strike some as a particularly challenging proposition. However, it has been argued that all theoretical perspectives and therapeutic practices in mental health care have been established and are sustained by a variety of interests, and many of these extend beyond alleviating the mental distress and improving the general wellbeing of those who use mental health services (Johnstone, 2000; Bostock, Noble & Winter, 2012). Moreover, it is important to recognise that simply discerning the interests that may be implicated in the establishment and maintenance of a supposedly self-evident feature of the present is not sufficient to displace what is currently accepted as obvious, universal or natural. Indeed, not only are interests, motives and affiliations an acceptable and arguably unavoidable aspect of mental health care but they can also be powerful motivating factors that can direct and sustain continued research and critical investigation into the various theoretical perspectives and therapeutic practices that are employed to understand and respond to mental distress. Therefore, in so far as it suggests the need to politicise the seemingly self-evident features of contemporary mental health care, Foucault's history of the present is not simply concerned with detailing how a plurality of interests may be implicated in the emergence and maintenance of those features as self-evident. Rather, it is also concerned with attempting to determine the potential influence of those interests, both within and beyond the clinical encounter, and the multiplicity of ways in which they may be obscuring, marginalising and even opposing the interests, concerns and needs of those who use mental health services.

Transformation

As a productive framework in which to situate the critical capabilities of mental health nurses and thereby contribute to the development of a critically orientated mental health nursing practice, the history of the present necessitates both the historicisation and politicisation of the theoretical perspectives and therapeutic practices that characterise contemporary mental health care. In particular, it seeks to destabilise any approach to mental distress that is currently regarded as obvious, universal or natural by critically considering the multiplicity of interdependent historical processes and political interests that have established and that continue to sustain that which is uncritically accepted as self-evident. In doing so, the history of the present can be understood as enabling a space of possibility, or what Foucault (1990d) refers to as 'a space of concrete freedom' (p36), in which mental health professionals can begin to think differently about those features of mental health care that are regarded as obvious, universal or natural. Indeed, the disruption of such apparent self-evidence by critically considering the historical and political interests that are implicated in its establishment and maintenance is central to bringing about the transformations in thought that can engender meaningful transformations in practice. For example, while not underestimating the considerable challenges that can be associated with attempting to transform any supposedly self-evident feature of the present, Foucault (1990b) makes it clear that:

> A transformation that remains within the same mode of thought... can merely be a superficial transformation. On the other hand, as soon as one can no longer think things as one formerly thought them, transformation becomes both very urgent, very difficult, and quite possible. (p155)

While the history of the present can be employed to disrupt the seemingly self-evident features of contemporary mental health care, and thereby engender a space of possibility in which to consider alternative ways of understanding and responding to mental distress, it does not specify what transformations in thought or practice should follow such a disruption. In seeking to resist the characterisation of his work as prescribing what people should think or how they should act, and to refute the suggestion that he provides anything that resembles a general programme of theoretical and practical reform for others to implement, Foucault (2002a) states: 'I wouldn't want what I may have said or written to be seen as laying any claims to totality. I don't try to universalize what I say...' (p223).

Indeed, while the traditional tendency in any area of human inquiry has been to generalise from singular, contingent and arbitrary events so as to establish universal principles and practices that are 'just-and-true-for-all' (Foucault 1991c: 68), the history of the present should be understood as being concerned with moving in the opposite direction. That is, Foucault's work begins with supposedly obvious, natural and therefore universal principles and practices and seeks to disclose how these apparently universal features of the present are a product of a multiplicity of singular, contingent and arbitrary historical and political events; in doing so, it seeks to disrupt these seemingly universal principles and practices so that what people think and how they should act is no longer regarded as self-evident. Rather than telling people what to do, Foucault (2002a) makes it clear that his project 'is precisely to bring it about that they "no longer know what to do", so that the acts, gestures, discourses that up until then had seemed to go without saying become problematic, difficult, dangerous. This effect is intentional' (p235). Foucault was aware that the manner in which his work sought to disrupt those features of the present that are commonly regarded as self-evident, without then prescribing what subsequent transformations in thought or practice should occur, could be a source of frustration and irritation for some (Foucault 1990c: 15, 2002a: 237). His refusal to prescribe what people should do, however, is a reflection of his insistence that such critical work ought to be conducted by those who are directly involved in and affected by the specific problems and possibilities that exist within a given context, rather than by any 'reformist' intellectual or organisation that claims to speak on their behalf (Foucault 2002b: 288). For example, in discussing who is best positioned to effect meaningful change in any area of human practice, as well as highlighting the multiple challenges involved in effecting those changes, Foucault (2002a) maintains that they are more likely to occur:

> ... when those who have a stake in that reality, all those people, have come
> into collision with each other and with themselves, run into dead ends,
> problems, and impossibilities, been through conflicts and confrontations –
> when critique has been played in the real, not when reformers have realized
> their ideas. (p236)

This does not mean that his textual, scholarly research – and his historical studies in particular – cannot be employed to destabilise the seemingly self-evident features of a particular area and to consider critically what subsequent transformations in thought and practice should occur. However, he insists that what he has to say throughout his work should be understood as 'propositions' or 'game openings' in which people can selectively use aspects of that work to inform their own critical thinking and reflection in the particular contexts in which they are situated; they are not 'dogmatic assertions' that have to be accepted or rejected 'en bloc' (Foucault 2002a: 224).

The history of the present therefore requires that the historicisation and politicisation of contemporary mental health care and critical considerations about the potential transformations in thought and practice that might follow are conducted by mental health nurses themselves in the varied contexts in which they work. However, this is not to say that this critical practice cannot make productive connections with and draw on the work of critical networks and allies within, for example, psychiatry, clinical psychology and the service user/survivor movement (Double, 2006; Bracken et al, 2012; Corstens et al, 2014; Cooke, 2017). Indeed, while highlighting the degree of critical and collective activity that may be necessary to displace the seemingly self-evident features of the present and yet stressing the need to incorporate into that activity 'the voices' of those who have traditionally been marginalised and excluded, Foucault (2002b) proposes:

Years, decades of work and political imagination will be necessary, work at the grass roots, with the people directly affected, restoring their right to speak. (p288)

In order to engage in this work, mental health nurses will therefore not only be required to collaborate meaningfully with the diverse groups that comprise the service user/survivor movement, and to become receptive to the critiques of the approaches to mental distress – such as the technological model – that have come to dominate mental health care (Wallcraft, Read & Sweeney, 2003; LeFrançois, Menzies & Reaume, 2013; Russo & Sweeney, 2016). Rather, it will also be necessary to gain an awareness of those alternative approaches to mental distress that have been presented and promoted by service user/survivor groups – such as trauma-informed and social, materialist models (Beresford et al, 2016; Sweeney et al, 2016) – and begin to consider critically how these approaches can be incorporated into a responsive, proactive and critically orientated mental health nursing practice.

Conclusion

There is a recognition that mental health nurses need to possess sophisticated critical thinking and reflective capabilities in order to provide informed, effective and responsive mental health care, and to do so in an evidence-based, collaborative and recovery-focused way. This chapter has suggested that those capabilities can be productively situated within the context of the general methodological approach that can be discerned across Michel Foucault's work (and within his historical studies in particular), which he refers to as the history of the present. In doing so, it has been proposed that the history of the present can be understood as that which can contribute to the development of a critically orientated mental health nursing practice by emphasising the need to both historicise and politicise the theoretical perspectives and therapeutic practices that characterise contemporary mental health care.

In particular, this critical activity necessitates a consideration of the multiplicity of interdependent historical processes and political interests that have established, and that continue to sustain, the seemingly self-evident status of any feature of contemporary mental health care. While the destabilisation of these seemingly self-evident features of the present can produce a space of possibility in which mental health nurses can begin to consider alternative ways of understanding and responding to mental distress, Foucault's work does not determine what transformations in thought and practice should follow. Rather, it emphasises the need for mental health nurses to conduct this critical work themselves, in meaningful collaboration with critical allies within psychiatry, clinical psychology and the service user/survivor movement, in order to develop a critically informed mental health practice that is responsive to the interests, concerns and needs of those who use mental health services.

References

Alpers RR, Jarrell K, Wotring R (2011). The importance of nursing history: a method of inclusion. *Teaching and Learning in Nursing 6*(4). 190–117.

Bentall RP (2010). *Doctoring the Mind: why psychiatric treatments fail.* London: Penguin.

Beresford P (2010). *A Straight Talking Introduction to Being a Mental Health Service User.* Ross-on-Wye: PCCS Books.

Beresford P, Perring R, Nettle M, Wallcraft J (2016). *From Mental Illness to a Social Model of Madness and Distress.* London: Shaping Our Lives.

Bostock J, Noble V, Winter R (2012). Promoting community resources. In: Newnes C, Holmes G, Dunn C (eds). *This is Madness: a critical look at psychiatry and the future of mental health services.* Ross-on-Wye: PCCS Books (pp241–251).

Boud D, Keogh R & Walker D (1985). Promoting reflection in learning: a model. In: Boud D, Keogh R, Walker D (eds). *Reflection: turning experience into learning.* London: Kogan Page (pp18–40).

Boyd EM, Fales AW (1983). Reflective learning: key to learning from experience. *Journal of Humanistic Psychology 23*(2): 99–117.

Boyle M (2011). Making the world go away, and how psychology and psychiatry benefit. In: Rapley M, Moncrieff J, Dillon J (eds). *De-Medicalising Misery: psychiatry, psychology and the human condition.* Basingstoke: Palgrave Macmillan (pp27–43).

Bracken P, Thomas P, Timimi S and 26 others (2012). Psychiatry beyond the current paradigm. *British Journal of Psychiatry 201*(6): 430–434.

Brookfield SD (2001). *Developing Critical Thinkers: challenging adults to explore alternative ways of thinking and acting.* Milton Keynes: Open University Press.

Busfield J (2015). The pharmaceutical industry and mental disorder. In: Coles S, Keenan S, Diamond B (eds). *Madness Contested: power and practice.* Ross-on-Wye: PCCS Books (pp90–110).

Campbell P (2013). Service users/survivors and mental health services. In: Cromby J, Harper D, Reavey P (eds). *Psychology, Mental Health and Distress.* Basingstoke: Palgrave Macmillan (pp139–151).

Coles S, Keenan S, Diamond B (2015). Introduction. In: Coles S, Keenan S, Diamond B (eds). *Madness Contested: power and practice.* Ross-on-Wye: PCCS Books (ppvii-xvi).

Cooke A (ed) (2017). *Understanding Psychosis and Schizophrenia.* Leicester: British Psychological Society.

Corstens D, Longden E, McCarthy-Jones S, Waddingham R, Thomas N (2014). Emerging perspectives from the Hearing Voices Movement: implications for research and practice. *Schizophrenia Bulletin 40*(suppl4): S285–294.

Cromby J, Harper D, Reavey P (eds) (2013). *Psychology, Mental Health and Distress.* Basingstoke: Palgrave Macmillan.

Deleuze G (2001). *Difference and Repetition.* London: Continuum.

Dewey J (2012). *How We Think.* Mansfield Centre, CT: Martino Publishing.

Double DB (ed) (2006). *Critical Psychiatry: the limits of madness.* Basingstoke: Palgrave Macmillan.

Fook J, White S, Gardner F (2006). Critical reflection: a review of contemporary literature and understandings. In: White S, Fook J, Gardner F (eds). *Critical Reflection in Health and Social Care.* Maidenhead: Open University Press (pp3–20).

Foucault M (2006). *History of Madness*. Abingdon: Routledge.

Foucault M (2002a). Questions of method. In: Faubion JD (ed). *Power: the essential works of Foucault 1954-1984 volume 3*. London: Penguin (pp223–238).

Foucault M (2002b). Interview with Michel Foucault. In: Faubion JD (ed). *Power: the essential works of Foucault 1954-1984 volume 3*. London: Penguin (pp239–297).

Foucault M (2001). *Madness and Civilization: a history of insanity in the age of reason*. London: Routledge.

Foucault M (2000a). The order of things. In: Faubion JD (ed). *Aesthetics: the essential works of Foucault 1954–1984 volume 2*. London: Penguin (pp261–267).

Foucault M (2000b). Madness and society. In: Faubion JD (ed). *Aesthetics: the essential works of Foucault 1954–1984 volume 2*. London: Penguin (pp335–342).

Foucault M (1998a). *The Use of Pleasure: the history of sexuality volume 2*. London: Penguin.

Foucault M (1998b). *The Will to Knowledge: the history of sexuality volume 1*. London: Penguin.

Foucault M (1991a). *Discipline and Punish: the birth of the prison*. London: Penguin.

Foucault M (1991b). Nietzsche, genealogy, history. In: Rabinow P (ed). *The Foucault Reader*. London: Penguin (pp76–100).

Foucault M (1991c). Truth and power. In: Rabinow P (ed). *The Foucault Reader*. London: Penguin (pp51–75).

Foucault M (1990a). *The Care of the Self: the history of sexuality volume 3*. London: Penguin.

Foucault M (1990b). Practising criticism. In: Kritzman LD (ed). *Michel Foucault: politics, philosophy, culture: interviews and other writings 1977–1984*. New York, NY: Routledge (pp152–156).

Foucault M (1990c). The minimalist self. In: Kritzman LD (ed). *Michel Foucault: politics, philosophy, culture: interviews and other writings 1977–1984*. New York, NY: Routledge (pp3–17).

Foucault M (1990d). Critical theory/intellectual history. In: Kritzman LD (ed). *Michel Foucault: politics, philosophy, culture: interviews and other writings 1977–1984*. New York, NY: Routledge (pp17–46).

Holme A (2015). Why history matters to nursing. *Nurse Education Today 35*(5): 635–637.

Ion RM, Beer MD (2003). Valuing the past: the importance of an understanding of the history of psychiatry for healthcare professionals, service users and carers. *International Journal of Mental Health Nursing 12*(4): 237–242.

Johnstone L (2000). *Users and Abusers of Psychiatry: a critical look at psychiatric practice* (2nd ed). London: Routledge.

LeFrançois BA, Menzies R, Reaume G (eds) (2013). *Mad Matters: a critical reader in Canadian mad studies*. Toronto: Canadian Scholars' Press Inc.

Lewenson SB (2004). Integrating nursing history into the curriculum. *Journal of Professional Nursing, 20*(6): 374–380.

Madsen W (2008). Teaching history to nurses: will this make me a better nurse? *Nurse Education Today, 28*(5): 524–529.

McKeown M, White J (2015). The future of mental health nursing: are we barking up the wrong tree? *Journal of Psychiatric and Mental Health Nursing 22*(9): 724–730.

McKie A, Naysmith S (2014). Promoting critical perspectives in mental health nursing education. *Journal of Psychiatric and Mental Health Nursing 21*(2): 128–137.

Mezirow J (1991). *Transformative Dimensions of Adult Learning*. San Francisco, CA: Jossey-Bass.

Middleton H (2015). The medical model: what is it, where did it come from and how long has it got? In: Loewenthal D (ed) *Critical Psychotherapy, Psychoanalysis and Counselling*. Basingstoke: Palgrave Macmillan (pp223–238).

Moloney P (2013). *The Therapy Industry: the irresistible rise of the talking cure and why it doesn't work*. London: Pluto Press.

Morgan G (2006). *Images of Organization* (4th ed). Thousand Oaks, CA: Sage.

Newnes C (2012). Histories of psychiatry. In: Newnes C, Holmes G, Dunn C (eds). *This is Madness: a critical look at psychiatry and the future of mental health services*. Ross-on-Wye: PCCS Books (pp7–27).

Paul R, Elder L (2014). *Critical Thinking: tools for taking charge of your professional and personal life* (2nd ed). New Jersey, NJ: Pearson Education.

Rapley M, Moncrieff J, Dillon JM (eds) (2011). *De-Medicalising Misery: psychiatry, psychology and the human condition*. Basingstoke: Palgrave Macmillan.

Roberts M (2018) *Understanding Mental Health Care: critical issues in practice*. London. Sage.

Roberts M (2015). *Critical Thinking and Reflection for Mental Health Nursing Students*. London: Sage.

Roberts M (2005). The production of the psychiatric subject: power, knowledge and Michel Foucault. *Nursing Philosophy* 6(1): 33–42.

Russo J, Sweeney A (eds) (2016). *Searching for a Rose Garden: challenging psychiatry, fostering mad studies*. Monmouth: PCCS Books.

Shim R, Koplan C, Langheim FJP, Manseau MW, Powers PA, Compton MT (2014). The social determinants of mental health: an overview and call to action. *Psychiatric Annals* 44(1): 22–26.

Smail D (2014) *Power, Interest and Psychology: elements of a social materialist understanding of distress*. Ross-on-Wye: PCCS Books.

Sweeney A, Clement S, Filson B, Kennedy A (2016). Trauma-informed mental healthcare in the UK: what is it and how can we further its development? *Mental Health Review Journal* 21(3): 174–192.

Taylor BJ (2010). *Reflective Practice for Healthcare Professionals: a practical guide* (3rd ed). Maidenhead: Open University Press.

Thompson S, Thompson N (2008). *The Critically Reflective Practitioner*. Basingstoke: Palgrave Macmillan.

Wallcraft J, Read J, Sweeney A (2003). *On Our Own Terms: users and survivors of mental health services working together for support and change*. London: Sainsbury Centre for Mental Health.

Whitaker R, Cosgrove L (2015). *Psychiatry Under the Influence*. New York, NY: Palgrave Macmillan.

8 | The ideology of recovery in contemporary mental health care

Alastair Morgan

In this chapter I want to argue that recovery functions as an ideological concept in contemporary mental health care. I am not arguing that people don't recover and I respect the multiple meanings and ways of recovering from experiences of mental distress. What I am interested in is a critique of a discourse of recovery that, while ostensibly valuing choice and empowerment, functions in contemporary healthcare as a means of masking fundamental inequalities, lack of choice and increasing coercion. Therefore, my critique is aimed at this discourse, not at any individual person's narrative or experience of recovery.

The concept of recovery in mental health care developed from the late 1970s as a discourse initially mapped out by service user movements and representatives (Chamberlin, 1978; Deegan, 1993; Coleman, 1995). These movements emphasised a social rather than clinical definition of recovery that focused on aspects of personal growth, meaning attributed to mental distress and recovery both from distress and from the invalidation and stigma associated with using mental health services. The recovery concept brought together both a regathering of critical psychiatric efforts following the retrenchment of psychiatry in response to the critical voices and campaigns of the 1960s and early 1970s and a new emphasis on consumer discourse and individual identity rights. Seminal early texts emphasised the process of service user-led rather than professional-led care (Coleman, 1995).

This social concept of recovery nevertheless arrived on the clinical scene at the same time as a renewed optimism around clinical treatment that moved psychiatry away from the concepts of chronic illness that underpinned models of psychiatric rehabilitation. Of particular importance was the growth of attention to early intervention in psychosis and a focus on a new wave of psychiatric drugs synthesised for use with psychosis and depression (Marshall & Rathbone, 2011). The 1990s was also marked in popular culture by an increasing fascination with the potential of psychiatric drugs to mould and improve the psyche and to make us 'better than well' (Elliott, 2004; Kramer, 1997).

The 1980s and 1990s also marked a period of mass de-institutionalisation across Western countries, resulting in the shutting down of the old asylums and the shunting of people into the community, alongside a period of right-wing cuts to public services and a discourse of personal responsibility. The fight against institutions, which had been a radical force in the 1960s and 1970s, became part of a general whittling away of state provision and social responsibility (Scheper-Hughes, Lovell & Schob, 1987; Crossley, 2006).

The discourse of recovery, which needs to be seen as a cluster of concepts rather than a singular concept, arises through a force field of differing and contradictory developments (Stacey & Stickley, 2012). It carries the radical legacy of the critical political movements of the late 1960s and early 1970s, alongside an emphasis on individualism and choice, and all this in a climate of a paring away of state provision in healthcare.

What is recovery?

Given these multiple and conflicting strands to the origins of the recovery movement, it is not surprising that it is hard to pin down a concept of recovery. Indeed, it is important to acknowledge and respect the vagueness of the concept as a reflection of its multiple and often conflicting meanings and affiliations. Turner (2002: 29) writes of recovery as an 'idea, a movement, a philosophy, a set of values, a policy and a doctrine of change'. Slade and colleagues (2008) acknowledge that recovery has a range of meanings, some of which are incompatible with each other. Leamy and colleagues (2011) similarly write of recovery in terms of a process and a 'life orientation'. Anthony (1993) offers the oft-quoted, succinct but little discussed definition of recovery as a:

> ... deeply personal, unique process of changing one's attitudes, values, feelings and/or roles... a way of living a satisfying, hopeful and contributing life even with the limitations caused by illness. (1993: 529)

Anthony's definition, so often cited by students, is highly controversial as it contains an implicit acceptance of the concept of 'illness' that was the very ontological issue at stake in the battles around psychiatry in the 1960s and 1970s. The definition completely bypasses a central and critical debate in the history of mental distress and aligns recovery with a social approach to a medical problem.

Nevertheless, despite these disputes about the nature of recovery, it is clear that all recovery literature emphasises a range of shared key components. Recovery is an active process that involves self-definition and development. It is therefore fundamentally about growth, and thus the repeated and now rather hackneyed reference to the 'recovery journey'. Recovery relies on the narratives and expertise of people who have experienced mental distress. Therefore, recovery approaches prioritise individual self-understanding, narrative and meaning. At its best, this means that conceptualisations of mental distress are left pragmatically open; it is up to the person to define their own understanding of their experiences, and healthcare services should work with that self-understanding. All recovery approaches emphasise the centrality of hope and occasionally align a discourse on hope with a generalised, religiously unspecific concept of spirituality. Finally, and most importantly in a UK context, is the emphasis on social inclusion (Repper & Perkins, 2009; Repper & Perkins, 2003). There is a social element to people's recovery, and recovery cannot be conceptualised as a purely individual endeavour.

This nest of concepts enclosed in the overarching umbrella of the recovery name leads Leamy and colleagues (2011: 199) to write that recovery, as a conceptual framework, is a 'network, or a plane, of interlinked concepts that together provide a comprehensive understanding of a phenomenon or phenomena'. My contention, in opposition to this notion, is that recovery should be understood as a super ideology, and that nested within the ideological concept of recovery are a number of other ideological concepts. Concepts such as hope, growth, strength and 'lived experience' have an aura of authenticity and genuineness that leaves them invulnerable to critique or inspection. If we invoke 'hope' as a prerequisite to positive healthcare relationships, how can there be any critique? However, I want to claim that it is precisely in this language that a form of a 'jargon of authenticity', to use Adorno's phrase (2003), rears its ugly head. Before moving on to the details of my critique, it is necessary first to outline the concept of ideology that I am relying on.

What is ideology?

My use of the term ideology and the notion of an ideology critique stems from a Marxist understanding of the concept. There is a liberal tradition of understanding ideology as simply a collection of ideas or an ever-changing political narrative that attempts to explain and understand the social world (Freeden, 2003). However, the Marxist use of the term moves beyond deploying it as a descriptor of a series of ideas and specifically relates particular ideas to a social whole by asking whose interests are served by them (Eagleton, 1991). For example, for Marxist critics, ideas such as justice and equality are deployed in discourses in order to serve the interests of those with power.

There are five broad elements to the concept of ideology as outlined by Marx in a range of writings and then deployed by the Marxist tradition (Marx, 1988; Horkheimer, 1973; Gramsci, 1999). I will outline these below as these five elements will structure my critique of the recovery concept.

1. **Mystification or masking** – ideologies mask reality; they outline a state of affairs that is a way of hiding material realities. Marx's key example is the idea of free and equal commodity exchange that masks the exploitative reality of unequal labour relations. Capitalist markets are termed 'free' when they are really exploitative and dominating.

2. **An inversion of reality** – ideologies invert reality; they turn the world the wrong way round. In *The German Ideology* (Marx & Engels, 1988), Marx gives the example that humans produce the materials of their life but, as commodities, these objects come to rule over us as alien and external. He writes:

> If in all ideology men and their circumstances appear upside-down as in a *camera obscura*, this phenomenon arises just as much from their historical life-process as the inversion of objects on the retina does from their physical life-process. (Marx, 1988: 164)

An example of this in psychiatry is that many writers have argued that the claim that psychiatry is developing more and more evidence-based practice that offers better treatments is an ideological inversion of a reality where treatments on offer fail and mental illnesses proliferate (Bentall, 2009; Whitaker, 2010).

3. **Socially necessary illusions** – ideologies are socially necessary illusions; they enable the stability of society. Functionalist accounts of power would see this aspect of ideology in a positive light – Parsons argues that such 'illusions' are necessary for a stable order (Lukes, 1986). Marxists tend to view them as means of stabilising an unjust order (Horkheimer, 1973).

4. **Naturalising accounts** – ideologies naturalise social processes. The Marxist theorist Georg Lukács terms this process 'reification' – the way that human and social processes that are the product of the struggles of history are treated as natural facts (Lukács, 1971). We often hear statements such as the 'market will decide' – a statement that 'reifies' the social processes that constitute a market economy into a natural entity above, beyond and impervious to human action. In this way, the 'market' is perceived to function like natural fluctuations in the weather, and we cannot question or criticise its operations.

5. **Truth content of ideologies** – for Marx, ideologies always point beyond themselves to the possibility of a reality that could fulfil the idea of the debased concept. Thus, although the concept of freedom often functions as an ideology to serve particular class interests, it nevertheless contains the promise of a better future. An example of this, for Marx, is religion. Marx believes that religion masks and distorts, serves the interests of the ruling class and naturalises states of affairs that are more properly treated as social. However, he also writes that religion is the 'sigh of a soulless world'; within the religious hope for a better world lies a truth, but a truth that will only be attained if that hope can be turned towards revolutionary purpose in this world rather than the next (Marx, 1988: 64).

In the following critique, I will take each of these aspects of the concept of ideology and apply them to the way that recovery functions in contemporary mental health care.

Recovery as mystification

What is being mystified, masked, covered up or no longer discussed by the hegemony of the recovery discourse? First, we can consider the way in which discourses around recovery, positivity and strengths can very rapidly become a 'duty to be well'. Although recovery originated as a social concept rather than a clinical state, it has increasingly been aligned with strands from positive psychology that emphasise notions of resilience and redemptive narratives that downplay suffering and distress. Slade (2010) has explicitly aligned a notion of recovery with that of positive psychology and has described a recovery journey as moving from 'foundering and languishing' to 'flourishing (by developing valued social roles)' (Slade, 2010: 3). However, there is little description of the content of such states of languishing and flourishing and Slade doesn't acknowledge how fulfilling functioning social roles might play into forcing people back into employment and deadening roles in social life that contributed to mental distress in the first instance. Slade (2010: 4) proposes a 'validated approach' of 'training for optimism' that requires the individual to focus on transforming negative thought patterns into positive internal messages and external behaviours, leading to 'flexible thoughts and resilience' (Slade, 2010: 4). In this process of self-fashioning, there is no acknowledgement that mental distress is a product of social pressures, environments and experience, not just a shaping of thought patterns. Slade (2010: 9) prescribes the right kind of recovery story that can be told by arguing that narratives need to emphasise the 'transformation of a bad experience into a good outcome and the imposition of a coherent structure'. Narratives must be coherent, redemptive and uplifting; they cannot include accounts of suffering.

In her withering attack on positive psychology, *Smile or Die*, Barbara Ehrenreich (2009) has called this kind of wellness discourse a 'mandatory optimism'. This kind of individualised, mandated optimism instructs people to be positive whether they are or want to be or not. Ehrenreich (2009) argues that such positivity is not only regarded as normal but also as normative. Any person that doesn't fit in with such a narrative of redemption is difficult, stuck or, to use the terms of positive psychology, 'languishing'. This 'mandatory optimism' feeds into the contemporary hegemony of cognitive behavioural approaches that focus on people changing how they think rather than addressing the reality of their social situations. The outcome of such an inculcated optimism is that, if your life situation does not change, then you have singularly failed to adequately engage in recovery and change your thoughts. Basically, it's your fault. Feelings of hope that are always tentative and based on an uncertain yearning become reified into a forced positivity that will not allow any critical voice to emerge.

Davidson and Roe (2007) have proposed three reasons why people might not engage with recovery in the correct manner. First, they argue that the person has failed to 'differentiate the illness and its effects from the remainder of his or her life' (Davidson & Roe, 2007: 469). The implicit message here is that mental distress has no meaning in relation to one's life and recovery proper can only begin if one accepts that one is ill according to psychiatry's terms. Second, they argue that some people can be too overwhelmed by illness to engage in recovery. This argument has some force, but it appears to accept a purely clinical concept of recovery and consign a group of people to a 'medical treatment only' approach. Finally, they argue that some people choose not to recover; they just don't want to help themselves. They write that these people are analogous to 'people living with lung cancer who continue to smoke' (Davidson & Roe, 2007: 468).

Recovery becomes totally aligned with a discourse of neoliberal self-government and self-management that focuses on positivity, flexibility and resilience. This self-fashioning involves reifying your feelings and thoughts in order to instrumentally produce the supposed outcome of a happy state. Marcuse (2002) wrote about this mode of self-reification in *One Dimensional Man*. It is a way of turning your own thoughts and emotions into fixed things, which Marcuse termed a 'pure form of servitude' (Marcuse, 2002: 36). It remains a form of servitude even if the person does not experience this as reification and considers his or her own emotional life as something 'pretty, clean, mobile...' (Marcuse, 2002: 36).

Emotions and feelings are treated as possessions, in a form of individualism that MacPherson (1988) describes as 'possessive individualism'. In 'possessive individualism', the individual thinks of themselves as essentially the owner of their own capacities and feelings, which have nothing to do with society or the context of their life, and which can then be taken 'to market', so to speak. The interaction of individuals in communities is an exchange and negotiation of feelings and emotions as commodities (MacPherson, 1988: 3). Illouz (2007) has written about 'emotional capitalism', where intimate life and emotions are turned into objects of calculation that can be captured quantitatively. This gives rise to what she terms a new 'emotional ontology', where 'emotions can be detached from the subject for control and clarification' (Illouz, 2007: 36). She further explains how this emphasis on emotional labour and work on the self oscillates between a demand for happiness and the production of 'suffering selves'; it produces identities that are defined by what they lack and are simultaneously impelled to work on the project of an empty self-realisation (Illouz, 2007: 108–110).

The individualised nature of this understanding of recovery is important to stress here. In the recovery approach, the individual is the source of growth, hope and meaning. Society is seen as a network of resources that are potentially enabling rather than constraining. This can be clearly seen, even where recovery attempts to emphasise its social aspects through the concept of social inclusion. Spandler (2007) has written about the shift in public policy in the UK in the early 2000s from discourses that focused on social exclusion to a discourse around inclusion. This discourse on social inclusion was key to many of the messages around recovery in the UK (Repper & Perkins, 2003). Although the emphasis on inclusion rather than exclusion frames a discourse in a positive and empowering manner, it tends to downplay the constraining and limiting effects of social structures. Recovery planning looks at society and social structures as a series of potentially life-enhancing opportunities rather than life-limiting and unjust structures. Spandler (2007) puts this well when she writes that:

> The policy shift to 'inclusion' can make invisible the social structures and divisions which generate and sustain exclusion and create an obsession with the choices and responsibilities of the individual rather than the constraining context in which they live. (Spandler, 2007: 4)

As Spandler notes, there is no acknowledgement here that it is very often the same 'inclusive' society that is generating the pressures and injustice that lead to mental distress in the first place.

Recovery is a mystification because it covers over the social and material causes of mental distress by emphasising an empty notion of hope and positivity that in reality is tied to a concept of successful functioning and 'fitting in'. RD Laing famously noted that the first requirement for a training psychiatrist was an understanding and appreciation of despair (Laing, 1990). In contemporary discourse around recovery, notions of suffering and despair are made invisible and, even worse, blamed on the person experiencing the distress.

Recovery as an inverted representation

Recovery functions as a distorted and inverted representation of the state of mental health services. Mental health services set themselves up as champions of hope, choice and empowerment. At the heart of any mental health trust lies a series of philosophy statements about service user choice in treatment and co-producing care (Mental Health Task Force, 2016). This emphasis on choice, diversity of provision and co-producing care occurs at the same time that coercion has increased exponentially in mental health care in the UK.

The most significant development in mental health services in the UK in the past 10 years has been the introduction of enforced community treatment under the Mental Health Act 2007. People who have been detained under section 3 or some forensic sections can be put on community treatment orders (CTOs), which allow them to be recalled to hospital for up to 72 hours if they are not complying with the conditions of their order (Department of Health, 2008). Although the person cannot be forcibly treated in the community, the formal conditions require a person on a CTO to make themselves available for treatment, on pain of being returned to hospital, where they can be forcibly treated. A number of other conditions can be applied at the discretion of the individual's responsible clinician (usually their psychiatrist), including that they must take their medication as prescribed, must live in a specified place and must not use illegal drugs (Department of Health, 2008).

Supervised community treatment was introduced in England and Wales against a background of much controversy and united opposition among healthcare professionals and service users, organised through the Mental Health Alliance (Mental Health Alliance, 2005). The background evidence for the effectiveness of CTOs was extensively reviewed by Churchill and colleagues (2007) and found to be lacking. They found no evidence for any reduction in readmission rates or length of hospital stay, and no improvement on a range of patient satisfaction measures. The most rigorous recent randomised control trial in the UK, carried out by Burns and colleagues (2013), also found no evidence that CTOs reduce readmission rates and concluded that, in the absence of such evidence, CTOs are an unethical imposition. As Burns and Dawson (2009) write, there are serious questions about how ethical such a treatment can be when it is implemented without any evidence base at all.

What is therefore of deep concern is the readiness with which CTOs have been accepted as an established and extensively used tool in the armoury of the mental health services and how rapidly they are becoming an unquestioned part of the picture. In a survey of 533 psychiatrists in England and Wales, most said they found CTOs useful (Lawton-Smith, 2010). However, we shouldn't be fooled into thinking that larger societal pressures and forces do not continue to play a role in the implementation of such legislation. One of the most concerning aspects of the implementation of CTOS has been their acknowledged disproportionate use with people from black and minority ethnic backgrounds (Social Care Institute for Excellence, 2007).

The latest Care Quality Commission (CQC) report on the application of the Mental Health Act details a bleak picture of increasing use of formal detentions; there was a 10 per cent increase in 2014/15, the highest ever year-on-year rise (CQC, 2017). At a time when coercion has increased in mental health services and more and more people are subject to formal powers both within hospital and without, the mental health services are representing the picture as one of increased choice, hope and empowerment.

Recovery as a socially necessary illusion

The illusion of recovery-orientated services is needed in order to mask the reality of continuing and increasing coercion. Recovery becomes a brand that enables healthcare providers to mask the expansion of coercion in mental health care. It is interesting to note that in many of the recovery documents and literature, there is little discussion of the issues of coercion and power (Morgan et al, 2015). As Edgley and colleagues (2012) note, this recovery paradigm chimes with the climate of individual choice, self-management and responsibility. However, such a discourse of choice feeds into an ideology that emphasises notions such as shared decision-making and co-production without acknowledging and thinking through the reality of coercion and inequalities of power.

In this context, recovery becomes a form of marketing, serving to mask continuing inequalities while allowing a discourse around increasing liberalisation and humanisation of care to continue.

A further significant factor in the success of the recovery concept is that it masks the central dispute and debate in mental health around the ontological status of mental distress. Adherents of recovery principles can range from traditional critics of psychiatry who disagree with an illness concept of mental distress to those who accept illness and even disease models of mental distress. Thus, the central point of philosophical dispute in the 20th century arguments over psychiatry, namely the ontological status of mental distress itself, is masked and covered over in a 'postmodern pragmatism' (Morgan, 2008). Such a postmodern pragmatism asserts that it doesn't matter what our beliefs are about fundamental ontological issues as we can develop care that meets people's needs according to their way of defining themselves.

The fact that recovery is a heterogeneous concept helps with this pragmatic downplaying of differences (Davidson & Roe, 2007). Pilgrim (2008) has identified three broad strands within the overarching recovery model and these three strands often stand in fundamental contradiction to each other philosophically. First, there is the notion of a biomedical recovery based on longitudinal research that demonstrated a heterogeneity of outcomes with severe mental distress and stresses a notion of a remission of symptoms. This is a more traditional concept of medical recovery and is illness based. Second, there is a social model, focusing on community inclusion, social skills, social inclusion and employment. Pilgrim (2008) terms this a model of successful rehabilitation from a previous impairment. The social model could be illness based or it could be more focused on social causes of distress. Finally, there is a model of recovery from social invalidation – namely, that what the person is recovering from is not an illness but the effects of psychiatric treatment and stigmatisation. Traditionally, this has been an approach that has been hostile to any illness-based model.

When approaching Pilgrim's very helpful tripartite division of the concept of recovery, it is interesting to note that these three strands have increasingly merged into a discourse that prioritises notions of illness rather than challenging such concepts. Although recovery began, as we saw earlier, as a user-led challenge to psychiatric conceptualisations of distress, illness-based models are becoming increasingly hegemonic. This can be most clearly seen in campaigns that attempt to challenge the invalidation of mental health conditions. Mental health campaigns such as Time to Change focus exclusively on stigma as a problem with an individual remedy; it does not campaign to revoke the legislation on community treatment orders or against increasing coercion. Such campaigns often promote a message of equivalence between physical illness and mental illness, positing that there is no difference between being mentally unwell and physically unwell. This message is promulgated as a means of challenging stigma but serves to reinforce the notion of mental illness as straightforwardly biological in its origins. The central battle of critical approaches in the 1960s and 1970s has been reduced to an acceptance of illness models, even within a discourse that supposedly represents critical perspectives.

The result of this flattening out of critical options and alternatives is an 'us-and-them mentality'. Critical perspectives on recovery are labelled as backward and reactionary; you are either a believer or an infidel. Importantly, this labelling of critics as negative unbelievers has been challenged in recent years by groups such as Recovery in the Bin, which have taken a critical service-user perspective on the discourse of recovery and analyse it precisely in terms of its entanglement with notions of successful functioning in a capitalist economy (Recovery in the Bin, 2015).

The 'truth content' of recovery

It is important to note that Marx's critique of ideology is dialectical. It is dialectical in the sense that concepts are not seen as fixed and stable in meaning but as internally contradictory and pointing beyond themselves to other possibilities. There are, within any ideological concept, possibilities that are positive and can be mobilised, given different social circumstances. Therefore, it is important to acknowledge that there are many important features of the recovery concept and the recovery movement in mental health care. In his famous critique of religious belief as ideological consolation, Marx calls religion the 'sigh of the soulless world' (Marx, 1988). It is important to recognise that such a 'sigh' registers a form of critical opposition even in its capitulation, and as Marx writes: 'Religious suffering is, at one and the same time, the expression of real suffering and a protest against real suffering' (Marx, 1988: 64). What he means here is that in religious concepts of the suffering Christ, there is a protest against unequal material conditions in the world but that protest misfires because it is turned towards salvation in another world; thus, religion loses its critical function and becomes a 'moral sanction' and 'solemn complement' to the injustices of daily life in capitalist societies (Marx, 1988: 64). Recovery has become just such a 'moral sanction' in contemporary mental health care; mental health services vaunt pietistic concepts such as growth, hope and spirituality against a backdrop of a growth in coercion and lack of any critical attack on the injustices in psychiatric care.

Nevertheless, within the principles of recovery, there is an important set of 'truths' that would be part of any positive mental health care system. The emphasis on narratives and service-user voices, the opposition to diagnostic labels, the emphasis on choice and opportunities for hope and growth, the opposition to therapeutic and prognostic nihilism and the recognition of peer-led services are all essential components of a truly progressive mental health system. However, it has become increasingly apparent that 'recovery' as a critical concept is highly compromised due its ideological use in contemporary mental health care. In the concluding section of this chapter I will explore whether recovery can ever function again as a critical concept and, if not, what kind of critical voices are needed in its stead.

Recovery as a critical concept

Is it possible to rescue a concept of recovery from the emasculation and co-option described above? Can recovery retain or regain its critical focus or should we dispense with any notion of the recovery concept in mental health care? Recovery in the Bin (2015) has very usefully set out a critique of recovery that emphasises being 'unrecovered' as a political self-definition that rejects any concept of recovery that defines people's wellness according to imposed definitions of social functioning and acceptance of medical labels. Importantly, it stresses that any recovery movement must acknowledge the existence and extension of coercion in mental health care and address this coercion as part of its practice. It opposes the forced telling of 'successful stories' and the integration of peer support into traditional frameworks of medical care. It further notes the differential discrimination and use of force on specific groups in society, and in particular black and minority ethnic people. If elements of recovery are to survive, then they can only do so through engaging with these principled and critical discussions of empty concepts such as hope and positivity.

Harper and Speed (2012) have argued that what is needed is a historical reconnection of resistance and critical voices in mental health services. One of the issues with the recovery concept is the way it dislodged critical psychiatry from its link to earlier critical perspectives such as the inaccurately named 'antipsychiatry movement'. This enabled a united approach to be constructed but silenced important debates about the nature of mental distress and treatment. Harper and Speed (2012) point to the key 'rights-based' demands of the survivor movement that arose in the 1970s and 1980s and reconfigure those demands for a new set of challenges with the proliferation of mental health services and treatments.

A minimum requirement is to foreground the issue of coercion in mental health care. A statement that 'recovery is impossible whilst coercion exists' punctures the ideologies about choice and hope. The debate that is urgently needed is one about why coercion occurs, its legitimate bounds and responsibilities and the scandal of increasing use and forms of coercion in the mental health and welfare system.

References

Adorno TW (2003). *The Jargon of Authenticity*. London: Routledge.

Anthony WA (1993). Recovery from mental illness: the guiding vision of the mental health system in the 1990s. *Innovation and Research* 2(3): 17–23.

Bentall RP (2009). *Doctoring the Mind: is our current treatment of mental illness really any good?* New York, NY: New York University Press.

Burns T, Dawson J (2009). Community treatment orders: how ethical without experimental evidence? *Psychological Medicine* 39(10): 1583–1586.

Burns T, Rugaska J, Molodynski A, Dawson J, Yeeles K, Vazquez-Montes M et al (2013). Compulsory treatment orders for patients with psychosis (OCTET): a randomised control trial. *The Lancet* 381(9878): 1627–1633.

Care Quality Commission (2017). *Monitoring the Mental Health Act in 2015/2016*. London: Care Quality Commission. www.cqc.org.uk/content/monitoring-mental-health-act-report (accessed 10 April 2017).

Chamberlin J (1978). *On Our Own: patient-controlled alternatives to the mental health system*. New York, NY: Hawthorn Books.

Churchill R, Owen G, Singh S, Hotopf M (2007). *International Experiences of Using Community Treatment Orders*. London: Institute of Psychiatry.

Coleman R (1995). *Recovery: an alien concept*. Isle of Lewis: P&P Press.

Crossley N (2006). *Contesting Psychiatry: social movements in mental health.* Abingdon: Routledge.

Davidson L, Roe D (2007). Recovery from versus recovery in mental illness: one strategy for lessening confusion plaguing recovery. *Journal of Mental Health 16*(4): 459–470.

Deegan PE (1993). Recovering our sense of value after being labelled mentally ill. *Journal of Psychosocial Nursing 31*(4): 7–11.

Department of Health (2008). *Code of Practice: Mental Health Act 1983 (revised 2008)*. London: the Stationery Office.

Eagleton T (1991) *Ideology: an introduction*. London: Verso Books.

Edgley A, Stickley T, Wright N, Repper J (2012). The politics of recovery in mental health: a left libertarian analysis. *Social Theory and Health 2*(10): 121–140.

Ehrenreich B (2009). *Smile or Die: how positive thinking fooled America and the world*. London: Granta.

Elliott C (2004). *Better than Well: American medicine meets the American dream*. New York, NY: WW Norton & Co.

Freeden M (2003). *Ideology: a very short introduction*. Oxford: Oxford University Press.

Gramsci A (1999). *The Gramsci Reader* (D Forgacs ed). London: Lawrence & Wishart.

Harper D, Speed E (2012). Uncovering recovery: the resistible rise of recovery and resilience. *Studies in Social Justice 6*(1): 9–25.

Horkheimer M (1973). *Critical Theory – selected essays*. London/New York, NY: Continuum.

Illouz E (2007). *Cold Intimacies: the making of emotional capitalism*. Cambridge: Polity Press.

Kramer P (1997). *Listening to Prozac*. London: Penguin.

Laing RD (1990). *The Divided Self*. London: Penguin.

Lawton-Smith S (2010). *Supervised Community Treatment*. Briefing Paper 2. London: Mental health Alliance. www.mentalhealthalliance.org.uk/resources/SCT_briefing_paper.pdf (accessed 2 February 2012).

Leamy M, Bird V, Le Boutiller C, Williams J, Slade M (2011). Conceptual framework for personal recovery. *British Journal of Psychiatry 199*: 445–452.

Lukács G (1971). *History and Class Consciousness* (R Livingstone trans). London: Merlin Press.

Lukes S (1986). *Power: a radical view*. Basingstoke: Palgrave Macmillan.

MacPherson CB (1988). *The Political Theory of Possessive Individualism: Hobbes to Locke*. Oxford: Oxford University Press.

Marcuse H (2002). *One Dimensional Man: studies in the ideology of advanced industrial society*. London/New York, NY: Routledge.

Marshall M, Rathbone J (2011). Early intervention for psychosis. *Cochrane Database of Systematic Reviews 6*. Art. No: CD004718. DOI: 10.1002/14651858.CD004718.pub3 (accessed 10 April 2017).

Marx K (1988). *Selected Writings* (D McLellan ed). Oxford: Oxford University Press.

Marx K, Engels F (1998). The German ideology. In: McLellan D (ed). *Karl Marx: selected writings*. Oxford: Oxford University Press (pp159–192).

Mental Health Alliance (2005). *Towards a Better Mental Health Act: the Mental Health Alliance policy agenda*. London: Mental Health Alliance. www.mentalhealthalliance.org.uk/pre2007/documents/AGENDA2.pdf (accessed 29 May 2015)

Mental Health Task Force to the NHS in England (2016). *Five Year Forward View for Mental Health*. London: NHS England.

Morgan A (2008). *Being Human: reflections on mental distress in society*. Ross-on-Wye: PCCS Books.

Morgan A, Felton A, Fulford KWM (Bill), Kalathil J, Stacey G (2015). *Values and Ethics in Mental Health: an exploration for practice*. Basingstoke: Palgrave Macmillan.

Pilgrim D (2008) 'Recovery' and current mental health policy. *Chronic Illness 4*(4): 295–304.

Recovery in the Bin (2015). *RITB – key principles*. [Online.] Recovery in the Bin. https://recoveryinthebin.org/ritbkeyprinciples (accessed 10 April 2017).

Repper J, Perkins R (2009). Recovery and Social Inclusion: changing the mental health agenda. In: Brooker C, Repper J (eds). *Mental Health: from policy to practice*. Edinburgh: Churchill Livingstone (pp85–95).

Repper, J, Perkins R (2003). *Social Inclusion and Recovery*. Edinburgh: Balliere Tindall.

Scheper-Hughes N, Lovell AM, Schob T (eds) (1987). *Psychiatry Inside Out: selected writings of Franco Basaglia*. New York, NY: Columbia University Press.

Slade M (2010). Mental illness and well-being: the central importance of positive psychology and recovery approaches, *Health Services Research 10*(26): 1–14.

Slade M, Amering M, Oades L (2008). Recovery: an international perspective. *Epidemiologica and Psichiatrica Sociale 17*: 2.

Social Care Institute for Excellence (2007). *A Common Purpose: recovery in future mental health services – joint position paper*. London: SCIE. www.scie.org.uk/publications/positionpapers/pp08.asp (accessed 2 February 2012).

Spandler H (2007). From social exclusion to social inclusion? A critique of the inclusion imperative in mental health. *Medical Sociology 2*(2): 3–16.

Stacey G, Stickley T (2012). Recovery as a threshold concept in mental health nurse education. *Nurse Education Today 32*(5): 534–539.

Turner D (2002). Mapping the routes to recovery. *Mental Health Today* July: 29–30.

Whitaker R (2010). *Anatomy of an Epidemic: magic bullets, psychiatric drugs and the astonishing rise of mental illness in America*. New York, NY: Broadway Paperbacks.

9 'Ackin' it back t'brick with autoethnography, reflective practice and mental health recovery research

Tony Sparkes

In qualitative research, the initial and often highly personal questions that we demand answers to are constantly framed and reframed during the research process. It is reasonable to assert that this shilly-shallying reflects, at least in part, the concern that formal research questions can never fully cover the nuances that drive the researcher forward in their quest to make sense of some aspect of the social world. Moreover, and as Richards (2008: 1718) succinctly points out, 'We do not choose our topics accidentally and our motivation for researching them is often personal.'

If our motivations are indeed personal, then what techniques do we have at hand to better understand our decisions? Put another way, what practices can the researcher draw upon to make sense of their choice of topic? My line of thinking is not exclusively pitched at exploring macro-level choices in terms of the research topic itself but extends into micro-level selections that the qualitative researcher makes in the field. It is important to be clear here that my line of argument cares less about comparing X against Y (or some other entity), preferring instead to simply drill down into the relevance and qualities of X.

Taylor and White (2000) provide useful analysis in terms of professional sense-making. While they focus on the performative aspects of language and the work that language does in routine health and social care practice, they do not dismiss structural accounts or those analyses that are focused more on cognitive-emotional aspects. This chapter will focus upon the latter and draw on my experience of undertaking an empirical piece of qualitative recovery research during 2010/11.

As part of my Economic and Social Research Council-funded research, I spent seven months undertaking fieldwork with a social inclusion and recovery service in the north of England. My research question asked: 'What sense do mental health practitioners and service users make of recovery?' In this chapter, I draw on personal notes and fieldnotes and, while I accept my own vulnerabilities, I continue to uphold the confidentiality and anonymity of those that took part in the original study (Chang, 2016).

I set the substantive aspects out in two parts: the first part explores the context that instigated the topic of study; the second part is my attempt to make better sense of why I attended to certain events while in the field. Towards the end of the chapter, I will make a case for autoethnography and reflective practice to be indivisible and suggest a relatively novel approach to research. Before this, however, it will be useful to offer a little more exploration of the intersection between qualitative research, autoethnography and reflective practice.

Qualitative research, autoethnography and reflective practice

Ridgeway (2001: 336) claims that 'qualitative inquiry is the appropriate approach when knowledge is sought concerning complex, little-understood personal, interpersonal and social processes'. This perspective is reiterated by Slade (2010: 6), who comments on the inductive tradition within recovery research and its compatibility with 'an emphasis on individual meaning and experience'. Indeed, the advantages of qualitative methodologies to the study of recovery processes are well documented in the empirical literature (Davidson et al, 2008). Such perspectives guided my early thinking in terms of recovery research and I was keen to learn about how service users and mental health practitioners accounted for recovery in their routine, day-to-day lives.

In 2009, as part of my 'social science training' as a PhD student, I was introduced to autoethnography. As a practising mental health social worker, I found the fundamental premise of autoethnography made sense and, as with Chang's (2016) description (below), the resonance with reflective practice is deafening. Of course, the resonance is only complete in so far as the social worker's identity is aligned with that of the social scientist rather than the social technician:

> … qualitative research method that uses a researcher's autobiographical experiences as primary data to analyse and interpret the sociocultural meanings of such experiences. The ultimate goal of autoethnography is to connect 'the personal' with 'the social'. (Chang, 2016: 444)

Autoethnography has grown up. It has weathered the early criticisms levied against it and has developed into an 'avant-garde' form of qualitative research, attracting interest from a range of academic disciplines (Wall, 2016: 1). The journey has not been easy, and qualitative research itself is frequently side-stepped due to its perceived lack of scientific rigour. It is a contested approach, with critiques ranging from solipsistic navel-gazing and self-indulgence (Burnard, 2007; Denzin & Lincoln, 2017), through to out-and-out claims of scholarly lethargy (Delamont, 2007). That said, autoethnography can potentially offer insights that are evocative and analytical, personal and scholarly, descriptive and theoretical (Burnier, 2006). Autoethnography is not therefore a panacea against reductionist enquiry or scientific imperialism (of a kind that I shall later refer to as 'formulaic') more generally, but an approach that offers some possibilities of knowing about the world that straddles the hinterland between art and science (Ellis, Adams & Bochner, 2011).

The Professional Capabilities Framework (PCF) underpins professional social work standards, and to be able to critically reflect on practice is an explicit domain throughout every level of professional activity (BASW, 2017). Reflective practice is core to continuing professional development (BASW, 2012a), part of the strategic statement for mental health social work (Department of Health, 2016), and a specific aspect of the role of mental health social work (Allen, 2014). The work of Schön (1983) and the practice concepts of 'reflection in' and 'reflection on' are assumed *de rigueur* to be, albeit rather uncritically (Newman, 1999; Bengtsson, 1995), champions of this capability. The relationship between reflective practice and autoethnography is blurry. It is also well-rehearsed in the literature, particularly in context of PhD work (Dowling, 2006; du Preez, 2008; Lake, 2015; Richards, 2015).

Between 1998 and 2009, I worked as a manager in a local authority community support team based in the north of England. This coincided with New Labour's reform of the mental healthcare system. During this period, the main planks of reform (Department of Health, 1998, 1999, 2000) introduced far-reaching structural and functional changes to the mental healthcare system, including the introduction of a plethora of new community mental health teams, such as assertive outreach, early intervention and home treatment teams. Pre-existing community mental health teams (CMHTs) were to retain their central role and be the 'mainstay' of the system (Department of Health, 2002: 3). New Labour first introduced its vision of recovery in 2001 (Department of Health, 2001). In addition, the mental health workforce underwent transformation under the government's New Ways of Working programme (CSIP/NIMHE, 2007) and the introduction of new categories of worker.

With only an undergraduate degree to my name and fearful of not having any professional power to advocate for the continuing work of my team, I undertook a masters (social work) programme in 2003. I returned to my team in October 2005, to the same role but with additional social work responsibilities. I didn't particularly want to be a social worker. The role seemed far too messy. I did, however, relish my role as line manager, probably because (in a utilitarian sense) I felt that supporting staff was the most productive way of supporting service users. All of that was about to change:

> Yesterday, Kym informed me that she has "acked it back to t'brick". She says she does a lot of DIY at home. Staff exchange a good deal of personal information during casual office talk. This is reciprocated with others joining in with supporting comments – or simply joining in with a different anecdote of their own. It is difficult not to participate in and I wonder what work this exchange or-self-revelation actually does? (Fieldnotes, Wednesday 28 July 2010)

Borrowing Kym's words, I ask you, the reader, to allow me to 'ack it back t'brick. I had little ambition to qualify as a social worker, and even less ambition to undertake doctoral study. All of this was a series of random incidents. Or were they?

Part 1

During the summer of 2005, support staff were renamed Support, Time and Recovery (STR) workers. There was no consultation. The former title of Community Support Worker was abandoned. While the state celebrated the introduction of the new role, others suggested that it was simply case of re-badging (Huxley et al, 2006: 36).

Staff team: We're all recovery workers now!

The above mantra was not an unfamiliar refrain in day-to-day office work, commonly used as a corrective and often chanted by staff in unison at whoever had made the error.

All well and good, but what *was* recovery? Was it about cure? Policy documents relating to the STR role (Department of Health, 2003, 2007) gave nothing away, and I clearly remember asking my line manager in a team meeting what recovery meant. Mick was a nurse and he was also manager of the local CMHT.

Mick: It's not rocket science. [Pause.] It's a key deliverable... [pause] part of the national roll-out programme.

Mick wore an inane grin most of the time, and particularly when he was uncomfortable. He was grinning now. I had previously learned that asking for elaboration was seldom productive as it was usually accompanied by more jargon and an invitation to 'think outside the box', or 'lead from the front'. Later, Mick offered an oblique suggestion of what recovery meant:

Mick: It will be a new way of working.

Tony: Well, that's fine. So, how do you want the team to work?

Mick: Much the same as now.

Very much like the Emperor's new clothes, a new way of working was imposed that seemingly didn't exist at all. Indeed, national guidance (Department of Health, 2003, 2007) set out an agenda for exactly what the local authority had been doing for the last 15 years. The imposition was important because it not only unravelled the work of the local authority in supporting people with the *effects* of mental ill health (that is, it undermined the notion of a social perspective), but it reaffirmed social problems as mental illness. I felt frustrated. What *was* recovery and what did it mean to me, to my colleagues, and to the people we supported? I asked Sarah (service user) what recovery meant to her as I supported her with her weekly shop.

Sarah: Ohhhh, I don't know!

Sarah shrugged and, with tobacco-stained fingers, continued to pick pieces of tobacco from the inside of her handbag and roll them into a larger collection before slipping the brown ball into a crumpled plastic money bag. In her defence, Sarah was probably thinking about her children. All but one had grown up and now lived in their own home. Sarah spent much of her time trying to tune into other worlds, pre-occupied with ideas of not being there for her children when they were younger. Multiple hospital admissions and months of chaotic living that had impacted on Sarah and her family's life. I did not know if Sarah would recover because, other than cure, I had no understanding of what recovery was either.

Ideas about turning points and hope are often reported in the recovery literature. Deegan (1988:14) suggests that they must be 'quickly followed by the willingness to act'. My personal (professional) turning point occurred in the middle of an NHS mandatory training course. I simply could not understand why the risk profile of an intravenous drug user diagnosed with schizophrenia would decrease over time.

Tony: But surely, over time, acquisition and injecting practices would at the very least keep the risk constant, if not increase it?

Tutor: No, it would decrease

Tony: But I don't understand. Why?

Tutor: Because it would!

I sensed a degree of frustration in the tutor's voice that was in danger of over-spilling. Travelling home later that day, I was so upset that I decided I did not wish to be trained; I wanted to be educated, so I set about trawling the internet to find academic institutions that would accept my proposal to research the issue of recovery in secondary mental healthcare. I applied to a university in the north of England, and even went for interview. But they wanted 'someone who could hit the ground running'. I wasn't too disappointed because their programme was tied to an evaluation of New Ways of Working (CSIP/NIMHE, 2007). My emerging perspective was more critical. I wanted to understand what recovery meant in terms of how it was talked about in day-to-day practice. Spurred on by this, I recalled how my previous university encouraged its students to ask 'why'? I made enquiries and, with a good deal of support, was accepted into their postgraduate programme – but I would have to wait a further year.

While I waited, I continued to read and made tentative enquiries with service users about how they understood the word 'recovery'. The broad response was that it meant getting better, but in the main it appeared that our conversations were at cross purposes.

I asked Colin. He was in his early 50s and had wanted to be an academic when he was younger. This was before he saw everybody as vampires and was compelled to keep them away by constantly smoking cigarettes. Colin hadn't got a clue what I was talking about. Disparities between service-user and service-provider references to recovery appear to be divergent and evidence appears to corroborate this (Piat, Sabetti & Couture, 2008).

Formal supervision sessions with staff on the topic of recovery were equally confused. What were they meant to *do* that was different? My own supervision records were not a lucrative source of help either. Recovery was rarely mentioned by my supervisor and I didn't mention it either. It featured only in a single record from 23 May 2008. The last paragraph reads:

> Tony is fully aware of the requirements to comply with NICE guidelines, the recovery model of working and all staff are compliant with eCPA, NCRS recording systems. Safety profiles are regularly updated. (Supervision notes, 23 May 2008)

Re-reading this, I note the assumptive leap that takes recovery from an unexplained concept to the status of a model. Indeed, a second assumption suggests that we both *knew* what the recovery model of working actually was!

While I was chasing ideas of what recovery meant, plans had been actioned to draw together all local mental health services under one roof. My team left our local authority office in January 2008. A rather stern looking assets manager from the NHS had visited the office previously and, using the tip of her Parker pen, had pointed at the items that we could and could not take. We left with one small desk fan and some personal stationery. I returned with a colleague during that week and shredded the team's history, other than any records I was legally obliged to keep. I remember feeling unfaithful and disloyal.

At the new office, we followed instructions and congregated in the designated office. I talked to the IT consultant and he showed us our new, individualised desks. The area manager came into the room:

Kevin: And who are you?

Sophie: We are the support team

Kevin: Well, you won't be here for long!

We looked at each other and, in embarrassed silence, busied ourselves in organising our workspaces. Later in the day I received a telephone call from my line manager.

Graham: Where are you all sitting?

Tony: Where the IT consultant said we were to sit.

Graham: I HAVE TOLD YOU WHERE TO SIT!

Tony: Do NOT speak to me like that!

I was being assertive with my own line manager! Me!! My pulse was racing, but I recall staying perfectly calm. It transpired that there was a second plan that only higher managers were aware of (Graham wasn't 'high' enough). The plan involved dividing the team across four different offices. The idea was integration. The practice was divisive.

Enough is enough! I felt frustrated and increasingly angry. If I and my colleagues were to be treated in such an undignified and uncaring way, then how would service users and their supporters fare? Later that evening, at home, I reflected and asked myself:

Where are we journeying to?

------

*I'm having a conversation in my head with Lisa, a work collea*gue.

Lisa: From what you have said, Tony, I am not encouraged. I do hope that you are in the minority in having these experiences. That said, I suspect your experiences have greater connection to the rough edges of managerialism (Learmonth, 1997). [Laughs]

Tony: It isn't funny, Lisa. I can accept this to a point, but it does not excuse it.

Lisa: No, it doesn't. But I do share your concerns and, at least in terms of values, things do not sit right. In many ways, this is the kind of gut reaction that, as social care professionals, we were always told not to ignore.

Tony: Absolutely. But don't forget, this is not just about our difficulties in making sense of recovery, it is about the way in which the NHS, or any other state agency for that matter, administer its power and authority.

Lisa: Ok. So, let's turn our attention to the idea of recovery itself and what it might mean.

Tony: I do feel something of a spoilsport. After all, I imagine that, when subjected to routine talk, who could honestly and compassionately deny that to refuse to embrace the idea of recovery is less than human (Holloway, 2013), a moral imperative if ever there was one. And from the early 2000s onwards, those professions involved in mental healthcare (for example social work, occupational therapy, nursing and psychiatry) have waxed lyrical about recovery and espoused some form of professional position statement on this topic.

Lisa: Yes, I understand that, Tony. At the same time, however, I find the connection strained and my nagging doubts are intersected by deeper concerns. For example, how can recovery be professionally embraced when there is so much debate over its meaning? I mean, let's say I'm a service user – was I ever asked about this journey? What about the detail? Who is travelling with me? When are we going? Will I like it when I get there? Can I change my mind and turn back?

Tony: I see what you mean, Lisa. So, you are questioning who owns recovery?

Lisa: Well, yes, up to a point. But I am also concerned that we are having a nebulous concept simply and uncritically foisted on us as the next good idea. For example, what if I don't want to travel on this road? What if I am content to travel alone, at my own pace? Perhaps what I find most annoying is thinking about the authority of the state to proclaim that we are on the road to recovery.

What I am left with Tony, is a sense of loss and social injustice. The loss isn't material. I think of it more as something intangible, something intrinsically part of me and whose quality I owned. It was part of my humanness or connectedness. Am I making sense here?

Tony: Ahhh… back to ownership again. So, in addition to whatever it is that recovery may mean, there is the thorny issue of recovery as a commodity. Part-owned and manipulated by other more privileged agencies. A 'brand' (Mind, 2008: 13).

Lisa: Well, I think that it becomes wholly-owned, not just part-owned. It becomes colonised (Russo & Beresford, 2015; Timander & Möller, 2016). But, I don't feel that you fully get this, Tony. It is not just about the issue of ownership; it is about state claims regarding its ownership of the 'self'. For example, if recovery concerns 'self-management', then at what point did I give permission for my 'self' to be used in this way? Fox and Ramon (2012) put this far better than me:

> We believe that the language and practice of recovery are best
> expressed when the responsibilities for deciding different treatment
> courses are shared between the professional and the service user.
> In such a process, the service user should receive full and unbiased
> information about the proposed course of action to make an informed
> choice to accept or decline the treatment offered. (p18)

Tony: You raise some interesting points but let me return to what I was saying earlier about social justice. Masterson and Owen (2006:30) indicate that professionally defined ideas of recovery may create an 'underclass' of people 'who do not recover'. Thus, to paraphrase Roberts and Wolfson (2004), recovery may [not] be open to all. How would long-standing social work values of social justice (BASW, 2012b) deal with this?

Lisa: In the first instance, I feel that there is a need to have the professional capacity to shift easily between clinical and personal accounts of recovery (Slade, 2009). This particular dichotomy is not the only way of explaining recovery. For example, recovery from and recovery in (Davidson & Roe, 2007), clinical and social (Secker et al, 2002), real and practical (Tilley & Cowan, 2011), scientific and consumer (Bellack, 2006), service-based and user-based (Schrank & Slade, 2007) are all broadly synonymous with the clinical-personal dualism. If, as health and social care professionals, we can achieve this undertaking, then we can be better able to listen and empower.

Tony: Yes, totally. But I am also mindful that the clinical-personal divide does not map squarely onto groups of people such as medics and social care workers, or practitioners and service users.

Lisa: Well, I am very glad you said that! Rule 1: don't make assumptions! However, I feel it is important that we have clarity because what are the consequences if I refuse to travel *your* road to recovery? Will you overtly or covertly coerce me? Will you penalise me with reduced or withdrawn services? Will your technologies record me as non-compliant, obstinate or treatment resistant? Or will you simply and additively repackage my clinical 'other' as having a disordered personality?

Tony: And I thought I could be cynical, Lisa!

Lisa: We have seen this already, Tony. We currently use six *different* computer systems. We assess, measure, record and categorise on all those systems. Maybe there will be two travellers on the road to recovery? One that aligns with Deegan's (1996) notion of what it means to be human, that validates human experience and potentially means whatever anyone says it means. The other...

Tony: Sorry for interrupting, Lisa, I think one of your postmodern rants is coming up. [We both laugh before Lisa continues]

Lisa: ... the other will be an abstraction, far removed from the lived experience. For those on the road to recovery, I would disconcertedly reflect that perhaps the only constant companion on the journey is a distorted and caricatured representation that is forever held within the cyberspace of an agency's hard-drive. Before the National Service Framework (Department of Health, 1999), travellers were awakened at 9am with a flick of the computer's on/off button and put to bed at 5pm (4:30pm on Friday) with a flick of the same switch. They were rarely disturbed at weekends. Both care and control are now available 24 hours per day, seven days per week, 365 days per year. The prescribed journey to recovery therefore threatens to obliterate the temporal and spatial boundaries afforded by our own existential realities and to conflate and confuse our own personal recovery journey. The 'deeply personal' (Walsh, 1996: 87) thus twists and turns into the deeply impersonal. Defiantly, Tony, my own perception of recovery emerges as conforming to the ticking of a very different clock.

Tony: Nice tirade, Lisa. But recovery is not necessarily the sole province of those who experience mental ill health and perhaps there is a genuine role for mental health professionals to collaborate with service users in their recovery.

Lisa: Oh, I agree with what you are saying to a certain extent but I must insist that collaboration can only be truly effective *if* that is what the service user feels would be of benefit for *their* recovery and however they may define it. Such is the political rhetoric surrounding recovery that the service user receives a paradoxical prescription to collaborate in what essentially belongs to them!

I mentioned this earlier, and I strongly feel that there is an important ethical question to be addressed here that concerns mental health practice. That is, if mental health services operate in full recognition of recovery as a *personal* journey, then what right do practitioners hold to assume that they are free to intrude into what Walsh (1996) refers to as the 'deeply personal'?

Tony: Well, I suppose this takes us into a conversation regarding whether mental health services can ever truly embrace the recovery perspective. Right?

Lisa: Absolutely, and that is my point. You are coming around to my way of thinking – at last. The issue is about mental health services embracing what *service users* define as recovery.

Tony: From my understanding, I think that the very least that services could do now is to promote an open relationship where ideas of recovery are discussed at the first point of contact between service users and providers. Without such discussion, collaboration carries the potential for interventions to be enacted with little respect for the individual and a great deal of assumption.

Lisa: Well, that would certainly be an improvement. But our desire to make sense of recovery will certainly need more work! Service-user narrative speaks of recovery journeys that are characterised by personal meaning (see, for example, Deegan 1988, 1996). They talk of recovery as a process, not an end-point or goal.

Tony: Absolutely, and it is intriguing that some methodologies acknowledge this, and then proceed to expose the same narratives to a range of reductionist analyses in order to excavate various themes, stages and components, with the ultimate aim of advising the best interventions going forward.

Lisa: … and I suppose our task as practitioners is to be aware of this and be mindful that there are other equally valid ways of accounting for recovery.

Tony: Undoubtedly. There are very real consequences that underpin practice. For example, themes and stages are often unproblematically reported in the literature as stable constructs and are variously presented as definitive versions of what counts as the recovery process. Orienting to recovery in this way constructs particular subjectivities and identities for mental health practitioners and service users and other ways of experiencing recovery become marginalised. For example, setting aside the claim that there are more than 49 definitions of hope (Schrank, Stanghellini & Slade, 2008), the theme 'hope' constructs a hopeful service user and by default also constructs a hopeless service user.

Lisa: We need to think about this!

Part 2

Sections of my fieldnotes are given to describing the research site, local environment and some of the more nuanced aspects of both. I am still unclear why my focus turned to these aspects, and why I felt compelled to offer this detail. The following is an example:

> The office base is relatively quiet when I arrive. Kirk is sat alone in the office looking at his computer screen. His purple-and-white, summery, short-sleeved shirt somehow seemed to be at odds with the cold, wet morning. As ever, the situation outside underestimates its own greyness and from my small window I can see grey-black sandstone walls, grey-black chimneys, broken aerials, battleship-grey mullions, black soil stacks and steel-grey skies. There are times when shades of darkness are impressive in their number and variety. In these parts, it seems like this is most of the time. (Fieldnotes, 8 November 2010)

I am however, influenced by some of the earlier work of Hester Parr (2000) and her notion of hidden social geographies, particularly in relation to mental health and the places and spaces in which certain identities are ruled in and ruled out. My attention is drawn to the fact that my research follows the above paper by over a decade, and it is poignant that, while Parr's more recent scholarly outings have concerned the relationship between social geographies and missing persons, missing people are also a theme in my fieldnotes. However, my subjects are not missing in Parr's sense of the word. Rather, they are missing because they have been removed from the landscape, their support centres 'modernised' and 'transformed' (Gilburt & Peck, 2014; NSIP, 2008).

Transformation however, does not stop at the structural boundary. There are transformational implications for service users, and what was once gifted to the local community by a wealthy benefactor has now become a public version of neoliberal social inclusion.

> Physically, service users no longer attend (or drop in) unless by invitation. The spaces within the outer walls are thus divided into smaller offices at the expense of larger communal areas. Outside spaces have ceased offering places to sit and chat. They now offer a car-parking space. It has become very business-like. (Fieldnotes, 24 August 2010)

But I am taken by surprise by the trajectory of transformation and the impact of information technology (IT).

> Following the team meeting, Kym spent some time discussing the referral and assessment processes with me. We talk in an office that is arranged galley-style. Space is organised to fit the four desk-top computers and four printers to the electricity supply that circumnavigates the room like a high-tech dado rail. Internet access is facilitated by more cabling, which shares the plastic dado rail and feeds into a large metal communications box mounted on the office wall. The glass door of the grey box allows the voyeur to peek into the dark interior. More cables, green flashing lights and the background hum of the cooling fans confirm that business is being taken care of. (Fieldnotes, 20 July 2010)

Earlier, I introduced the idea of choice and the inherent implication that choice is free and easy. While this certainly might apply to the choice of topic, the choice of research site itself is much less open. My choice of research site was influenced by Steve. I had known Steve on a professional level for many years and was keenly aware that he was an advocate of research and scholarly activity. Steve proved to be an excellent choice of 'gatekeeper', and an antithesis to the more negative accounts in the literature. For example, in their attempt to undertake qualitative work very similar to my own, Allbutt and Masters (2010) argue that front-line managers had a controlling influence over whom and what could be accessed and note the disempowering effects that research ethics procedures can have on service-user populations.

Prestart meeting – Thursday 15 July 2010

Tony: It is raining. Warm, summer rain. As I drive the few miles to my 10am appointment with Steve, I expected to be feeling apprehensive, a little nervous. Surprisingly, I am not any of these things.

Lisa: So, you've finally done it! What does it *feel* like? I am excited for you. You have worked so hard for this and now you are here, actually doing research!

Tony: Thanks. But as I say, Lisa, I just feel numb. I think the numbness is keeping me safe from the not-so-small matter that I don't feel like I know what the hell I'm doing!

Lisa: You'll be fine.

The main entrance to the offices is framed with a large metal and glass door that opens electronically. Clean, modern and totally impersonal. In the foyer, my advance was halted. My only possible progression was to talk to whoever was behind the reception glass. Luckily, Steve witnessed my arrival through the window and opened the second electronic door and invited me into the office.

I took a seat and he introduced me to Michael. Their conversation focused on the supervision of staff, although it was occasionally interrupted by Michael's request for housekeeping details and questions that related to security and confidentiality. Information technology was a sub-context in their exchanges and the amount of technology in the office (desktops, laptops, telephone, mobile telephones, wires, cables and switches) was surely impressive.

Lucy – Wednesday 21 July 2010

Lisa: How's it going?

Tony: Ok… I think. Some of my observations do unsettle me, though.

Lisa: How so?

Tony: I watched Sally and Ted undertake an assessment with a service user called Lucy. Lucy grappled with Mr Dog while inviting us into her home. After it had urinated over the front door frame, Lucy shoved the excitable animal into the kitchen and we went into the front room. We walked across a carpet that looked as though it had seen better days and sat on a similarly endowed sofa. Lucy talked about wanting to go to college and train as a hairdresser or beauty therapist.

Lisa: So, what's the problem?

Tony: Well, although most of the talk was about socially inclusive activity, I felt that the most important thing that Lucy said was something that was not recorded (or even heard by the assessment). Lucy said that she was 'tired of caring for other people' when that care was not shown back to her in return.

Lisa: Hmmm… without dismissing the emotional impact of Lucy's mum passing away, there is also a moral point here, isn't there? I mean, if you are living by the neoliberal mantra of 'no rights without responsibilities', then what about the reciprocity principle and the question around the state upholding any rights that it might have regarding Lucy, as a young person or as a (former) young carer.

Tony: Exactly. This is what I was focusing on. Maybe Lucy simply didn't know what she didn't know. But (far less excusable), the assessors should have known what they should have known. I was drawn to the agency's choice to sidestep Lucy's words and stick to the narrow remit of the assessment. It chose not to invite conversation from Lucy about her role as a young carer. It chose not to listen to Lucy's experience and her feelings. Instead, the assessment simply took a faint blueprint of what it was that Lucy would like to *do* going forward.

Lisa: Was that the end of the assessment? I mean, what happened next?

Lucy again – Friday 23 July 2010

Tony: I revisited Lucy a couple of days later with Kym. Lucy talked about things in terms of her 'not being confident' and I remain intrigued as to what this term means for those who use it and those who read it in the case notes. It doesn't mean anything!

Lisa: Yes, I see what you mean here

Tony: Lucy appeared no different to the previous day and showed similar levels of interaction. The front room and kitchen were sparsely furnished. All the furnishings seemed to be broken in some way.

Lisa: You mentioned this earlier. When you say that the furnishings seemed to be broken in some way, what do you mean? Why does this matter… to you?

Tony: Let me explain. But first, let me carry on. Back in the office, Kym logged onto the computer and accessed the agency's database and Lucy's record. Routine case-note entries from her counsellor mentioned recent family illness, loss and relationship difficulties, and I reflected on the supportive effects that some social networks can provide when adverse life events occur and why healthcare services routinely become involved with what are ostensibly social issues.

Lisa: … and the broken furniture?

Tony: My concern here is not just about stigma as it relates to mental ill health.

I was drawn to 'broken furniture' as an emblem for something else. It was more about the intersectionality of a number of vulnerable identities, ranging from young carer to service user. Poverty was at the forefront of my mind, the injustice, and the very idea of the struggle in people's lives.

Lisa: So, what did you do? What would you do differently?

Tony: I did nothing. To my shame, I did nothing. Like Lucy said, these 'things' need to be cared for. While I am mindful of the resonance here of Martin Niemöller's words,[1] speaking out is so much harder in practice. Schön's (1983) notion of reflecting in practice is fine, but some matters require careful consideration. Nevertheless, this learning was a significant part of my research back then and a more important part of my practice now. Challenging those in authority and ensuring that an individual's rights are upheld are of paramount importance, even if this simply means signposting the person or informing them about what is available somewhere else.

Lisa: And this has ramifications for recovery, right?

Tony: Absolutely. It is well-established that recovery is a contested concept (Hyde, Bowles & Pawar, 2015), and a key element of that debate is the argument that it can only ever be personally defined. I think it important to stress this point.

Lisa: So, what about the recovery model?

Tony: A myth I'm afraid! Sure, there may be different models and some models may be more persuasive than others. But a model is only a representation. What recovery actually means in practice will shift around and be completely fallible.

Lisa: Should I feel disappointed here?

Tony: No, absolutely not. Let me continue. If personal recovery is subjectively defined then it is what anyone says it is, whether this be social, medical, psychological, spiritual or any variation in between. In many ways, this is only part of the argument and it needs extension. By virtue of the fact that recovery is personally defined, then it becomes a *de facto* matter to situate it as a rights-based perspective on, or approach to mental healthcare.

---

1. Martin Niemöller was a German Lutheran pastor whose poem famously described the failure by German intellectuals to speak out in opposition to the Nazis' rise to power (for further discussion, see Marcuse, 2016). The poem appears in many versions, citing different groups. It typically begins, 'First they came for the Socialists and I did not speak out/Because I was not a Socialist...', and ends, 'Then they came for me – and there was no one left to speak for me.'

Lisa: This makes so much sense, because now the issue becomes more about getting people to articulate what recovery may mean to them, at the point it is talked about, as a way of empowering them?

Tony: Well, yes. That would be the focus and the ideal.

20 September 2010

I travel in my own car to visit Lucy with Kym as I have a private meeting afterwards. Lucy is quiet as Mr Dog snuffles his way around the front room where we sit. Lucy wants to do a hairdressing course but funding it is going to be impossible. Kym is trying to be practical and agrees that it will be difficult. Kym's disappointment resides in the lack of access and opportunity for Lucy to do this, especially as she is a young person who simply wants to get on in life. Maybe if she hadn't been a young carer then she could have got on earlier and quicker? Maybe.

Inclusion and mental health, both or neither? – Tuesday 24 August 2010

Tony: Hey, Lisa. This is important

Lisa: Yeah?

Tony: I went out with Kym to a local day-centre for children and we met with the service manager. Kym was on a fact-finding mission to learn about volunteering opportunities that the centre could offer and, at the same time, she was advertising the service and reiterating its social inclusion (and recovery) goals. Kym knew a service user who could possibly benefit from volunteering at the centre.

Lisa: So, why is this important?

Tony: Well, at one point during the meeting I reflected (in-action) about whether Kym saw herself as a social inclusion worker (and it just so happened that she worked in a mental health team) or whether she saw herself as primarily working within a mental health service that focused on social inclusion.

Lisa: And a) does this matter and b) the difference is...?

Tony: Oh, come on, Lisa! The difference is more than one of professional identity. The difference holds massive implications. For once...

Lisa: ... excuse me for interrupting, but the labels? What *exactly* is a social inclusion worker and what *exactly* is a mental health worker?

Tony: But, don't you see… this is exactly my point, Lisa. Sat in that office, on that day, I did not have an answer to your questions. Whatever these roles were, this experience undermined it. For a second, there was a gap, a space that could have been filled with anything. I have tried to recapture that moment ever since, but it has eluded me. Whatever it is, I suspect that the role is about supporting someone outside of orthodox mental health roles. It will be about relating to someone and their experiences in *their* terms. Very much like the second recovery task involving 'framing' outlined by Slade (2013: 8).

Lisa: [Laughs.] Yes, let's advertise for a rights worker! I have long had a problem with the term 'community mental health team' or 'community worker', because it is so aligned with the service. For example, it does not necessarily follow that professionals in that team have any particular knowledge of the local area and the communities, families and people that live there.

Tony: Yes, let's. And let's employ a social perspectives worker who does not just accept referrals from other mental health services.

The pop-up shop – Friday 23 July 2010

I attended a venue in the town centre with Kym. It is considered by the team to promote socially inclusivity as it invites all members of the public to participate. It also makes use of vacant space in the town centre and I guess it helps create a perception of hustle and bustle, of activity and of people moving purposefully along the high street

How is recovery talked about here? It isn't, at least not explicitly. An older lady came into the shop – Janie. She sat down at the communal table and, after making small talk, proceeded to get out her knitting. She was creating a football kit to clothe action figures in the colours of the local football team. A father and his young son came into the shop. Megan, one of the organisers, chatted to the couple about what was on offer. Individually, father and son had their picture taken wearing the local football team's home shirt. They were told that the image would join others and their faces would appear alongside fellow supporters in a model football stand.

Other knitters joined the table. Mary, Kym and I engaged a different craft. We wrestled with our pieces of A4 paper. Following the printed instructions, we tried to fold the paper into the shape of a football shirt. If we were successful, we could hang it with others on a makeshift washing line that was anchored across the shop. We managed – and then branched out into shorts.

Megan flitted about, cutting bits of paper here and snipping bits of card there. She was helping to make the model football stand. She had recently finished a fine art degree and was mucking in. The conversation around the table was about histories – personal and social histories. Janie talked about going abroad on holiday when she was younger. She didn't like it and has never been on holiday since. That was in the 1960s. Mary asked permission before taking a raisin from a bowl on the table. She chirped about making sure that her boys could look after themselves: that they could wash, cook, clean, polish and iron. She grinned smugly when she said that one of her boys was a pastry cook and he made the best pastry for miles around. She leaned over to Kym, smiled and, lowering her voice, spoke the words 'mental illness'.

Another lady came into the shop. She undid the fastener on her coat, rearranged her sari, and also produced a pair of knitting needles. She chatted with Janie and they organised who was knitting shorts and who would be knitting shirts. Janie talked about being placed in Scotland as service personnel during the Second World War. Mary talked about her boys and Gita laughed a lot as Megan continued to flit about, now arranging bits of coloured paper here and bits of coloured card there.

Lisa: So, is social inclusion part of recovery? 'Essential' as Repper and Perkins (2003: 136) would suggest? Or am I missing something here?

Tony: I suppose it could be, Lisa, but again it would largely hinge on what recovery meant for the person. I do agree with Ramon and colleagues (2009) and their claim that the relationship between the two is a particularly English one. Anyhow, I am not convinced that what I have just described counts as social inclusion, and I wonder if the transiency of the pop-up shop means it is too fragile to make such claims.

Lisa: This is difficult, isn't it. As with recovery, social inclusion is a difficult term to resist because, as Spandler (2007: 4) and Secker (2009: 4) both point out, it is 'self-evidently desirable', irrespective of the paucity of critique surrounding its usage and absence of clarity around who finds it desirable and in what ways. For example, if service users assert some resistance to be socially included, then it is suggested that such choices are actually erroneous, as they are based on the lived experience of mental distress, which fosters 'limited experience', 'narrow perspectives' and a 'limited knowledge of possible options' (Boardman, 2010: 32).

Tony: I can't believe you have just said that!

Lisa: I didn't.

A member of Art Space

Tony: Lisa, I had many of conversations, with lots of different people. This particular conversation was memorable and on reflection I think this is because the language used was the language of the recovery literature. My attention is caught by this because it was a rare exchange in which there was a sense of connection over the same concept.

Lisa: I am intrigued. Tell me more.

Tony: We had arranged to meet in the pop-up shop but my contact, a former service user, was late (she was next door 'nattering'). While I was waiting, I noticed the pop-up shop had changed its layout. It was now a gallery. The tables and chairs where knitters had previously sat and chatted had been removed. Open space had taken over. The open space was functional in that it allowed the viewer the choice either to stand back or to get up-close to the paintings, drawings and artwork on the walls. Megan stood behind a counter at the front of the shop, quietly chatting to people as they came in and browsed.

Lisa: This sounds just like a community that is almost the antithesis of stigma, where difference is the raison d'etre.

Tony: Very much so, but I guess it has its codes too. Anyhow, my contact arrived and we sat outside with our lattes, basking in the mid-day sunshine. People walked by on the main street as we talked. Our conversation was about recovery. It was an easy conversation; we took turns, and there was a willingness to be open enough to facilitate an exchange. Genuineness and honesty were elevated to a prominent position in our talk, as was the centrality of relationships. One person (a nurse) seemed to be of specific importance, and my contact talked about this person as facilitating a breakthrough in what was to be the start of their recovery. The breakthrough was described as a kind of realisation, of being conscious of one's situation.

My contact described her art work as a process of constructing and deconstructing; a process of constant revision and 'scratching off layers'. This was likened to a personal sense of recovery in which we agreed that 'repetitive processes discipline recovery'. It was *that* sort of conversation. The Prince of Wales' charities, she said, were one of the biggest helps in creating a structured environment for her self-development and, ultimately, her recovery. Our conversation had to be brought to a close, due to our respective afternoon appointments and we brought the chatter down to less lofty height as we walked back to Art Space, and I then returned to my car.

Lisa: I can see what she means in terms of structured environments and how this could have supported her recovery.

Tony: Yes, me too. The trouble is, of course, that this would not have worked for someone else.

Discussion and summary

'Ackin' it back t'brick was used in the title as a metaphor for a range of possibilities. There was a sense in which the phrase could refer to stripping back the meaning of autoethnography and reflective practice to expose their similarities, and then taking this alliance forward to explore what both of these processes contribute to the creation of new knowledge. Another use of the phrase could be to describe the process of unpacking some of the tensions and debates that cut across qualitative research more generally. 'Ackin' it back t'brick is not my phrase, however; as I mentioned earlier, these words belong to Kym. A further meaning could relate more closely to how I understood these words when I first heard them, when they were used to simply describe what she would be doing in order to get back to a basic structure before moving on to create something new and exciting. I find this particular reading resonates with my own understanding of the phrase.

Both autoethnography and reflective practice encourage a process that uses the self as an organising feature of the capacity to make sense of experience. Moreover, it is a process unlike any other that can lay claim to this particular method of constructing knowledge. During the process of writing and rewriting the first part of this chapter, I learned more about a range of values to which I did not, for whatever reason, give much consideration at the time. If I did, it was unconnected to me personally or professionally; nor, indeed, was it connected to what is set out as personal recovery (Slade, 2009). I argue that the growing realisation of the relevance of social justice is an important factor here. Indeed, it is pertinent that I use the word 'relevance' rather than 'importance' because what matters here is that the values are personally and professionally *relevant*. Moreover, there are multiple relevancies because each instance of injustice is nuanced and correspondingly takes on a different relevance.

From the same section of this chapter then, the very idea of critique is elevated to a relevance that I had hitherto not fully appreciated, whether this be by endeavouring to challenge assumption or by delivering 'choice' to service users via the learning emerging from that challenge. However, a reflective learning point is in the understanding that it is unlikely that the neoliberal rolling back of state support for vulnerable people will halt in my lifetime. To this end, it becomes pertinent to promulgate a sense of recovery as a rights-based agenda in mental health care.

In part two, the focus shifted from a concern about 'Why am I doing this?' to 'Why am I looking at this thing in particular?', ostensibly focusing the lens further down. Sections of this part orientated more around engaging with an understanding of the detail. I tried to find a balance between drilling down into a reflective consideration of why my attention may have been drawn this way or that way, while at times trying to let the description in my fieldnotes take the lead in this direction or that.

In the introduction to this piece, I discussed the relevance of qualitative research as a means to better understand what recovery may mean in health and social care. However, a broader comment is required to settle the score with positivist science and its claims to objectivity. The reductionist approach to measuring the human experience is on the wane, and post-World War 2 promises have simply not delivered the emancipation that was promised. If this blunt scenario introduces postmodern research vagaries, then by Denzin and Lincoln's (2017) age it also introduces autoethnography.

Assuming that Allott and Loganathan (undated) are adhering strictly to a Kuhnian account of paradigms (Kuhn, 1970), then they are arguing for a service-level transformation that makes a shift from one way of practising recovery to another, from the clinical to the personal. This represents the 'radical shift' (Adams, Daniels & Compagni, 2009: 43), or 'radical transformation' (Braslow, 2013: 785) articulated in the recovery literature. Yet, the Kuhnian account of paradigms is only one particular version. Wendel (2008) writes about Halloun's (2004) version of paradigms in which they are considered more as personal ways of making sense of the world. There is not one single paradigm shared by mental health practitioners (as the Kuhnian version would suggest); rather, I have many personal paradigms that have commonalities with the personal paradigms of other practitioners.

Social work is passionate about its value base, and rightly so. The struggle to find a voice for those who are vulnerable, to listen to someone's storied account of their experience and let them set out the terms of reference, does not always sit easily with dominant scientific paradigms. What is ruled in and ruled out in terms of legitimate knowledge and what counts as 'evidence' (Department of Health, 1999: 6) is under threat. Rhizomatic thinking (Deleuze & Guattari, 1987) offers a perspective through which to embrace the main points of this chapter. Underpinned by a rejection of traditional, arborescent ways of thinking where knowledge creation is hierarchical and linear, rhizomatic thinking offers an antithesis to formulaic research: a preference for 'boxed-out' rather than 'boxed-in' and the open pursuit of diversification (Alvesson & Gabriel, 2013; Alvesson & Sandberg, 2014). Autoethnography would complement this vision.

Conclusion

While I accept that there is healthy and much-needed debate to be had around the merits of autoethnography and its connection to reflective practice, the process of writing this chapter has cemented the notion that any scholarly disparity that is held to exist between autoethnography and reflective practice is illusionary and grounded more in the orientation of the lens-holder rather than the lens itself. Indeed, the implications and the effects of this approach are much more extensive than the sum of their parts.

The reflective use of the self to question, explore and better understand the decisions made ultimately turn back upon the author. To this extent, I fully concur with Lake's concluding comments on autoethnography in his own doctoral research, when he questions the orthodoxy of 'big science' against the personal and professional value of personal narrative, reflective practice and autoethnography.

I was unaware when composing those words that the reflection, thinking and development that occurred after my thesis was 'finished' were to be equally transformational for me, if not more so than 'doing the thesis'. I have made a voyage from being a natural science trained clinician to a medical educator who is increasingly troubled by the hegemonic influences of what West (2001: 206) terms 'big science', and embraces the value of personal narrative, reflective practice and autoethnography. (2015: 685)

References

Adams N, Daniels A, Compagni A (2009). International pathways to mental health transformation. *International Journal of Mental Health 38*(1): 30–45.

Allbutt H, Masters H (2010). Ethnography and the ethics of undertaking research in different mental healthcare settings. *Journal of Psychiatric and Mental Health Nursing 17*(3): 210–215.

Allen, R. (2014) *The role of the social worker in adult mental health services.* [Online.] Social Care Online. www.scie-socialcareonline.org.uk/the-role-of-the-social-worker-in-adult-mental-health-services/r/a11G000000CTDYqIAP (accessed 31 May 2017).

Allott P, Loganathan L (undated). *Discovering hope for recovery from a British perspective: a review of a sample of recovery literature, implications for practice and systems change.* Birmingham: West Midlands Partnerships for Mental Health. http://www.critpsynet.freeuk.com/LITERATUREREVIEWFinal.htm (accessed 31 May 2017).

Alvesson M, Gabriel Y (2013). Beyond formulaic research. *Academy of Management Education and Learning 12*(2): 245–263.

Alvesson M, Sandberg J (2014). Habitat and habitus: boxed-in versus boxed out research. *Organisational Studies 35*(7): 967–987.

Bellack AS (2006). Scientific and consumer models of recovery in schizophrenia: concordance, contrasts and implications. *Schizophrenia Bulletin 32*(3): 432–442.

Bengtsson J (1995). What is reflection? On reflection in the teaching profession and teacher education. *Teachers and Teaching: theory and practice 1*(1): 23–32.

Boardman J (2010). Social exclusion of people with mental health problems and learning disabilities: key aspects. In: Boardman J, Currie A, Killaspy H, Mezey G (eds). *Social Inclusion and Mental Health.* London: Royal College of Psychiatrists (pp22–45).

Braslow JT (2013). The manufacture of recovery. *Annual Review of Clinical Psychology 9*: 781–809.

British Association of Social Workers (2017). *Professional Capabilities Framework.* Birmingham: BASW.

British Association of Social Workers (2012a). *BASW Continuing Professional Development (CPD) Policy.* Birmingham: BASW.

British Association of Social Workers (2012b). *Code of Ethics for Social Work.* Birmingham: BASW.

Burnard P (2007). Seeing the psychiatrist: an autoethnographic account. *Journal of Psychiatric and Mental Health Nursing 14*(8): 808–813.

Burnier D (2006). Encounters with the self in social science research: a political scientist looks at autoethnography. *Journal of Contemporary Ethnography* 35(4): 410–418.

Care Services Improvement Partnership/National Institute for Mental Health in England (2007). *Mental Health. New ways of working for everyone: developing and sustaining a capable and flexible workforce.* London: CSIP/NIMHE.

Chang H (2016). Autoethnography in health research: growing pains? *Qualitative Health Research* 26(4): 443–451.

Davidson L, Ridgway P, Kidd S, Topor A, Borg M (2008). Using qualitative research to inform mental health policy. *Canadian Journal of Psychiatry* 53(3): 137–144.

Davidson L, Roe D (2007). Recovery from versus recovery in serious mental illness: one strategy for lessening confusion plaguing recovery. *Journal of Mental Health* 16(4): 459–470.

Deegan P (1996). Recovery as a journey of the heart. *Psychiatric Rehabilitation Journal* 19(3): 91–97.

Deegan P (1988). Recovery: the lived experience of rehabilitation. *Psychosocial Rehabilitation Journal* 11(4): 11–19.

Delamont S (2007). Arguments against auto-ethnography. *Qualitative Researcher* 4(February): 2–4.

Deleuze G, Guattari F (1987). *A Thousand Plateaus: capitalism and schizophrenia.* (B Massumi trans). Minneapolis, MN: University of Minnesota Press.

Denzin NK, Lincoln YS (2017). Introduction: the discipline and practice of qualitative research. In: Denzin NK, Lincoln YS (eds). *The SAGE Handbook of Qualitative Research* (5th ed). London: Sage (pp1–26).

Department of Health (2016). *Social Work for Better Mental Health: a strategic statement.* London: Department of Health.

Department of Health (2007). *Mental Health Policy Implementation Guide: support, time and recovery (STR) workers. Learning from the National Implementation Programme. Final handbook.* London: Department of Health.

Department of Health (2003). *Mental Health Policy Implementation Guide: support, time and recovery (STR) workers.* London: Department of Health.

Department of Health (2002). *Mental Health Policy Implementation Guide: community mental health teams.* London: Department of Health.

Department of Health (2001). *The Journey to Recovery: the government's vision for mental health care.* Department of Health.

Department of Health (2000). *The NHS Plan: a plan for investment, a plan for reform.* Norwich: the Stationery Office.

Department of Health (1999). *A National Service Framework for Mental Health: modern standards and service models.* Norwich: the Stationery Office.

Department of Health (1998). *Modernising Mental Health Services: safe, sound and supportive.* Norwich: the Stationery Office.

Dowling M (2006). Approaches to reflexivity in qualitative research. *Narrative Research* 13(3) 7–21.

Du Preez J (2008). Locating the researcher in the research: personal narrative and reflective practice. *Reflective Practice* 9(4): 509–519.

Ellis C, Adams TE, Bochner AP (2011). Autoethnography: an overview. [Online.] *Forum: Qualitative Social Research 12*(1). Art 10. http://nbn-resolving.de/urn:nbn:de:0114-fqs1101108 (accessed: 31 May 2017).

Fox J, Ramon S (2012). Recovery: bringing service users in. *Social Work and Social Sciences Review 14*(3): 10–22.

Gilburt H, Peck E (2014). *Service Transformation: lessons from mental health.* London: The Kings Fund.

Halloun I (2004). *Modelling Theory in Science Education.* Norwell, MA: Kluwer Academic Publishers.

Holloway F (2013). Recovery and medication: not quite a revolution: commentary on… from taking to using medication. *Advances in Psychiatric Treatment 19*(1): 11–13.

Huxley P, King S, Evans S, Davidson B, Beresford P (2006). *No Recovery Without Time and Support (or 'More Than Bowling Together'): evaluation of the introduction of support, time and recovery workers in three pilot sites.* London: Care Services Improvement Partnership/National Institute for Mental Health.

Hyde B, Bowles W, Pawar M (2015). 'We're still in there' – consumer voices on mental health inpatient care: social work research highlighting lessons for recovery practice. *British Journal of Social Work 45*(suppl 1): i62–i78.

Kuhn TS (1970). *The Structure of Scientific Revolutions* (2nd ed). Chicago, IL: University of Chicago Press.

Lake J (2015). Autoethnography and reflective practice: reconstructing the doctoral thesis experience. *Reflective Practice 16*(5): 677–687.

Learmonth M (1997). Managerialism and public attitudes towards UK NHS managers. *Journal of Management in Medicine 11*(4): 214–221.

Marcuse H (2016). The origin and reception of Martin Niemöller's quotation: 'First they came for the communists …' In: Berenbaum M, Libowitz R, Littell MS (eds). *Remembering for the future: Armenia, Auschwitz and beyond.* St Paul, MN: Paragon (pp173–199).

Masterson S, Owen S (2006). Mental health service user's social and individual empowerment: using theories of power to elucidate far-reaching strategies. *Journal of Mental Health 15*(1): 19–34.

Mind (2008). *Life and Times of a Supermodel: the recovery paradigm for mental health.* London: Mind.

National Social Inclusion Programme (2008). *From Segregation to Inclusion: where are we now? A review of progress towards the implementation of the mental health day services commissioning guidance.* London: National Social Inclusion Programme.

Newman S (1999). Constructing and critiquing reflective practice. *Educational Action Research 7*(1): 145–163.

Parr H (2000). Interpreting the 'hidden social geographies' of mental health: ethnographies of inclusion and exclusion in semi-institutional places. *Health and Place 6*(3): 225–237.

Piat M, Sabetti J, Couture A (2008). Do consumers use the word 'recovery'? *Psychiatric Services 59*(4): 446–447.

Ramon S, Shera W, Healy B, Lachman M, Renouf N (2009). The rediscovered concept of recovery in mental illness. *International Journal of Mental Health 38*(2): 106–126.

Repper J, Perkins R (2003). *Social Inclusion and Recovery: a model for mental health practice.* London: Bailliere Tindall.

Richards M (2015). Turning back to the story of my life: an autoethnographic exploration of a researcher's identity during the PhD process. *Reflective Practice 16*(6): 821–835.

Richards R (2008). Writing the othered self: autoethnography and the problem of objectification in writing about illness and disability. *Qualitative Health Research 18*(12): 1717–1728.

Ridgeway P (2001). Restorying psychiatric disability: learning from first person recovery narratives. *Psychiatric Rehabilitation Journal 24*(4): 335–343.

Roberts G, Wolfson P (2004). The rediscovery of recovery: open to all. *Advances in Psychiatric Treatment 10*(1): 37–49.

Russo J, Beresford P (2015). Between exclusion and colonisation: seeking a place for mad people's knowledge in academia. *Disability and Society 30*(1): 153–157.

Schön D (1983). *The Reflective Practitioner: how professionals think in action.* New York, NY: Basic Books.

Schrank B, Slade M (2007). Recovery in psychiatry. *The Psychiatrist 31*(9): 321–325.

Schrank B, Stanghellini G, Slade M (2008). Hope in psychiatry: a review of the literature. *Acta Psychiatrica Scandinavica 118*(6): 421–433.

Secker J (2009). Mental health, social exclusion and social inclusion. *Mental Health Review Journal 14*(4) 4–11.

Secker J, Membrey H, Grove B, Seebohm P (2002). Recovering from illness or recovering your life? Implications of clinical versus social models of recovery from mental health problems for employment support services. *Disability and Society 17*(4): 403–418.

Slade M (2013). *100 ways to Support Recovery: a guide for mental health professionals* (2nd ed). London: Rethink Mental Illness.

Slade M (2010). Mental illness and well-being: the central importance of positive psychology and recovery approaches. *BMC Health Services Research 10*(26): 1–14.

Slade M (2009). *Personal Recovery and Mental Illness: a guide for mental health professionals.* Cambridge: Cambridge University Press.

Spandler H (2007). From social exclusion to inclusion? A critique of the inclusion imperative in mental health. *Medical Sociology Online 2*(2): 3–16. www.medicalsociologyonline.org/oldsite/archives/issue22/pdf/mso_vol2_iss2.pdf#page=7 (accessed 31 May 2017).

Taylor C, White S (2000). *Practising Reflexivity in Health and Social Care: making knowledge.* Buckingham: Open University Press.

Tilley S, Cowen S (2011). Recovery in mental health policy: good strategy or bad rhetoric? *Critical Public Health 1*(1): 95–104.

Timander A, Möller A (2016). Recovery: experiences of resistance to disablism. *Disability in Society 31*(8): 1050–1063.

Wall S (2016). Toward a moderate autoethnography. *International Journal of Qualitative Methods 15*(1): 1–9.

Walsh D (1996). A journey toward recovery: from the inside out. *Psychiatric Rehabilitation Journal 20*(2): 85–89.

Wendel PJ (2008). Models and paradigms in Kuhn and Halloun. *Science and Education 17*(1): 131–141.

West L (2001). *Doctors on the Edge: gemneral practitiones, health and learning in the inner-city.* London: Free Association Books.

10 | Mental health workforce and survivor alliances: a personal story of possibilities, perils and pratfalls

Mick McKeown

This chapter draws on an anecdote from my past to explore the potential for creating and sustaining solidarity between social movement activists concerned with mental health and mental health services. My story connects with some of the tensions and turbulence of relations that can occur in the context of seeking political alliances between elements of the mental health care workforce and critically disposed service users and survivors. In terms of my own interest and involvement in such matters over the years, the central tale is certainly not my finest hour as an activist; far from it. I refer to it here in the spirit of learning from past mistakes. Perhaps these are the sorts of lessons that movement allies ought still to be interested in, as the important alliances at stake remain underdeveloped and fragile. The road to deeper and stronger solidarity is packed with positive, transformative possibilities but also fraught with perils for respective allies and maybe a few pratfalls along the way.

I begin with a number of caveats. First, I am concerned with constructive, democratic solutions and deliberative persuasion, not with the imposition of any ready-made blueprint for action, although it is action and activism with which I am most interested. I recognise the legitimacy and power of counter-arguments to the case I wish to make, including the right to dismiss or not to engage with it, in part or whole. Second, I hope the audience for these ideas includes both potential parties to the alliances I seek: that is, members of the workforce and survivors alike. The potential for discord that I speak of is, however, a hazard for this modest writing contribution; it might just as easily upset rather than appeal to different people. So, I wish to state my intention is not to add to existing upset and discontent, although I do aim to be provocative.

My personal view is that the mental health workforce, and my nursing discipline within it, should be more politically informed, active and appreciative of the criticisms furnished by an active service user and survivor movement

(McKeown, 2018, 2016a; McKeown, Wright & Gadsby 2018; McKeown, Wright & Mercer, 2017; McKeown & White, 2015). A big part of my concern is the assertion that the labour movement does not 'get' mental health as a political issue, beyond having an interest in defending services as we currently have them, such as demanding parity of funding with general healthcare. This is not a new argument; it was first brought to my attention by Peter Sedgwick in his book *Psycho Politics* (1982), published not long after the anecdotal events described here, although I didn't read it until a few years later. This was a text written in a time that presaged the period we are living through now, where right-wing assaults on the NHS and the wider welfare state precipitated some bold resistance on the part of the left and communities. This was exemplified in Liverpool where I lived and worked (and still do) by the left-populist politics of the Militant Tendency in local government. This radical grouping within the Labour Party increased its share of the vote in three successive elections and mobilised mass demonstrations on the streets of the city centre to protest against central government budget cuts and, towards the end, the disbarring of the councillors. The decade began with riots in Toxteth and Brixton and also witnessed the failed election campaign of Michael Foot, the courageous but similarly unsuccessful 1984–85 miners' strike and other major industrial disputes such as Grunwick's and Wapping, and closed with the Hillsborough football stadium tragedy.

In or out of Liverpool, Scousers were variously involved in all of these events and, through my involvement in the community and trade unions, so was I. My working career started as a nursing assistant on mental health wards in Fazakerley Hospital; I then did my general nurse training at the nearby Walton Hospital, before returning to complete mental health nurse training at Fazakerley (now renamed Aintree University Hospital). I joined the union[1] on my first day and, soon after attending a branch meeting, became a steward. We campaigned for Foot and supported the 1981 March for Jobs that set off from Liverpool Pier Head. We raised funds for the miners and hosted meetings at which they spoke in our workplaces and our communities. We supported the establishment of community, trade union and unemployed centres, which were sustained by local government grants, union funds and individual member's donations to the One Fund for All. We turned out for the budget demonstrations and eventually campaigned and raised funds for the disbarred councillors.

We shared in the pain of the Hillsborough families and survivors and, indeed, witnessed the physical and emotional consequences of that trauma in our daily work. A close colleague of mine who worked as a counsellor with Hillsborough survivors, including the bereaved families, succumbed to a mental health crisis of his own, eventually having to stop work in the NHS altogether. The extent to which the NHS and its unions were central to the unfolding politics and events was reflected in the fact that I was due to speak for my union on the platform of the

1. Confederation of Health Service Employees (COHSE), later subsumed into Unison.

local May Day Rally in 1989 which was postponed as a mark of respect after the events at Hillsborough.

If this was just a simple tale of combative workers and unions struggling for their economic and political rights, so far so good. At the time, we in the labour movement felt we were correct in our analysis of the political economy and were confident that our prescriptions for socialism and democracy would win out in the end. To a certain extent, our arguments have been vindicated, especially in particular terms, but the durability of what we called Thatcherism then and now call neoliberalism is somewhat depressing. The current popularity of so-called Corbynism appears to further vindicate a consistent attachment to labour values over all this time and offer a new gleam of optimism.

So, what is the problem?

There is, actually, a big problem, which I want to lead into with a reflection on some events from the earliest part of my working life. In the early and late 1980s, NHS staff and nurses were sporadically in dispute about pay and service cuts. One nursing dispute about job evaluation and grading resulted in nurses eventually winning one of the biggest (on average) pay rises in their history. Earlier disputes included an ambulance workers' strike and other intermittent industrial action, including short strikes with picketing of hospital entrances, including at Fazakerley and Walton, which were the hospitals covered by my union branch. Towards the end of the 1980s and into the next decade there was a concerted, but ultimately unsuccessful, community-based union campaign to save Walton Hospital from closure. For most of these disputes, the unions worked hard to ensure the public and local communities were behind the health workers, and this was usually a fairly straightforward state of affairs, with solidarity readily offered and relied upon.

One 'constituency' that was seemingly under-represented within these solidarity networks was mental health service users, or survivors, especially organised groups; this despite there being a number of such groups across Merseyside at the time. That said, one day, when I was in attendance on a picket of the Fazakerley Hospital entrance, I noticed that also present was a man who was currently a detained patient on the ward where I was working in my first job as a nursing assistant. For the purposes of this story, I will call him Bill. Through conversing as fellow pickets, I got to know Bill in a way I perhaps never would have done in a nurse–patient relationship within the limitations of the ward environment. As a fellow activist, Bill became known to me as a completely different person to Bill the patient.

Bill was in his late 50s, not that much older than I am now. At the time, I was in my early 20s. On the ward, Bill tended to keep himself to himself and didn't talk much with the care team or other patients. Reciprocally, the staff didn't appear to make much effort to engage Bill in conversation either, and he was seen in the system mainly as having needs for self-care, with a vulnerability to self-neglect.

He had spent previous periods of his life in the local asylum (as had a few of the staff), his appearance was fairly unkempt and in staff handovers he was sometimes referred to in the pejorative clinical-colloquial as a 'burnt-out schizophrenic'. With hindsight, this paints the care team in a bad light, but my recollection was actually of a well-staffed unit, with some incredibly decent and humane staff working in a fairly impoverished environment. Use of restrictive practices such as physical restraint was low and the wards were largely peaceful environments.

Despite the undoubted qualities of the team, the service was overwhelmingly 'medical model' and the frontline treatment was medication, whether the service users wanted it or not. As such, a substantial amount of nursing staff time was devoted to attempts to persuade compliance, rather than exploring people's lives or interests (although it wouldn't be fair to say this didn't ever happen). So, Bill's interior world and his political beliefs were largely unknown to the care team, and he was seen as something of a difficult patient or, in the language of the time, a 'social problem'.

On the picket line, it took a while to strike up a dialogue but we, as it turned out, were both intrigued by each other's presence and curiosity provided a spark for some very interesting chats. Bill was haughtily dismissive of my claims to be a 'socialist' and quizzed me to elaborate and back this up with deeper reasoning. My enquiries of him to explain his antipathy to socialism precipitated the revelation that he believed anarchism to be the superior philosophy, and therefore felt our conduct of the labour dispute was wrong-headed and doomed to failure. After much conversing and Bill's entreaties that I learn more (including bringing along and lending me a well-thumbed book of collected anarchist writings), we achieved something of a rapport. That said, when we continued our discussions in the ward setting, it was never quite the same. Either Bill was determined to maintain his distance within the ward setting or the requirements of my job role demanded that I focus on clinical/administrative matters.

To be honest, I think to some extent I saw our emerging relationship as an opening to develop other conversations about welfare and care provision, as much as valuing them in their own right. Unsurprisingly, Bill was having none of this and consistently refused to engage in talk about care and treatment issues, housing or benefits – often argumentatively. With hindsight and (I hope) greater maturity, I can see that these were entirely legitimate responses, especially from an avowed anarchist. But at the time I was confused by it and tended to regard Bill's responses towards me as inconsistent and possibly due to changes in mood.

Whatever the reasons, I never fully chased up the possibility of developing an ongoing activist relationship between Bill, me and my comrades in the local union branch. Looking back, this omission fascinates me as I think I would certainly act differently now. I am not really sure how to explain this, but I do think, on reflection, that my failure to act in this regard was indicative of broader problems in the relationship between the labour movement and survivor activism, which persist into the present day. Prime among such considerations is the aforementioned argument that the left does not have a sufficiently well-developed understanding of what a politics of mental health might look like. But also, at the time, I may have been wary of inviting Bill to a union meeting because I wasn't sure of the reception he might receive from fellow union activists, and, in turn, was concerned that there might be negative reactions towards me. Alongside this was a personal discomfort at the time with union structures and processes, hierarchies and meeting protocols, which allowed the easy get out 'Why on earth would anyone want to be at a union meeting who didn't need to be there?' Indeed, I am pretty sure that Bill would have refused any such invitation. I am conscious now that, either way, this smacks of paternalism and, if I'm honest, failures of insight, courage and solidarity on my part. I'm also conscious of a failure to think outside of the available structures and forums for a way to take forward any attempt at connecting the union with survivor activism.

My lack of confidence in my own union as a supportive place where any seeming outsider might care to be present is worth dwelling on briefly. In my experience, union activists spend quite limited amounts of time talking to each other, let alone to outsiders, about politics and political analyses of workplace issues. This is true of general political matters, and even more the case with regard to mental health politics. The fact that mental health is not discussed as a politicised issue is fairly unsurprising, as there is a deplorable lack of such interest across the board. The more general point, however, might surprise people who do not spend time in union circles but is explicable in terms of the overwhelming demands placed on grassroots activists' time responding to employer-defined or initiated issues, such as discipline, grievance and bargaining over local policies and disputes.

Union forums for debate are mostly attended by the most committed of activists – effectively, a substantial minority of the total membership – and there is little time to do justice to debating tricky issues. Arguably, the debate regarding a politics of mental health is one such issue, and working out the nuances of what this could look like would need a broadening of discussions to include other participants, beyond union activists and members. New union membership renewal and organising initiatives (Gall, 2009; Hyman, 2007; Jarley, 2005; Simms, Holgate & Heery, 2013) hold some promise for opening up the relationships and communication necessary to forge the sort of dialogue and alliances that could drive such an agenda forward.

Building reciprocal solidarity in the mental health context

Most of the practised organising approaches in the UK are arguably inward-looking and emphasise internal union connections, strengthening relationships between members, between members and activists, and between members, activists and officers. Other models attempt to extend union solidarity into local communities and forge connections with other progressive groups. This is sometimes referred to as reciprocal community organising, or social movement organising, and can be seen in notable campaigns such as *Citizens* groups agitating for living wages (Wills & Simms, 2006). These approaches hark back to an era when unions and workplaces were much more attached to specific locations and communities. Also, when the union is more strongly linked to community, then matters of legitimacy are less concerning; everybody sees the value of unions, whether a member or not. A major benefit for communities of such alliance building is that unions are relatively resource rich and can mobilise these resources into community campaigns. The biggest benefit for unions is that widespread community support for union interests legitimates union action, and this is ever more important in the public sector, where the employer is effectively the government, so there is always a political edge to disputes.

An influential approach to organising was developed over decades of practice by the mainly female technical workforce at Harvard University (Hoerr, 1997; Hurd, 1993). These workers built a union from scratch by focusing primarily on kindness and friendships, so providing the basis for what have come to be known as relational organising models. Such an approach to organising was put into practice in my union branch (Saundry & McKeown, 2013). In essence, it starts with building relationships rather than talking about workplace issues or potential union responses. By the time conversations turn to workplace grievances or demands, the connections between supportive workmates has been built and can be drawn on in more typical union activity. Interestingly, the Harvard workers, inspired by feminist ideals, retained their commitment to kindness in their dealings with the employer (Leery & Alonso, 1997). This does not mean they surrender their confidence, power or assertiveness; instead, they foreground their values by preferring calm, deliberative dialogue to angry posturing or argument. In their early negotiations with the university management, the Harvard workers secured democratic systems for ensuring the employee voice was heard from the grassroots up.

An important implication for the healthcare workforce of all this organising activity is the potential for alliances with critical service-user and survivor groups. Indeed, one of the first community union organising campaigns that the Harvard workers turned to once they had secured their rights within the university was in the nearby hospital. Their slogan was 'Pro patient, pro union'. Such developments are at the heart of more recent public-sector union organising activities that I have been involved in through my own union, Unison. The other main UK public-sector union, Unite, has developed a network of community branches in a similar spirit. Trade unionists, however, cannot always assume that there will be public support for union actions in the workplace or the community. Community–union solidarity is hard won and has to be worked at.

With colleagues, I have written at length about the value and the potential problems of organising in the mental health context (McKeown, Cresswell & Spandler, 2014; McKeown, 2016b). My union has some very progressive policy on alliances with service user groups and there are many people in the union who really appreciate the intricacies of this and the sophistication needed to transcend tensions between the workforce, service users, refusers and survivors in this tricky political territory (Unison, 2011). A fully formed progressive politics of mental health has yet to be realised and variable understandings of each other's perspectives has resulted in problems in even successful conjoint campaigns. Arguably, what might begin as a staff-related struggle makes more sense and gains legitimacy when it becomes a fight that views staff and service user problems as wrapped together. Recognition of this demands we seek to form alliances grounded in mutual recognition and respect.

Trade unionists who are mental health workers need to address issues of power imbalances within services, not reinvent them in alliances; we need to be open to all allies, critics as well as appreciative groups, and we need to remember to challenge negative media portrayals of service user allies, even when this plays into wider community support for workers. On the latter point, a union strike in Manchester in 2007 gained traction in the public eye when the media recycled narratives of the workers being the last line of defence against dangerous individuals, or that they ministered to disempowered, socially incompetent people in the community. Clearly neither stereotype was true to the active and able survivor supporters of the industrial action (McKeown, 2009). Similar tensions have to be worked out between more broadly framed disability social movement groups and mental health activists (McKeown & Spandler, 2015).

Back to the future?

Reflecting on my encounters with Bill, I believe that if those events in my early career as a nurse and union activist had occurred more recently, against a backdrop of a union movement more committed to progressive models of organising, the outcome might have been different. One possibility is that Bill and I might have developed a deeper, more comradely relationship and this solidarity might have led us to interesting dialogue within and outwith the union branch in which we worked out implications for a new politics of mental health. In doing so, we could have drawn on a mutual interest in the anarchist-inspired notion of prefiguration – how we might shape the world we would like to see in the course of striving to achieve it. We would both have been able to engage with Sedgwick's book, which, among other things, vindicates Bill's criticisms of the socialist left and offers a path to a new politics of mental health that makes the most of both anarchist and socialist thinking. Reciprocal community organising would have enabled connections with service user and survivor groups in the community and joint activism within each other's campaigns; it would have promoted dialogue between workers and progressive mental health activists. Ultimately, a new politics forged in such a way would envision alternative forms of care provision that are better for both service users and staff and would effectively link socio-political understandings of mental health and society as a whole.

While exercising our imagination, we also need to contemplate some of the possible pitfalls. All parties may enter discussions and dialogue and joint actions in good faith, but problems may arise because of variable commitment to the process, or disagreement over ends or means. A consequence of this would be a sort of imperfect solidarity. This would be more likely if there was insufficient effort put into organising dialogue and debate, or if workers reverted in their activist alliances, even unconsciously, to prevailing workplace cultures and power imbalances. The lack of a reflective politics of mental health can be a chicken-and-egg scenario; either it derails discussions early on or differences constrain the collective capacity to formulate the necessary ideas for such a politics to emerge. Here it is worth revisiting Sedgwick, who suggests the commitment to an ethos of prefiguration is a way out of such pitfalls (Moth & McKeown, 2016; Spandler et al, 2016). This means that relationships and communication within alliances demand careful and concerted effort. They need to be worked at and nurtured, and not abandoned at the first sight of turbulence (Church, 1995, 1996). Careful dialogue is deliberative, is given sufficient time and ideally reflects care for each other, even when differences are asserted (Barnes, 2012).

One of the many lessons for me from my encounters with Bill, confirmed across subsequent years of attempting to do a better job of forging alliances, is that the place in which dialogue takes place is important. So too are the efforts made to ensure the conditions for constructive dialogue are established. Shifting the setting in which conversations take place from clinical to activist environments makes for better, more respectful relationships, allowing richer, more fruitful dialogue, including the discussion of the political and the personal. Thus, I have been fortunate to play the role of ally[2] to a number of self-organised groups concerned with mental health politics. One of these, a radical group in Liverpool called ReVision, has worked alongside local trade union activists and other critical groupings such as the Social Work Action Network (SWAN). ReVision also received a grant from The Edge Fund[3] to bring together trade union and service user activists in creative writing workshops, with the ultimate aim of forming personal connections to sustain solidarity.

ReVision have developed their own manifesto and contributed to the drafting of SWAN's Charter for Mental Health[4] (Kinney & Wilson, 2016). With other local service user and survivor activists, ReVision also played a key role alongside trade unions in the Save Our Sanity (SOS) campaign, which successfully defended cuts to day services and also ushered in fresh dialogue about how best to deliver such services in the future. This campaign also involved connections and solidarity with similar campaigns elsewhere in the country, with activists from Cambridge and Salford attending meetings and protests in Liverpool (Moth, Greener & Stoll, 2015). These initiatives and struggles, although imperfect in many ways, demonstrate the

2. See Russo, Beresford & O'Hagan (2018) for a critical discussion on the notion of allies in this context.

3. The Edge Fund for radical change https://edgefund.org.uk/

4. SWAN Charter for Mental Health http://socialworkfuture.org/attachments/article/172/SWAN%20 Mental%20Health%20Charter.pdf

potential of solidarity alliances and the start of work to develop ideas that could form more progressive demands on mental health services and wider society. Some of the imperfections in these and other efforts may be a result of plunging into struggle without having spent sufficient time and energy in forging the alliance beforehand. Needs must, especially in neoliberal times, but the legacy of decades of survivor activism also point to some strategies for laying more solid foundations for political alliances.

Truth and reconciliation

One of the impediments to alliances between the mental health care workforce and users and survivors of the system is the history of and on-going harm inflicted in and by that system. Arguably, a powerful feature of these harms, extending hurt of different sorts to both service users and staff caught up in the system, is the epistemic nature of the injustices therein (Fricker, 2007; Russo & Beresford, 2015). With Helen Spandler, I have revisited a previous call from the survivor movement for a form of truth and reconciliation process within mental health services (Spandler & McKeown, 2017). We see a grassroots truth and reconciliation approach as a potential stepping stone to the sort of dialogue necessary to establish more genuine and powerful solidarity among workers, service users and survivors. Along the way we hope to begin the process of healing some of the harms implicit in the mental health system as we know it. This in and of itself would appear sufficient grounds for attempting such an initiative.

We have discussed this idea in meetings of critical scholars and mental health activists, such as conferences convened by Mad Studies and the Critical Voices Network Ireland, with both positive and critical reaction (McKeown, 2016c; Russo, 2017). With Jan Wallcraft, who initiated an earlier petition for truth and reconciliation in psychiatry, we organised a fringe meeting to discuss this with Unison activists at their health delegate conference in Liverpool in 2017. This meeting exceeded our expectations for how well delegates would receive the ideas we presented, and we will be following this up in future dialogue with the union.

Conclusion: trust the tale

DH Lawrence once famously declaimed: 'Never trust the artist, trust the tale.' In the mental health field, matters of trust and tales are important in many ways, and connect with the ideas developed in this chapter. Narrow, biological psychiatry, legitimated and administered via a coercive legal framework, delivers alienating and violent experiences and outcomes, as we see in numerous testimonies, not least in the pages of this book. The very narratives that sustain psychiatric hegemony are a big part of the problem and their existence and effects constrain and deform the stories that many service users and staff are able to tell about themselves.

Union renewal campaigns are a potential opening for thinking about alliances with mental health service users and survivors and doing something constructive to build them. In the different context of attempting to organise nurses in a union in a Californian hospital managed by Catholic nuns, it is interesting to see how an element of the organising campaign illustrates a connection to epistemic concerns (Reich, 2012). Traditional organising methods were not gaining any traction in a place where the Catholic workforce and surrounding community respected the nuns and their vocational ideals and remembered their solidarity with striking farm workers in a previous labour dispute, when some nuns were jailed for supporting the strikers. The current workforce, however, were left in a bind: respect for the nuns was not helping them address important differences about pay and other aspects of their employment. The nuns' support for the unions did not extend to those within their own hospital, where the workforce was expected to be vocational, meek and selfless. The success of the organising campaign turned on the unions foregrounding moral issues about what is right and fair, with the implication that the nuns were on the wrong side of this debate.

To me, this turning of epistemic tables is also open to activists in the mental health context. The stories we tell or buy into effectively legitimise psychiatry, or aspects of it. A new politics of mental health is an alternative story (a different way of knowing, a morality tale, or episteme) and can be constructed through attention to a range of stories told from different perspectives. A prefigurative process of dialogue and testimony is one way of achieving this and, in turn, laying the foundations for future alliances. Thus, truth and reconciliation may be the way to inject more trust in hearing and respecting each other's tales. From there, we ought to be better placed to engage in care-full interaction that might help us arrive at an insightful and workable, progressive politics of mental health and sustain more authentic solidarity to take into important struggles. This feels like a goal worth striving for.

Bill's tale is now part of my own, but its influence at the time was held back by my own inability to fully trust it and appreciate its value. The beauty of our humanity is that we are able to learn from mistakes and do better next time. I met Bill in the course of a struggle I defined at the time largely from a worker perspective. I have come to appreciate over the years something that activists down the ages have always known: that any dispute worth winning has to extend its appeal and benefits to a much wider constituency. If we define our demands narrowly, we only ever win narrow victories. My lesson from a combination of insights from Bill and Peter Sedgwick, and countless others, is that the transformation of psychiatry and society can be one and the same thing.

To contemplate such change is to engage in an ongoing struggle, a struggle that arguably can't be won, or the victory won't be worth having, unless we take it on in an authentic alliance. Nye Bevan's (1952: 170) views are salutary: we need to both enjoy the struggle and recognise 'that progress is not the elimination of struggle but rather a change in its terms'.

References

Barnes M (2012). *Care in Everyday Life: an ethic of care in practice*. Bristol: Policy Press.

Bevan A (1952). *In Place of Fear*. London: Heinemann

Church K (1996). Beyond 'bad manners': the power relations of 'consumer participation' in Ontario's community mental health system. *Canadian Journal of Community Mental Health* 15(2): 27–44.

Church K (1995). *Forbidden Narratives: critical autobiography as social science*. London: Routledge.

Fricker M (2007). *Epistemic Injustice: power and the ethics of knowing*. Oxford: Oxford University Press.

Gall G (2009). *The Future of Union Organising: building for tomorrow*. Basingstoke: Palgrave Macmillan.

Hoerr J (1997). *We Can't Eat Prestige: the women who organized Harvard*. Philadelphia, PA: Temple University Press.

Hurd RW (1993). Organizing and representing clerical workers: the Harvard model: In: Cobble DS (ed). *Women and Unions: forging a partnership*. Ithaca, NY: ILR Press (pp316–336).

Hyman R (2007). How can trade unions act strategically? *Transfer* 13(2): 193–210.

Jarley P (2005). Unions as social capital: renewal through a return to the logic of mutual aid? *Labor Studies Journal* 29(4): 1–26.

Kinney M, Wilson T (2016). Putting the politics back into 'psycho': grass-roots consciousness raising in Liverpool. *Critical and Radical Social Work* 4(3): 391–396.

Leery E, Alonso J (1997). The women who organized Harvard: a feminist model of labor organization? [Online.] *Monthly Review* 49(7). https://monthlyreview.org/1997/12/01/the-women-who-organized-harvard (accessed 29 June 2018).

McKeown M (2018). No concession without demand. *Journal of Clinical Nursing* 27(13–14): 2521–2522.

McKeown M (2016a). Stand up for recalcitrance! *International Journal of Mental Health Nursing* 25(6): 481–483.

McKeown M (2016b). Educate, agitate, organise! The democratic challenge facing workers and survivors. *Asylum: the magazine for democratic psychiatry* 23(2): 21–22.

McKeown M (2016c). Can we put the hurt behind us? *Asylum: the magazine for democratic psychiatry* 23(4): 8–9.

McKeown M (2009). Alliances in action: opportunities and threats to solidarity between workers and service users in health and social care disputes. *Social Theory and Health* 7: 148–169.

McKeown M, Cresswell M, Spandler H (2014). Deeply engaged relationships: alliances between mental health workers and psychiatric survivors in the UK. In: Burstow B, LeFrancois BA, Diamond SL (eds). *Psychiatry Disrupted: theorizing resistance and crafting the revolution*. Montreal, QC: McGill/Queen's University Press.

McKeown M, Spandler H (2015). Solidarity across difference: organising for democratic alliances. In: Spandler H, Anderson J, Sapey B (eds). *Distress or Disability? mental health and the politics of disablement*. Bristol: Policy Press (pp271–286).

McKeown M, White J (2015). The future of mental health nursing: are we barking up the wrong tree? *Journal of Psychiatric and Mental Health Nursing* 22(9): 724–730.

McKeown M, Wright K, Gadsby J (2018). Introduction: making a critical case for mental health nursing. In: Wright K, McKeown M (eds). *Essentials of Mental Health Nursing*. London: Sage (ppxxii–xxix).

McKeown M, Wright K, Mercer D (2017). Care planning: a neoliberal three card trick. *Journal of Psychiatric and Mental Health Nursing 24*(6): 451–460.

Moth R, Greener J, Stoll T (2015). Crisis and resistance in mental health services in England. *Critical and Radical Social Work 3*(1): 89–101.

Moth R, McKeown M (2016). Realising Sedgwick's vision: theorising strategies of resistance to neoliberal mental health and welfare policy. *Critical & Radical Social Work 4*(3): 375–390.

Reich A (2012). *With God on Our Side: the struggle for workers' rights in a Catholic hospital*. Ithaca, NY: ILR Press.

Russo J (2017). It's not about past hurt: it's about the way you call for alliances. *Asylum: the magazine for democratic psychiatry 21*(4): 14–16.

Russo J, Beresford P (2015). Between exclusion and colonisation: seeking a place for mad people's knowledge in academia. *Disability & Society 30*(1): 153–157.

Russo J, Beresford P, O'Hagan M (2018). Commentary on: Happell B & Scholz B (2018). Doing what we can, but knowing our place: being an ally to promote consumer leadership in mental health. *International Journal of Mental Health Nursing* 27: 440–447. [Online.] *International Journal of Mental Health Nursing* 9 July. https://doi.org/10.1111/inm.12520 (accessed 27 August 2018).

Saundry R, McKeown M (2013). Relational union organising in a healthcare setting: a qualitative study. *Industrial Relations Journal 44*(5–6): 533–547.

Sedgwick P (1982). *Psycho Politics*. London: Pluto.

Simms M, Holgate J, Heery E (2013). *Union Voices – tactics and tensions in UK organizing*. Ithaca, NY: ILR Press.

Spandler H, McKeown M (2017). Exploring the case for truth and reconciliation in mental health. *Mental Health Review Journal 22*(2): 83–94.

Spandler H, Moth R, McKeown M, Greener J (2016). Editorial: psychopolitics in the twenty first century. *Critical & Radical Social Work 4*(3): 307–312.

Unison (2011). *Working with Local Communities to Fight Cuts and Privatisation: a practical guide*. London: Unison.

Wills J, Simms M (2006). Building reciprocal community unionism in the UK. *Capital and Class 82*(Spring): 59–84.

11 | Standing at the cliff edge but very safely belayed

Benny Goodman

This story is a (sociological) reflexive deliberation on my inner conversations and personal choice of action. It is about the 'personal trouble' of being male, overweight (around 12 stone) and short (five feet, four inches on a good day) in an otherwise very privileged life. It touches on the idea of 'masculinities' (note, not gender identity per se) and how they help shape my creation of my self-concept and hence a subjective sense of health and wellbeing and the personal actions I take in everyday life. Thus, it is about acknowledging the 'subjective' within society, and the power of *affect* (Fox, 2015) for the individual. It is about the construction of masculinities that, once internalised, has left for me with long-lasting and continuing feelings of falling short (no pun intended) of the 'body normal', let alone a 'body ideal' (Price, 1990). If I can feel this and survive, I do so perhaps *because* of my social privileges. I can feel very fortunate that, no what matter what I experience about my own weight and body image, I have not experienced the despair that can be anorexia.

I'm British, white, male, affluent, heterosexual, not a mental health nurse (although I am a nurse lecturer) and nor have I ever been a 'service user' of any mental health service, all of which might make me underqualified to discuss any mental health issues 'from the inside'. This chapter is therefore very much written from this perspective only. These ethnic, patriarchal, class and heteronormative 'privileges' also have the potential both to help me construct a certain sense of self (a subjectivity) and position me into a lifeworld (Habermas, 1981) that faces very few challenges to ego or sense of wellbeing. They might also have the potential to make it easy for my lifeworld to be colonised by the systematic distorted communication (Habermas, 1981) of certain power groups, due to the lining up of those interests, rendering my own critical reflexivity problematic. This is because many of the most powerful people in the UK are white, male, affluent and heterosexual and have the opportunity to shape social, economic and political narratives and structures according to their values and interests (Scambler, 2012), which fortunately align with my own. However, my adoption and continuing development of the 'sociological imagination' (Wright Mills, 1959) facilitates a critique of wider 'social forces' – such as class, patriarchy and heteronormativity – although it has been a very long personal journey, starting in 1982, which is the year I first started reading any sociology.

A more sociological underpinning to this narrative is provided by Margaret Archer (2000, 2003, 2012), who provides a rich theory of how our 'reflexive deliberations' – our 'inner conversations' – operate within the matrix of Structure/Agency/Culture. This chapter will not delve into this theory, but a reading of Archer would help practitioners better understand the complexity of human action. Another more literary source is George Orwell (1933, 1937). In both *Down and Out in Paris and London* and *The Road to Wigan Pier* (part 1), rich descriptions can be found of how human agency (food choices, for example) were mediated by position in the social structure (eg. unemployed miners) and working-class culture(s) in the north of England at that time in history. Orwell uses a 'sociological imagination' before Wright Mills (1959) really clarified the concept.

I am pulled up sharp by the realisation of the power of the effect on their experiences of the subject positioning of those who do not share my privileges. A sociological analysis also exposes the complicity of care systems that have some of the character of 'total institutions' and that can dehumanise through 'mortification of the self' processes (Goffman, 1961). This might seem obvious to some, but my nurse education in particular often led me to act *and think* as a normative agent of neoliberal individualism (Gadsby, 2015), which locates health, illness and disease firmly within a biomedical individual self and seeks solutions to misery, illness and disease *within* individuals rather than acknowledging that they arise also from social and political action.

Following on from Archer (2000, 2003, 2012), I acknowledge my own reflexive deliberations as a 'communicative reflexive', my dominant mode of reflexivity, which seeks consensus and considers how others think and feel before I act. Reflexive deliberations mediate between the objective facts of social conditions and one's personal projects and concerns. Communicative reflexivity, I theorise, results in my decision-making and acting, which can be characterised as 'going with the flow' and which, in an obesogenic environment, results in health behaviours that lead to weight gain. In my case, this is not a dangerous outcome per se.

In addition to critical sociology aiding an analysis, cognitive psychology is also an ally. Daniel Kahneman (2012) gives us the concept of heuristics – that is, 'mental short cuts'. This is the normal function of human thinking, which requires the reduction of cognitive loads and thus engages in short cuts or 'heuristics' that allow us to quickly come to conclusions about the world around us. Confirmation bias is one such commonly discussed heuristic and results in the seeking out of evidence that confirms a pre-existing theory while ignoring contradictory evidence. The 'affect heuristic' suggests emotion is important in guiding judgments and decisions and also acts as a mental short-cut to aid quick decision-making. As Fox (2015: 2) argues: 'Alongside reasoned choices and decisions, what humans *feel* has a part to play in producing the world.'

Conscious reasoning, in this view, is therefore mediated by heuristics.

This goes against the grain for me. I like to think I make rational decisions based on cold, hard analytical thinking (Kahneman's System 1), but it could be that my decades-long struggle with weight gain and my life-long 'struggle' with being short is rooted in 'emotion': the surface raft of rationality hides the deeper seas of *affect*. Knowing at some level that I figuratively and literally do not 'measure up' to *socially constructed* male norms may well be an emotional driver underpinning my daily actions around food choice and exercise.

However, this is not part of my self-concept; it is not supposed to be this way. I come now to think that I've never really accepted the reality of being short and overweight and that this has manifested in myriad subtle ways in my life choices. I also realise that this is the first time I've written that down.

The writing of this story initially focused on the weight issue, but during the writing the height 'issue' has had to be acknowledged as also a problematic. I also acknowledge that, set alongside the experiences of many other people lacking my privileges, this potential 'poor me' story is self-indulgent. I've never had to face the harsh realities of being 'mentally ill' and thus, what do I know?

I need no emotional comforting beyond the 'self-medication' administered over the years in what others might term 'maladaptive coping'. I am fortunate, I have prospered, but this realisation is juxtaposed against the many who have not, or to a lesser extent. I have no lessons for mental health students beyond my story and a consideration of how one's place in the social structure and the positive health assets (Scambler, 2012) one enjoys may be protective against the development of substance abuse, eating disorders, anxiety and depression and suicide.

An analogy comes to mind. Rock climbing has been an aspect of my life ever since joining the Royal Navy mountaineering club for a weekend in North Wales back in 1975. This was before 'sticky boots' were widespread and before modern, comfortable harnesses facilitated 'belaying' – that is, being held securely with rope. So, it was that I found myself up a rock face on the mountain of TryFan, wearing combat boots, scrambling for a foothold and wondering where the next handhold would be. Always just out of reach, it seemed to me. Well, of course they were, given how 'stumpy' (the Royal Navy description of me) I was. I was both terrified and exhilarated. Many years later, I was standing on the granite cliff edge at Bosigran in West Cornwall, staring down to what looked like a steaming, boiling sea many metres below. The only thing between death and a glorious day climbing was the rope belay. If I wished to be free from the rope, all I had to do was unclip and go. A very simple action. I never thought about doing it, but it was very clear how easy it could be. It was, again, both terrifying and exhilarating. Other climbers had been killed at this spot, perhaps for taking one too many risks.

It's a cliché but being on the edge is where life becomes more precious and transient. Is that why we go there? What is wrong with jigsaw puzzles? I still own a motorcycle and have more than flirted with substance use. I might be what some have referred to as 'neophile' (Haidt, 2012); not for me boring tradition, custom and practice. I want to look over the edge, but perhaps I have always known that it is safe for me to do so. However, I have a psycho-social 'belay': a suite of 'positive health assets'. It is perhaps why substance use never became 'addiction', why my relationship with food never became an eating disorder and why being pissed off with being short and overweight has never descended into depression.

Health assets

Graham Scambler (2012) takes a sociological approach to understanding patterns of health inequalities. He postulates that each of us experience flows of health assets in our lives. The assets are usually weak or strong 'across the board'; they have particular impact at critical junctures in our lives; they have a cumulative effect over the life course, and subjective evaluation of our assets may have a compensatory affect over the objective reality (objectively, poor income, but subjectively, money does not matter). He argues there are seven assets that flow in our lives: material, biological, psychological, social, spatial, cultural and symbolic.

The 'material' health assets (wealth, income) are, however, 'paramount'.

If I conduct a quick inventory of the flows of health assets in my own life, I note, and would argue for the protective effects of, positive health assets across the board: that they were positive at birth and early childhood, adolescence and middle age (critical junctures) and that they are having a positive, cumulative affect as I grow older. Generally, my subjective evaluation of most health assets has been positive, bar the biological, in which I have always felt I was dealt a poor hand. This sounds terribly self-indulgent and self-pitying, especially if you know that I was born with no physical disabilities at all (apart from congenital cataracts). Yet I have to acknowledge the lifelong wish to be taller and the two-decade-long wish not to be overweight.

Overall, though, this suite has been a strong belay, saving me from tipping over the edge in any dangerous way. My inner conversations never were that of Archer's (2003) 'Fractured Reflexive', whose inner disorientation in the world often prevents positive action being taken. My culture was protective, my position in the social structure was protective and thus my personal actions were never self-destructive.

If the positive assets have been protective, what other techniques have I employed to stay at the edge and never go over it?

Self-tracking, self-policing

My reflexive deliberations lead me to analyse my own lifeworld and an instance of that is the personal data tracking I undertake as part of the process of the 'quantified self'. An aspect, of course of doing so (self-tracking) is the health reason: I don't want to develop type 2 diabetes. Another aspect is tracking progress or otherwise in my main sporting activity, now that climbing is a bit much: cycling. But I also have to acknowledge it is also for aesthetic reasons, which is, on the face of it, a pathetic reason for a nearly-60-year-old, short, bald, overweight man.

I acknowledge how my subjectivity is constituted by culture, that culture runs through *myself*. This leads me to consider issues such as obesity/fatphobia and the misery of body image: body reality v body ideal. This discussion is normally reserved for young women. I have been protected by white male privilege from feeling their pain and distress, which may result in the status of user of mental health services. If there is a lesson for mental health students here, it is one of addressing the socio-political context and the structural transformations of society that highly structure, while not determining, personal stories.

The suite of positive 'health assets' are protective. I don't need or seek counselling, but it occurs to me that, if even I can feel this way, then it may be an indication of the thoroughgoing level of 'dis-ease' with bodies prevalent in Western society. With fewer health assets, might I have fallen prey to maladaptive coping as an answer to body alienation?

I self-police using self-tracking as part of a strategy to become something I am not, in an attempt to achieve body ideals I know I should reject out of hand.

For me, the socio-political context is crucial, the biopolitics of it all. I contend that the 'neoliberal imaginary' has colonised the lifeworld of too many people, including me. Gadsby (2015), in his discussion of the 'UnRecovery Star', mentions an 'onslaught of neoliberalism in mental health, in which people are to be made individually responsible for difficulties which would be better thought of as originating in society'. This includes the happiness (Gadsby, 2017), mindfulness, resilience and wellbeing 'industries' that individualise problems and solutions rather than seeking structural changes. The critique is a take on Erich Fromm's (1955) *Sane Society* and Herbert Marcuse's (1964) *One-Dimensional Man*. Fromm's reversal of psychiatry is pertinent here – what if culture/society is insane? What if society is selling unrealistic, unhealthy, unattainable body ideals – a process speeding up with advent of the digital and quantified self? 'Insane' and unattainable social masculinities are always in the background, so that my subjective self, pointing accusatory fingers at itself, never quite 'measures up' socially and literally.

Personal tracking

It is Monday morning on 23 January and I weigh myself: 12st 4 lbs and 30.1 per cent body fat. I have (of course I do, as I'm a middle-class 'worried well') a set of scales that is electronic and wirelessly linked to my fitbit app on both smartphone and ipad. I am the same weight as last Monday. I have watched my weight fluctuate during the week and return to where it started. Another week has passed with no progress. In fact, I have put on between five and six pounds over the Christmas period. I have returned to wearing the fitbit after a six-month absence in a bid to increase my physical activity. This week I have, every day, passed the 10,000-step target, and have recognised again the motivating effect of this constant tracking, as a few times I have forced myself to go out for a walk on a cold January evening. The non-weight loss is disappointing, to say the least. I have also recently signed up for Public Health England's 'One You' health campaign and have downloaded their drink tracker app. This shows that, for the past three weeks, I am averaging 19 units per week, including two or three drink-free days. I have not tracked food intake and that has to be the next step, but as I've done this before, I am not convinced it will do anything other than provide data. There is something else going on; I have a clue (sedentary job – cold and dark evenings so not conducive to my cycling), but it is not the whole story.

I am the 'quantified self' (Lupton, 2016) engaged in 'lifelogging, personal informatics, personal analytics' and I agree that these 'practices, meanings, discourses and technologies associated with self-tracking are inherently and inevitably the product of broader social, cultural and political processes' (Lupton, 2016: 1). I can guess at what these broader social and political processes are, but at the level of *affect*, I have to grapple daily with a gnawing *feeling* of body dissatisfaction. I think I have a handle on what the 'influences, discourses, technologies and power relations and systems of thought' (Lupton, 2016: 1) may be, but do I have the power to resist, to feel differently or to uncover why I subject myself to this daily routine?

The sociological imagination

Wright Mills' *The Sociological Imagination* (1959) is a key work in the sociological literature and provides a way of thinking about our experiences as individuals in society at any given point in time. The argument is that, to fully understand ourselves, we have to apply the 'sociological imagination' to our 'personal troubles'. The relevance is that this takes us beyond making an overly *simplistic analysis* of the health behaviours, experiences and decisions of patients, clients and, of course, ourselves. If our analysis is too simplistic, then we come up with partial answers to healthcare issues at best and irrelevant, judgmental or dangerous answers at worst.

Wright Mills (1959: 3) wrote: '...men (sic) do not usually define the troubles they endure in terms of historical change.' We are 'seldom aware of the intricate connection between the patterns of their own lives and the course of world history'; we may not 'possess the quality of mind essential to grasp the interplay of man and society, of biography and history', and so we 'cannot cope with their personal troubles in such ways as to control the structural transformations that lie behind them' (p4).

So, what is a 'trouble'? These occur within the individual's immediate experience and relationships. They relate to the individual self and to those areas of social life of which the individual is immediately, directly and personally aware. The description of what the trouble is and what the solutions are comes from the individual and occurs within the scope of their 'social milieu'. A trouble is a private matter and such troubles arise when we feel our values are threatened.

My personal trouble is the distance between body reality and body ideal as defined by certain masculinities that I have internalised as well as critiqued. My subjectivity includes distorted visions of male physical identity that play out in affect and compensatory behaviours.

In applying the sociological imagination, I take Wright Mills' questions and try to analyse historical changes and connect my own life with broader historical developments. Importantly, I try to control structural transformations that result in the 'dis-ease' I feel.

What is a 'structural transformation'?

If we think of society has having 'structures', which vary from society to society and within the same society over time (history), we may begin to understand that society 'works' when individuals, groups, communities and populations decide to act out their relationships with one another and in doing so create (and are created by) social 'structures'. Relationships between people both evolve as humans live their lives and then also act as structural patterns for others to follow. In the jargon, these are 'generative mechanisms' working 'behind our backs' (see the work of Roy Bhaskar (1975) and 'critical realism' as social theory, which underpins Margaret Archer's work (2008)). This process of 'evolution' and 'pattern' changes over time and between societies. Thus, an individual is both shaped by these (structural) patterns of living and, in living their life, in turn shapes the patterns (structures). Our lives are thus 'structured' but not *determined* by these structures. Archer (2008) refers to morphogenesis (process of change) and morphostasis (stability) and ponders why this occurs. Why are some of us pattern followers and why do some of us break free? Her answer is that 'reflexive deliberations' mediate between structure, culture and the exercise of personal agency.

In my case, what social structures are there, what cultures am I embedded within, that lie beneath my personal troubles and my choice of action?

To help answer that question, Wright Mills argued that:

> ... what (people) need... is a quality of mind that will help them to use information and to develop reason in order to achieve lucid summations of what is going on in the world and of what may be happening within themselves... this quality...[is] the sociological imagination. (1959: 5).

Linked to my perceived lack of height is being overweight. So, what information do I have about weight gain – rate, prevalence, risk groups, epidemiology, aetiology, social determinants? To fully understand why my own BMI is not within the 'normal' range, I'll need to examine social structural changes and cultural shifts over my lifetime and how they are embodied within me.

These social structural changes involve and include my own socio-economic status, which make the purchase of goods and services aimed at both weight gain (eg. wine and malt whisky) and weight loss (carbon fibre bicycles and cyclo-touring holidays in France) easier and thus set up an opposing binary; the abundance of fossil fuels to use for energy, instead of food (eg. cars replace cycling and walking); the easy availability of calorie-dense, high-sugar, processed foods; the reduction in occupations that require the expenditure of physical energy and my own choice of a sedentary occupation, and the marketing of body ideals and products aimed at men. The cultural changes include modes of masculinity that include a 'health culture', the social meanings, price and availability of alcohol, and the increasing sexualisation of body presentation for both men and women.

So, to what degree have I been responsible for gaining this weight? I lived through a time when the public's understanding of diet was perhaps rudimentary and constrained by availability and the social norms that construct perceptions of a 'healthy' diet. I have experienced 'socialisation', which involves learning the values, norms and beliefs regarding food of a certain culture. During my younger adult days, to what degree was vegetarianism popular and/or promoted as a healthy option? We need to consider what a healthy diet is and how the public get to know. In addition, to what extent is the abundance of sugar, in the form of high-fructose corn syrup, implicated in this? My early life would have been guided by social norms and what shops could provide, as well as cost, of course.

I have to also to acknowledge the potential psychological process of 'future discounting', the role of affect, the role of pleasure, and the physiological – dopamine/serotonin/endorphin responses all operate at this point in time, in this society. I am a free agent but not a rational one, maximising utility based on means/ ends calculation. My actions are highly structured without being determined. As a consensus seeker (communicative reflexive), I tend not to rock the boat in social situations. Therefore, as part of a culture (the Royal Navy in particular) that valued drinking highly, I was not about to be the odd one out.

My *personal trouble* is weight gain but it is also a *public issue,* as the whole UK population has gained weight. So, we need to connect changes in social structures and historical events to my personal story to fully understand my current health and the decisions I know can and cannot make in managing my weight. The role of sugar in the diet is an issue; what is the history of the dietary advice regarding fat and sugar? I may well have been consuming sugar in amounts that seemed normal and, indeed, were hidden. This could be part of what is called an 'obesogenic environment' in which we are all immersed and have been for several decades. What did I believe and think about sugar in my diet? To what degree did rational thinking about the risk to weight from eating a 'normal' UK diet feature in my buying, cooking and meal-preparation decisions?

'The sociological imagination enables its possessor to understand the larger historical scene in terms of its meaning for the inner life' (Wright Mills, 1959: 5).

This is what Wright Mills refers to when he argues that:

The first fruit of this imagination...is the idea that the individual can understand his own experience and gauge his own fate only by locating himself within his period, that he can know his own chances in life only by becoming aware of all those individuals in his circumstances. (p5)

Wright Mills and public issues

These are matters that go beyond the local environment of the individual and their inner life. They result from the 'organisation' of many such situations into the structure and institutions of society. The countless individual social milieux overlap and create society at points in history. An issue is a public matter; issues threaten values held by the public. When this happens, there may be public debate about what that value is and what really threatens it.

To adapt Wright Mills to my ends:

When... only one man is [overweight], that is his personal trouble, and for its relief we look to the character of the man, his skills and his immediate opportunities. When... 15 million... are [overweight], that is an issue, and we may not hope to find the solution within the range of opportunities open to any one individual. The very structure of opportunities [for not being overweight] has collapsed. Both the correct statement of the problem and the range of possible solutions require us to consider the economic and political institutions of society and not merely the personal situation and character of a scatter of individuals. (1959: 9).

What the individual fat man (out of the 15 million) experiences is often caused by structural and cultural changes in society. When global economics means that high-fat, high-sugar-loaded foods can be produced very cheaply (a structural change), then we have a plethora of fast-food outlets and supermarkets selling cheap, calorie-dense food. To be aware of the idea of social structure and to use it is to be able to trace links among a great variety of individual social milieux, and that, as Wright Mills states, 'is to possess the sociological imagination' (p11).

I am not the only man who is overweight. Therefore, my personal issue is also a public issue for society. To fully understand one's life means understating how society has changed and the opportunities and threat to health that arise as a consequence. It means understanding that personal agency, the freedom to act, operates within particular social structures that constrain action as well as provide enablements.

Understanding obesity using the sociological imagination links the personal trouble of weight gain with the public issue of whole population shifts in BMI, within the context of the obesogenic environment. A fuller understanding of 'fatness' goes beyond overly simplistic equations of calories in = calories out and simplistic exhortations to 'eat less, move more'.

Weight gain and obesity as a wicked problem

On one level of analysis, weight gain for the individual is a simple cause-and-effect, linear relationship: calories in, balanced with energy expenditure, equals weight stability. Framed this way, this can be thought of as a tame problem. To lose weight we have to change the balance between calories in and energy expenditure. We can objectively measure the problem with BMI and calorie counting. The focus and unit of control is the individual's physiology and behaviour, which may be amenable to behaviour-change technologies and educational approaches. Failure to lose weight is seen as being down to failure to apply behaviour-change techniques or, more subtly, failure to apply relevant 'nudges'. Obesity is individualised, biomedicalised and subject to scientific analysis based on physiology and metabolism studies. It shares this with the dominant forms of institutional psychiatry as critiqued in this book.

However, an approach that acknowledges the social and political determinants of health recognises that obesity is a multi-factorial, 'wicked problem' arising out of a complex of various systems that include the individual's physiological system, the food manufacture, distribution and marketing systems, our urban landscapes and travel systems, changing occupational structures and the political economy of profit-based, techno-food capitalism. Christakis and Fowler (2007) suggest network phenomena are relevant to the 'biological and behavioural trait' of obesity and that social ties may be important in the spread of obesity among communities.

We have to understand subjectivities and how culture flows in and through self and that self is both constitutive and constitutes culture and society. These construct for us our lifeworlds, our taken-for-granted and background assumptions, values, attitudes, social patterns, norms, mores and beliefs. Constructs such as obesity and fatness need to be contextualised in a social world in which there also exist eating disorders and wider problems of body image, a context in which there are vested interests and powerful discourses at play that shape our subjectivities and lifeworlds.

An individualised, biomedical, reductionist, mechanistic, linear world view allows arguments about the health properties of individual foodstuffs to be framed in terms of the consumer's individual responsibility for health. This allows debates about sugar taxes to be framed within nanny-state versus individual-responsibility tropes. It also allows the efficacy of sugar taxes to be framed within the 'calories-in versus energy-out equation' so it can be stated with conviction that certain foodstuffs in and of themselves are not harmful to health and thus the consumer should be the ultimate arbiter. This allies itself with both the neoliberal imaginary and the liberal humanist self. Both philosophies delineate clear boundaries of responsibility and agency for the individual and allow market solutions, health education and consumer choice to be touted as the only and best solutions. The ease with which we understand individual responsibility within a linear cause-and-effect world allows us to elide a social determinants of health understanding into a 'lifestyle drift' solution beloved of many health policy advocates, especially those in the political arena.

A Facebook exchange nicely illustrates this phenomenon. Responses to a post, 'It's poverty, not individual choice, that is driving extraordinary obesity levels' (Cohen, 2018), included:

> It is a matter of education with food, along with people being able to take the necessary, time and steps to get this done.
>
> I'd prefer to think it is something to do with accountability. If you can stuff your face with all the foods you love (and are marketed to love, eg. sugar rich) without have to personally take the consequences, then a fat bugger you will be. You only have to see the glee on people's faces as they take a moment from tucking into their cakes, fizzy drinks, pasties, Greggs pies and Domino pizzas to rejoice in a new miracle pill that will take them back to their trim selves without having to change their pork life. If you want to change the arc of the obesity epidemic then people need not only to be re-educated about food but re-educated to understand that it is their responsibility and not that of an overstretched (forgive the pun) NHS.

Why do I not do the 'rational thing' for health?

Mental health nurses engage with people in their social contexts. An argument can be made that behavioural decisions that have health impacts are influenced by the psycho-social context in which people find themselves and not just by their rational understanding of risks and benefits, derived from education. This context includes the actions of those with vested interests, cultural expectations and myriad health messages and information that form the basis of educational initiatives.

An assumption might be made that education equals knowledge and that knowledge equals action based on a rational analysis of risks and benefits. As a lecturer in nursing, I know the 'facts'. I know the physiology, the biochemistry, the dopamine and serotonin responses; I've read about metabolic adaptation syndrome, the Barker thesis, insulin resistance and the Glycaemic Index.

I know from experience as well as from the literature that the 'education = action' relationship is a false assumption. If my weight reflected my knowledge, I'd be as thin as a whippet.

While it is the case that certain health-risk behaviours, such as smoking, are reducing, and certain causes of death, such as cardiovascular disease, are also reducing, we face increases in obesity and diabetes. It appears that, although we know what a healthy diet is and that moderate exercise is beneficial, we continue to make consumer choices about food and other consumer products and pay little attention to the health consequences. The myriad health messages appear to have only a modest effect on many groups in society. For example, 2012 figures suggested that 33 per cent of men and 45 per cent of women do not achieve recommended levels of physical activity in the UK (Public Health England, 2014). Therefore, we need to think about why people appear to ignore healthy messages in a consumer society.

Standing at the cliff edge of health, why do I buy consumer products that are deleterious to health and avoid healthy goods and services? When we choose a particular product or service, it seems that its health benefits are not our first criterion; in fact, we may discount health as irrelevant. My purchasing decisions are not based on 'utility maximisation', meaning the availability, price and quality of a product and the degree to which it meets a fundamental need. Utility is the degree of satisfaction one gets from the purchase of a good or service, but this is not the underlying mechanism.

One hypothesis is that the mechanism at play (behind our backs?), for some of us, at least, is that we are more interested in status and differentiation in our purchasing decisions than we are in health. My decisions to climb rock faces and to engage in 'now gratification' could be based on deeper feelings. Could it be that my own physical status is on view to anyone and thus, objectively, I fail to live up to structures of idealised masculinity, and climbing gives me back that status, as well as being pleasurable in its own right?

Back in 1798, Thomas Malthus argued, interestingly, with reference to status and social judgements:

> The cravings of hunger, the love of liquor, the desire of possessing a beautiful woman will urge men to actions, of the fatal consequence of which, to the general interests of society, they are perfectly convinced, even at the very time they commit them. Remove their bodily cravings, and they would not hesitate a moment in determining against such actions. Ask them their opinion of the same conduct in another person, and they would immediately reprobate it. *But in their own case, and under all the circumstances of their situation with these bodily cravings, the decision of the compound being is different from the conviction of the rational being.* (My added emphasis)

Although I am not predisposed to agree with an 18th century preacher, I can spot the beam in my own eye. Objectively, I would counsel my risk-taking self not to try to compete with other men; that height, although in one sense an objective fact, is a mere social construction that cannot be put right by prowess on the rock face, or in any other arena. Of course, another retort is that rock climbing is not about any deeper meaning at all; it is about the surface 'affect' – it feels good. Am I in danger of over-psychoanalysing common behaviour?

However, the rational human actor model is here rejected. Instead, it might be the case that action, behaviour and choices are affected by the nature of social relationships within what might be called consumer capitalism. One theory is that consumerism is driven by unconscious, sublimated, repressed desires fuelled by such discourses as the pseudo satisfier, dissatisfaction manufacturing and convenience constructing (Stibbe, 2009). This draws on Freudian psychoanalytical theory about the unconscious and the interplay of ego states. The discourses might be open to empirical verification – that is, we can describe them and test them in actuality – but unconscious desires remain theoretical while also providing some explanatory power.

Another theory is that behaviours are driven by the need to differentiate between ourselves. The theory suggested by Heath and Potter (2006) is that people buy 'stuff' to feel superior, whether that is cooler, better connected, better informed, more discerning, morally superior or just plain richer (2006: 106). Brand identity in consumer capitalism is about establishing differentiation. That is why branding is important. It also reduces the 'cognitive load', making purchasing decisions easier.

A third theory is that 'status anxiety' (de Botton, 2004) results from the desire for differentiation, to be higher on the social scale, and from the attendant anxieties that result from how one is perceived by others. This may relate to the 'psycho-social comparison thesis' (Abbot, 2007), which suggests that people (short, fat men?) compare themselves in small groups to referent others (tall, thin men?), and where they feel disadvantaged, they experience, or sublimate, negative emotions injurious to health. In my case, that might mean having to daily establish masculinity through risk taking (sport, drugs, sex) to compensate for being short, overweight and bald.

Wilkinson and Pickett (2009) posit another mechanism, that of psychosocial comparison, and argue that inequality within countries also has pernicious effects. These include eroding trust and increasing anxiety and illness. They identify 11 health and social problems (from physical health to child wellbeing) and argue that for each one, outcomes are significantly worse in more unequal countries. More recently (Wilkinson & Pickett, 2018), they followed up their analysis to argue that more equal societies reduce stress, restore sanity and improve everyone's wellbeing.

Products, goods and services in consumer capitalism are not neutral objects devoid of social meanings (Baudrillard, 1970). Fred Hirsch (cited in Heath & Potter, 2006) differentiated between *material* goods, such as bread and steel, and *positional* goods, such as status and property. Positional goods are zero-sum – that is, we can't all have them but we all want them. An example would be a house in a 'nice area'. Veblen goods might be positional goods, as they help to differentiate and position people in the social hierarchy. A Veblen good is one whose price rises with the demand for it, because of its exclusivity and appeal as a status symbol. The 'sign value' (Baudrillard, 1970) of Veblen goods indicates exclusivity, superiority, differentiation and high status. A Louis Vuitton bag is a Veblen good, as is an Aston Martin. I have to admit that, reflecting on the climbing equipment I owned and the way I wore it at the cliff edge, I was clearly feeling that exclusivity, superiority, differentiation and status. We were 'rock climbers', not mere mortals having a day out at the Cornish coast.

Positional goods signify and enable membership of an exclusive club. Conformity and distinction go together; one conforms to the standards of the distinct class in order to differentiate from the 'other'. Consumption is thus driven by differentiation and status seeking. The value of a good comes from a sense of superiority associated with membership of a club. This may apply as much to dreadlocks and hip hop as to Louis Vuitton bags and Beethoven. Does the 'sign value' of a good signal this sense of differentiation? I have pictures of me in climbing gear at classic climbing locations. I also have pictures of me in motorcycling gear and on various bikes, and latterly on bicycles during my frequent long-distance cycle rides in France. In each, I am establishing membership of a club, differentiating myself from 'ordinary' men, but also claiming 'uber' masculinity. The photographs, the clothing, the branding and the equipment are all part of the show; they have 'sign values'. This is not *necessarily* injurious to health.

What all of this suggests is that many decisions have much more to do with personal assessments of social status and the drive to differentiate oneself from some social groups (in my case, short, fat men) and identify with other, more valued, aspirational groups (tall, thin men). This analysis may not apply to material goods that have physical triggers and rewards, such as the dopamine response associated with sugar. Yet even those goods might have a positional sign value. For example, teenagers buying high energy drinks might be doing so to signal to others their membership of a distinct social group, as well as to obtain the physical stimulus they provide.

Masculinities, illness and obesity

Cecil, McCaughan and Parahoo (2010) described male participation in cancer support groups and the impact cancer has on masculinities. This small, qualitative, pilot study, which was conducted in Belfast, involved semi-structured interviews with eight men with a history of cancer who were no longer being actively treated (ie. they were not receiving chemotherapy or radiotherapy). Whereas most studies of men with cancer that looked at issues of masculinity have been on prostate and/ or testicular cancer and have tended to focus on *sexual ability* and *activity*, this study identified more sociological issues of concern that also present challenges to masculinity and to male identity.

Three issues seem pertinent for these men surviving cancer in Northern Ireland:

- money worries – perhaps their role of 'breadwinner' is undermined
- their other roles in life and how cancer changes that
- body image – their virility and strength might be challenged.

Cancer is, of course, not the same as being overweight, but the subjective experiences of these men might be able to tell us something about masculinities. These are the subjective experiences of *this* group of men, and we can see that, for them, cancer not only brings about physical changes but also challenges the very idea of what it is to be a man. Are these men feeling a loss of control and power over their jobs, their lives and their women? In the context of testicular and prostate cancer, the loss of sexual function, or perceived loss, perhaps diminishes them both in their own eyes and in the eyes of wives and girlfriends.

But what do we think being masculine actually means for other men? Are these ideas fixed in society? Raewyn Connell (2005) discusses what being masculine means and considers that it is a dynamic concept: namely, what it means to be a man is not fixed and can change over time and across a society. Masculinity is about where one sits in a power structure, and therefore there is more than one masculinity. So, we must be careful to understand that a change in health status may be subjectively different for the metrosexual man, for example, living in central London. Connell also refers to a 'world gender order in which men continue to have power over women'. A cancer diagnosis for a man will of course impact on his family and partner, and if they are feeling challenged in the most fundamental aspect of their identity, this may well impact on their ongoing relationships. We might ask whether we have a set of norms and patterns for the 'correct' social response to these challenging issues.

Gender identity intersects with class and ethnicity in myriad ways and so, to more fully understand subjectivity and health behaviours, we need to consider these aspects as well. As already noted, my personal intersections of gender, class and ethnicity have, I believe, placed me in a more privileged position than others.

This anonymous post from the US raises the issue of obesity, ethnicity and class in the relationship between men and their doctors, arguing that condescension, arrogance and rudeness from some doctors may also be class and racially based:

> The problem is, a LOT of doctors are rude, condescending assholes who may be very good scientists and diagnosticians but are HORRIBLE at customer service! For a lot of men – including myself – going to a 12:15 appointment but not being seen until 2 and then being told a whole lot of stuff that I already know AND having to deal with medical arrogance is insufferable!
>
> Add to that that I'm *fat, African American* and *working class* and multiply the rudeness factor x 20. I know I'm going to be accused of being a fat pig and a glutton and will be branded as a liar if I comment on what I eat – I know the doctor won't give a damn if I give him/her an accurate description of how I got fat in the first place – and I know that I will be blamed, guilt tripped, shamed and not listened to – why would I want to subject myself to that bullshit (AND have to pay a $20 co pay!). If I want to be insulted for being fat, I can find some neighborhood elementary school kids who will do it for free! (Emphasis added)

Here the writer illustrates obesity as a 'fatphobia' or as a personal moral failing, which might be the default position of some healthcare professionals. Being fat could be seen as not taking responsibility. This view downplays or challenges the idea of an obesogenic environment. It buys into the cultural/behavioural explanation for health – ie. that illness arises because of your cultural habits and behaviours (eating junk food and smoking for example) – and it also forms part of the moral underclass discourse, which focuses on the failings of people themselves and locates the origins of illness in their ignorance and fecklessness.

So, being a man in a particular subculture can be dangerous: you take risks occupationally, which you might not be able to avoid, for example, in the construction industry, and you take risks with lifestyle choices because that upholds your idea of masculinity. Not going to the doctor because a) they are a different class and b) 'that's not what men do' and c) you cannot afford the time or money further places you into a place of risk of undetected health problems.

Implications

Health and illness are to be thought of as arising from social structure as well as, if not more than, biology. The knowledge that weight gain results not just from the individual's choice of diet but also from the socio-political environment should indicate that nursing has a public health and socio-political role. Health education is not just an individual issue, based on a biomedical understanding; health has much wider determinants. The concept of an 'obesogenic environment' suggests just that. Therefore, strategies that will assist people to move towards health must take into account the social and political context in which they live. Society has to change, as much as the individual. Individualised models for change that ignore this will have less chance of success. The nurse must become, like the social scientist and the liberal educator, an agent for social change.

Nurses work with individuals and thus understand that illness that at first may seem self-inflicted, out of free will, may result from the person's social milieu. Blaming of the unpopular patient, the obese, the self-harmer, the drug addict, the alcoholic is not only poor practice but is theoretically myopic. That is to say, it does not understand the wider determinants of health. This realisation should change the language and the practice of nursing into a more open, less judgmental stance towards the patient. Discourses that *always* focus on individual failings, psychiatric diagnosis or organic disease are *partial* discourses and may miss something vitally important in understanding our actions.

If people 'cannot cope with their personal troubles in such ways as to control the structural transformations that lie behind them' (Wright Mills 1959: 4) then the profession of nursing must be a force to transform the social structure that results in public harm and personal troubles.

This last statement is a normative (value-laden) description of nursing and is therefore open to critique. Without the sociological imagination, however, this question would not even be raised.

To summarise:

- Health and illness both derive from socially structured human agency, societal as well as biology.

- The patterns, experience and causes of health and illness have to be understood in the context of history, social structure and culture.
- The meanings that people attach to health and illness not only are built by social structure but go towards creating social structures.
- Professionals need to acknowledge the complexity of health and illness and adopt a more open, non-judgmental viewpoint.
- There is a social/political and public health role for nurses.
- Models for change have to go beyond individualised, psychiatric, biomedical understandings of health and illness, and realise that 'education' is not a universal panacea.

Progress

At the time of writing (February 2018), I'm no lighter. I was much fitter, having completed a nine-week couch-to-5K training programme early in 2017. I also undertook another big cycling trip of 1,500 km in France in July 2017, involving four Alpine stages of the Tour de France and finishing off in Provence on the iconic Mont Ventoux. This trip saw me lose at least 14 lbs in weight. As it happened, I experienced angina at the top of Mont Ventoux, and on my return to the UK underwent an angioplasty. I regained all the weight I lost in just over six months.

I should not be surprised. The Cornish obesogenic environment (which includes pasties, craft beer and clotted cream) and my love of good food and wine and now forced sedentary living as I undergo cardiac rehabilitation involving medications, have worked their magic. My privileged health assets are not enough to prevent the return of the weight. I will not be depressed, I will not be anxious. But I will acknowledge that a good deal of my emotional and cognitive loading every single day will be about aspirations towards a leaner, fitter male self, better equipped to compete in a 'man's world'. I know this is useless, I know it is not necessary, I know on one level it is stupid. I'll tell myself that just a bit more planning and the application of willpower will sort it, at the same time that I'll tell myself this is untenable, unrealistic and a complete waste of my time. If my personal trouble was, say, habitual and problematic cocaine use or depression instead of the privileged obsession with weight (and height, it seems!), this realisation would be frightening. I'll engage in more adaptive and maladaptive coping mechanisms; I'll wallow in dopamine rushes;, I'll engage with the 'What the hell effect' and blame that. I'll argue against behaviour change techniques as a justification for my own failure to live up to my body ideal. Mindfulness and resilience will be held up as two imposters in glorious justification of another week gone by with little change. The 'pleasure principle' will be indulged, its fires stoked as a compensatory measure.

My inner conversations, my reflexive deliberations, have more recently involved a degree of 'fractured reflexivity' (Archer, 2012) due to the challenge to my cardiac status and its implications for the ongoing masculine body ideal, which is just not tenable.

I will not be seeking the assistance of counsellors, of psychoanalysts or of mental health services. My privileges, which include socioeconomic status, social relationships and positive cultures, I believe are still very protective. However, I do recognise that standing on the edge has become more real somehow… and that precarity of existence recognises no one as special. We can all fall.

References

Abbot S (2007). The psychosocial effects on health of social inequalities. *Critical Public Health 17*(2): 151–158.

Archer M (2012). *The Reflexive Imperative in Late Modernity*. Cambridge: Cambridge University Press.

Archer M (2008). *Realist Social Theory: the morphogenetic approach*. London: Routledge.

Archer M (2003). *Structure, Agency and the Internal Conversation*. Cambridge: Cambridge University Press.

Archer M (2000). *Being Human: the problem of agency*. Cambridge: Cambridge University Press.

Baudrillard J (1970). *The Consumer Society: myths and structures*. London: Sage.

Bhaskar R (1975). *A Realist Theory of Science*. London: Verso.

Cecil R, McCaughan E, Parahoo K (2010). 'It's hard to take because I am a man's man': an ethnographic exploration of cancer and masculinity. *European Journal of Cancer Care 19*(4): 501–509.

Christakis N, Fowler J (2007). The spread of obesity in a large social network over 32 years. *New England Journal of Medicine 357*: 370–379.

Cohen M (2018). It's poverty, not individual choice, that is driving extraordinary obesity levels. [Online.] *The Conversation*. https://theconversation.com/its-poverty-not-individual-choice-that-is-driving-extraordinary-obesity-levels-91447?utm_source=facebook&utm_medium=facebookbutton (accessed 2 July 2018).

Connell R (2005). *Masculinities*. Berkeley, CA: University of California Press.

De Botton A (2004). *Status Anxiety*. London: Penguin.

Fox N (2015). Emotions, affect and the production of social life. *British Journal of Sociology 66*(2): 301–318.

Fromm E (1955). *The Sane Society*. London: Routledge.

Gadsby J (2017). The Layard Report: *The Origins of Happiness*. How science can transform our priorities. [Online.] *Critical Mental Health Nurses' Network*; 23 January. https://criticalmhnursing.org/2017/01/23/the-layard-report/ (accessed July 17 2018).

Gadsby J (2015). The Recovery Star meets the UnRecovery Star. [Online.] *Critical Mental Health Nurses' Network*; October 2015. https://criticalmhnursing.org/2015/10/19/the-recovery-star-meets-the-unrecovery-star/#more-350 (accessed July 17 2018).

Goffman E (1961). *Asylum: essays on the condition of the social situation of mental patients and other inmates*. London: Random House.

Habermas J (1981). *Theory of Communicative Action: vols 1 and 2*. Boston, MA: Beacon Press.

Haidt J (2012). *The Righteous Mind*. London: Penguin.

Heath J, Potter A (2006). *The Rebel Sell*. Chichester: Capstone.

Kahneman D (2012). *Thinking Fast and Slow*. London: Penguin.

Lupton D (2016). *The Quantified Self: a sociology of self-tracking*. Bristol: Polity Press.

Malthus TR (1798/1976). *An Essay on the Principle of Population*. New York, NY: WW Norton & Co.

Marcuse H (1964). *One Dimensional Man*. London: Routledge.

Orwell G (1937). *The Road to Wigan Pier*. London: Penguin.

Orwell G (1933). *Down and Out in Paris and London*. London: Penguin.

Price B (1990). A model for body-image care. *Journal of Advanced Nursing 15*(5): 585–593.

Public Health England (2014). *Everybody Active, Every Day*. London: Public Health England.

Scambler G (2012). *GBH: greedy bastards and health inequalities*. [Online.] https://grahamscambler.wordpress.com/2012/11/04/gbh-greedy-bastards-and-health-inequalities/ (accessed 20th February 2018).

Stibbe A (2009). *The Handbook of Sustainable Literacy*. London: Earthscan.

Wilkinson R, Pickett K (2018). *The Inner Level*. London: Penguin.

Wilkinson R, Pickett K (2009). *The Spirit Level*. London: Penguin.

Wright Mills C (1959). *The Sociological Imagination*. Oxford: Oxford University Press.

12 | On the borderlands of care: towards a politics of welcoming

Erica Fletcher

> To survive the Borderlands
> You must live *sin fronteras*
> Be a crossroads. (Gloria Anzaldúa, 2007)

Within this nonlinear narrative, I trace the porous, problematic forms of care surrounding myself, my older sister, who experienced mental distress, and a patchwork public mental health system. I also consider what it means to live in Houston, USA, a site of slow violence – a city exploited yet nurtured by industries of petroleum, medicine and space technology – and how it shapes our experiences of suffering (Nixon, 2013; Tuana, 2008). Drawing from postcolonial scholarship, radical ecopsychology and my own mixed cultural background, I write against what Vimalassery and colleagues (2016: 1–2) describe as 'colonial agnosia', against the sense that 'colonialism is simultaneously everywhere and nowhere'. In small ways, I trace the 'persistent violence of colonial displacement'. I seek to comprehend the many small ways we suffer from the ideologies that have given colonialism pervasive powers. I explore the borderlands of care where relationships fracture and our bodies reject systemic demands for particular forms of rationality and logic. Together, separately, we resist and uphold the diagnostic and prescriptive regimes that have perpetuated destructive notions of sovereignty over our bodies and lands.

Affirming a narrative of interdependence against and alongside our counsellor's prognosis of codependence, I sought to validate my inclination that the micro-aggressions enacted within medical and educational bureaucracies, memories and premonitions, climate change as mental duress, personal visions and fears are all valid ways of describing the wounds inflicted by structural violence and inadequate social support (professional or communal). They are small pathways for my sister and I to recognise the mutual suffering we endured and work together to craft stories that can weave together. Our relationality, our sisterhood, our ability to care for each other open us up to new ways of being together, beyond social pressures to establish financial or residential independence from each other. Rather, our interdependence helps us begin a slow healing process.

More broadly, this chapter responds to tensions between the emerging field of Mad Studies, which largely critiques epistemologies and methodologies of psy disciplines through an intersectional feminist lens, and the older field of psychopolitics, which tends to take a Marxist framework to uphold the importance of providing social services against the neoliberalisation of the helping professions (Cresswell & Spandler, 2016). I join this conversation from a post-colonial perspective to ask, what are the limits of a Mad Studies approach to noncoercive treatment in a neoliberal city whose gaps in the social services do not allow for me to engage with my sister in the way she would prefer? I centre my discussion on the immediacy of what is at stake – my sister's physical safety – even while I question my own actions and beliefs as a young scholar who began her academic career as a Mad Studies ethnographer.

In small, everyday solutions, we found workarounds and moments of subversion that made sense to us. More broadly, these small decisions allude to an uneasy alliance that can be made between a field of scholarship that seeks to trouble, even dismantle the psy disciplines and one that seeks to uphold and rehabilitate them. Within a politics of welcoming both disciplines and the strange, novel scholarship that emerges from their intersections, my experience as a caregiver helps me affirm an uneasy third space between these fields.

Despite our internal contradictions and divergent opinions about what should be done, we find our own way through the tempest together. Against colonial agnosia, beyond a biopsychiatric approach to treating mental disorder, we do our best to recognise communal loss and welcome reclamation. To illustrate our haphazard navigation of tricky mental spaces, I purposefully conflate time, space, and imagination so they layer upon themselves in unusual ways (Reid, 2014). I collapse time boundaries in my autoethnographic writing; past, present and future meld into a hybrid stream of consciousness. I switch between first and second person narration. I draw promiscuously from popular media – blog posts and journalism articles – and from academic scholarship and personal experience (Anzaldua, 2015). My citations allude to the body of work from which I draw, but I purposefully do not define the terms used or the full context of the scholar's work. I aim to suggest kinship, rather than perfectly incorporate their theories and commitments into my own. In this way, I seek to advance messy texts of postcolonial scholarship as a tenuous bridge between Mad Studies and psychopolitics.

When you approach the floodwater's edge, drink a tea of valerian root, lemon, chamomile and honey. If that does not work, try some wine. You will soon find that madness is an underworld of fears and fantasies that can no longer be veiled. You will be a doula for your sister, travelling with her through her altered mental states. When you can stand it, you will bear witness to her sadness, her mourning the passing over of three generations in your family, her concerns about a dystopian future. You will hurt her as you both navigate the florescent halls of well-intentioned bureaucracies. Attend family counselling sessions; she participates in them for your sake too. Help her fight against a diagnosis that does not represent all that she is, all that she could be. If only there could be a quiet place for her to exist, to live beyond the fray, the heat of Houston's sprawl, where plants and animals could be her antidote.

Shroud yourself with busyness. Publish or perish. Craft a myth that encompasses you both, even the city itself. Turn the ethnographic gaze back on yourself, on that which will bring shame to your family. Neoliberalism turns your family's suffering and dishonour into a sentimental book chapter (Tamas, 2009; Rodriguez, 2017). And yet, perhaps these words resist this end as well.

My sister and I live in the colonised land of Houston, Texas, the fourth largest city in the United States of America. We live on the borderlands between madness and sanity, within industrialisation and assimilation. We mourn our losses on this toxic land, the displacement of our family, the uprootedness of inhabiting a global capital of petrochemical refinery and trade (Harper, 2004; Wingard, 2013). We walk in circles back to each other. We find a way to spin our stories again and again.

In 2016, my sister Jessica and I landed in a windowless office of a well-intentioned psychiatrist in Houston's public mental health care system. Dr I, a middle-aged, sharply-dressed psychiatrist, listened to our struggles, pieced together from my recollections what other psychiatrists had suspected, noted my sister's silent rage, her noncompliance, her anger with the situation into which I had dragged her, her anger with me. She diagnosed Jessica with type 1 bipolar disorder.

It hurts to type those words – the diagnosis – knowing they have a troubling power to them; knowing that they most certainly can never represent what came to us; knowing she will read this. I have misinterpreted her reflexes, her response to grief. She will feel badly for the suffering she has caused me. She will tread lightly because she cares for me, because she has always supported my academic career, because she knows I must profess my truth. Even so, these words could cause her harm. They could become warped or distorted.

My sister and I do not speak in diagnostic terms, except perhaps when I am upset or frustrated with her or when I am speaking to someone who I know will not understand me – or her –anyway. When it is just us, I refer to those troubled times as 'tricky spaces' – times in Spring 2016 when she saw in binary, spoke too quickly, incomprehensibly, stared vacantly, paced barefoot, felt background 'noise' – a controlling haze of fears and directives – or spoke so slowly it seemed like her thoughts had been lost in the effort to speak them at all. In the summer, the hottest on record, she had classic, undeniable symptoms of psychosis – rapid speech patterns, inhibition, nonlinear thought, instant shifts from elation to devastation.

I am not my own. I am not myself, and neither is she. Together, separately, we dissolve, resist, reform, respond to the misfortune and ills that come to us. Codependent? Interdependent? We ask ourselves, each other. We argue – an occurrence that rarely happened in our childhood. She has not slept for days, and so neither have I. She does things she has never done in front of me. I will keep her secrets, but they hurt me too. 'Maybe I like getting into trouble. Maybe I am trouble,' she taunts me. There is something wild in her eyes. She tells me I am not helping her – that she should have never told me that her mind had started to shift again. As if she could keep it from me. As if it were something she could keep from everyone else.

As children, we found ourselves thrown into a family rife with diasporic tensions – migration, assimilation – and again the cycle repeats. My mother, a descendant of Taiwanese indigenous peoples, immigrated to Brazil as a child to escape the longstanding effects of the Japanese encroachment on the island and the US-backed White Terror that followed it. She was raised in a Buddhist family and converted to Christianity as a young adult, near the time she graduated from dentistry school. At an English-speaking church, she met our father, an American immigrant. He had also grown up in Brazil after his father moved his family there to set up the first computer systems in the city of São Paulo. There our parents married and soon after immigrated to the United States, where our father studied aerospace engineering. As toddlers, we settled into a mouldy apartment complex in Texas, near the National Aeronautic and Space Administration's Johnson Space Center, where our dad would eventually work as an engineer. The cloudy night sky glowed orange and purple outside our apartment. We learned about the moon and stars, but they seemed foreign to us. Our parents joined a fundamentalist Baptist church in the era of the Religious Right and the Moral Majority. Our mother, who could not practise dentistry in the US as she had in Brazil, taught us a conservative Christian curriculum at home – she taught us to shun the world of sinful delights and temptations.

We were still young girls when spells of great sadness and confusion began to come to our mother. After a year of caring for our grandmother, who was dying from cervical cancer at the age of 57, our mother was heartbroken after she passed.

Our mother's episodes of madness grew and clouded over our adolescence, as did her divergent realities. Despite these challenges, or because of them, she managed to convince our father to break from the fundamentalist church. She became more and more distrustful of people around her and grew to rely on me for emotional support. I was 15 when paramedics and the police took her away from our home. I saw how poorly psychiatric staff treated her at an academic hospital, in the same university system I would later attend as a graduate student. Our mother was eventually diagnosed with bipolar disorder and schizophrenia but refused the diagnoses and any psychopharmaceutical medication. As with many others, her 'symptoms' fell uneasily between the two states and sometimes, many times, she was perfect 'able' to serve as a homemaker (Luhrmann & Marrow, 2016). She stubbornly believed that the world had conspired against her. I was the only one who believed that there was something fundamentally true in her assertion.

Later, my sister's state-sponsored counsellor would ask us both to draw out our family trees, with markers denoting who was dead or alive, which relationships were strained. She asked us to explain our origins. She let me borrow her book on codependency (Mellody, Miller & Miller, 2003). She was genuinely interested in our past, I am sure. Eventually, she came to refer to our background as 'cultural issues'. She was not wrong, exactly. I am sure she had been trained in cultural competency (Hester, 2016). But she would never be fully culturally competent, and our family's past can never be distilled down to a tree and marks for divorce, separation or disavowal. Such classification systems – these family trees – have always been tools of anthropologists, the colonisers (Behrouzan, 2016; Fanon, 2008; Anzaldúa, 2015; Metzl, 2009; Burstow & LeFrancois, 2014).

I lived only 20 miles away from my mother and studied at the University of Texas Medical Branch's Institute for the Medical Humanities. My dissertation was a loosely veiled attempt to understand her non-consensus realities, to legitimate her madness, to validate my own critique of her forced treatment. I moved away from Texas for almost a year, to conduct ethnographic research with The Icarus Project, a grassroots network of mad activists (Icarus Project, 2013). When I returned, I lived at my parents' place for a couple weeks before returning to Galveston Island to finish writing my dissertation. A month after I graduated, my mother died suddenly of a massive stroke, in September 2015. She was 52 years old. I was inconsolable.

Four years before my mother died, I began to hold within me a deep sense that the time of her departure would be coming shortly. I began my mourning. Or maybe I was just suffering from imposter syndrome, a common occurrence for naïve graduate students. Sometimes I would take antidepressants and do my best to slog through graduate school. The feeling of doom was not logical, I was told. A friend in medical school, who planned to go into psychiatry, diagnosed me with catastrophic thinking and magical thinking – typical of depressive states. And, for a time, such a prognosis would give me peace. 'Of course, my fears are just that. Irrational. Nonsensical,' I told myself. But that proclamation did not sit well with me either.

The summer before my mom died, I started to feel as though my sister was entering a frenzy. She was having the best summer of life, she claimed. There was something in her voice – in her separation from the world – that irked me. I told my partner that I felt Jessica could go mad. He reassured me that she would be just fine. In hindsight, he said what I needed to hear at the time. And he was wrong as well.

My thoughts played out these episodes for a lifetime, as they had done when I was a child. I began wondering if my preoccupation with madness, my resistance against and capitulation to the psy disciplines, had contributed to my sister's breakdown. My inability to 'help' my mother through her madness had presented itself once again in my sister – the cycle of loss and codependence that would not end. If the biological ties that bind us had an undeniable fatality to them, would I too become incomprehensible to those who loved me? Perhaps the illness would not come to me – but a life drowning in others' madness seemed too much to bear as well. 'That is just me catastrophising again,' I would tell myself gently, hopefully. Maybe it is still naïve of me to think I can create an ecological narrative that is big enough to encompass all of my family's glimpses into nonconsensus realities. But what else can I do?

My sister's grief over our mother's death came more slowly and violently than mine. As the seasons changed, Jessica learned that she was pregnant. She felt scared and unprepared emotionally, relationally and financially for her and her husband to care for a child. She had been deliberately unemployed for over two years and her savings from her time as an engineer in the oil and gas industry had dried up. She lived in a noisy, gentrified neighborhood, and she could not sleep deeply. On Christmas night in 2015, we talked in hushed tones about getting an abortion before it was too late. A couple days later, she made up her mind to end the pregnancy. Texas, a state that made national headlines for cutting funding for reproductive health, has strict abortion laws – laws that would only become more strict the next year. She breathed deeply, refusing complete sedation as an older physician performed the operation. After the procedure, we had lunch at a 24-hour diner, one we had frequented in college. We smiled at each other from across a booth and shared a strawberry pie for dessert. I drove her back to the house she had been renting with her husband and two other roommates. I did not realise how deeply defeated she would come to feel (Luhrmann & Marrow, 2016). Looking back, her story seems to have checked off almost all of the social predictors of psychosis, but I am not sure that this form of knowing would have helped us.

Two months after the procedure, one of her roommates called me on her behalf and I cut short a weekend trip to San Antonio, driving back past wildflowers that had come early that year. I found her in a state I had never seen her in before. Later, Jessica told me that she remembered my embracing her as she cried, mourning our mother's loss for what felt like the first time. She felt as though I held her for a long time – it was less than five minutes. Her perceptions of time grew further and further distorted. She came to my place for a restless, fitful night. She wanted to walk outside – sound amplified in my studio apartment. She wanted to investigate what she felt were the sounds of war. Houston felt like a menacing whirl of grime and alienation. She was scared. She was angry at me for wanting her to stay inside. She grabbed a knife. We fought with words, bodies, minds. The next day, my dad and I took her to the Emergency Department of the nearest public hospital. She was uninsured. Despite my research into peer support and mutual aid, I was at a loss for what else I could do. I was traumatised too.

Over the year, time played tricks on me as well. Time became something that was not my own. It escaped me; I could not make plans; I could not achieve the goals I had set for myself as a 25-year-old scholar. I was supposed to shop out my book proposal and publish my dissertation on radical approaches to mental health as a monograph. Instead, Ben Taub, Harris Health's neuropsychiatry clinic and their Strawberry Clinic in Pasadena, St Vincent's student-run, free clinic in Galveston, National Alliance for Mental Illness meetings and the Harris Center for Mental Health and IDD became my field sites and battlegrounds. I felt the forces of the psy disciplines around us. I worried about how our engagement with such social services would affect us both. Caregiving had a way of clearing my schedule, limiting my capacity to do more than just care for my sister and mourn.

Every week I receive an automatic notification from this book group's email thread, asking me what I have accomplished. 'Does keeping my sister out of the hospital for a few sleepless days count as an accomplishment?' I wonder. Journalling, taking fieldnotes of our maddening interactions, saving paperwork from our visits with healthcare professionals – it seems as bizarre as attempting to get my sister to fill out paperwork to get her social services while she was still in altered, paranoid state. A pile of primary sources grows. Memories shift and morph with time and distance (Jones & Kelly, 2015). My archive is a mess (Cvetkovich, 2003). I am a poor historian.

Flash floods came to Houston that year. Eight people drowned on Tax Day. Ten thousand homes were flooded. Our bayous, drainage ditches and flood ponds were not enough to curb the toxic flow. In response, Mayor Sylvester Turner apologised to residents and hired Stephen Costello as the city's first chief resilience officer.

Costellos's job was to listen to complaints from displaced residents. Little was done to improve the city infrastructure (Satija, Collier & Shaw, 2016). Houston was resilient. The rusting urban beast was too big to fail. And Hurricane Harvey was far beyond our horizon of possibilities.

When the world is too much for you, sink into your bed; let it be a cave to lick your wounds at night. Hold your partner close as you grapple with your sister's becoming someone else. Tell yourself that her journey through this underworld is not like your mother's madness; that her becoming will not be like your mother's in breadth or scope. Forgive yourself for your missteps, for the moments when you did not show your sister or your mother the kindness and respect they deserved. Emerge when you can, if you can. Be careful of those who cannot carry your secrets well.

Over the summer months, Jessica found herself in tricky spaces – some worse than others. The friend who was hosting her at the time would text me when the world was shifting too quickly around her. Having tapered off psychopharmaceutical medication after her first mental break near the beginning of the year, Jessica wanted to explore a new ontology as someone who experiences intense spiritual awakenings, wide emotional valences, time distortions and energy fluctuations, without the mediation of traditional psychiatric treatment. I worked around her wish not to be hospitalised as much as I could, but the basics of her life became my struggle in patience. She was listless and slow speaking throughout parts of the day. At other times, she became animated, zealously pursuing trains of thought and laughing uncontrollably. I would ask her to take a shower or eat a meal I had prepared or to change. She would look at me as though she did not understand the sounds coming out of my mouth. As if the sounds themselves were pointed arrows pricking her skin. I started clapping, at times, to get her attention, to help her focus on the task at hand. Now, looking back, I am sure that the claps hurt her or scared her. But the sounds would bring her back into herself, even just for a moment. She would finish chewing some of her food.

Revisiting the literature on the Open Dialogue model spurred me to initiate family dinners with my dad and sister that year (Seikkula & Olson, 2003). I didn't tell them about Mikhail Bakhtin's theories on dialogism, and it didn't matter to them anyway. The food and a sense of duty was enough to bring us together. We tried to have a meal together every week, especially when the tricky spaces became more frequent. She would eat silently, as my dad and I made small talk, hoping our words could smooth over the awkwardness we all felt about the situation. More often than not, we would have dinner every other week, and as things stabilised, once a month. We did not have the capacity to come up with a larger plan to work together. We could only be this much engaged when we were all still coping with the shock of what had come to us. I am sure Open Dialogue can work, with enough guidance and social support. But I was often tired and felt rather alone in trying to bring our family together. My attempts at communication often failed.

A friend of Jessica's started a small discussion group on Facebook Messenger about helping her. They were worried that she was suicidal. A friend who was living abroad at the time added me and Jessica's partner in the thread and listed suggestions for ways Jessica could find help through medication and counselling. One of them suggested alternative healing practices – an idea that was quickly shot down by most everyone else in the thread. Another one suggested sliding-scale counselling at Legacy Community Health, a nonprofit organisation nearby that had a six-week wait time. Six weeks felt like an eternity at the time, and Jessica would have to set up an appointment herself. In her current state of cognition, that would have been a Sisyphean task. Explaining to her friends that Jessica did not want either medication or talk therapy felt exhausting. I told them that we had already come up with wellness actions plans that she had used until this point, but that she was not in a state to implement them now. I was doing what I could to respect her decision not to have treatment, yet I felt both attacked as though I was not doing enough to help her and also abandoned by those who claimed to care for her. [It was around that time that she walked out of my house and rode the buses in an altered state. I could not bring myself to stop her.] They were too far away to do the work of being in community with her or too busy with their own lives to take off time from work to be with her. I cancelled my Thursday classes. These friends' physical absence made me feel even more alone. Open Dialogue only works when everyone makes crisis a priority, when there is an adequate safety net to keep those in need housed and fed.

In the days leading up to her hospitalisation in September 2016, I found myself alone again with her. My partner was out of town, and hers was gone as well. I was working as a visiting assistant professor at the University of Houston. I spent the humid nights with her when I could.

What felt like a long time later, in just a few days or weeks, she was back at my house, and this time there was really no support from those who knew how to be with her through her altered frames of mind. I called a crisis intervention hotline and talked to a woman. Maybe her name was Pamela? She asked me why Jessica did not want to take medication, how long she had been out of work and staying with a friend. Pamela, like the social worker at the emergency walk-in clinic we visited a few weeks previously, reiterated the various mechanisms for hospitalising my sister.

After a few more hours of watching Jessica's mental states deteriorate and fearing that she might soon start walking the streets of my neighborhood, I decided to go with the cheaper option of calling a crisis intervention trained (CIT) officer through the Houston Police Department. Taking her to a mental health court would have cost me $150 and a lot more time. I was operating on little sleep and needed to prepare for the four classes I was teaching that week. I called 911, knowing that I had failed my sister by not honouring her wishes. A uniformed officer came to our house in a police car. I asked him if the CIT officers would come. He said that only a couple of CIT officers were on call for the whole city and that he was the only response. Jessica's eyes widened even further when she saw him. She did not know what to do.

A few minutes later, a red CIT van, converted from an ambulance, showed up as well. I guess they had not communicated with each other. Now, there were four officers to we two. They asked me a battery of questions once they realised they would get very little, if anything, from my sister. An older man in a red polo shirt asked Jessica if she was suicidal or homicidal. There was no attempt at subtlety. In her listless state, she could barely form one-word responses. Her hair was long and unkempt. A chemical heat pricked at our skin. They noted that she had not showered in days. They did not have the time to wait for her truncated speech. I said what needed to be said for them to take her away. They wrote what they needed to write to get her treatment. I knew she did not understand what was happening to her, that I had done a violence to her. I knew she would not trust me for a time. They gave me an option to attend the mental health court hearing that would commit her to the Harris County Psychiatric Center. They would code her 'ASIAN' on their medical records. At least she was beautiful and underweight. She would not be criminalised. They would treat her well, unlike other patients (Rosenthal, 2016). I declined the offer to attend the hearing. I was so very tired, and I had a class to teach that afternoon.

Pamela called me back when I was at my office to follow up with me before she left her job at the hotline for the day. I told her what happened, grateful that she cared enough to check in with me. Maybe calling back is standard practice. But it felt reassuring, nevertheless. Her soothing voice on the line had been more help than anything else I could find at the time.

In the middle of September 2016, Jessica was housed for a week in a lock-down psychiatric ward for people with dual diagnoses at the Harris County Psychiatric Center. I stood in line waiting for an Indian family with a dozen small plastic containers of food to pass through security's metal detectors. I went up to the third floor and took a left down a long hallway. A brown-skinned, middle-aged woman from Jamaica, a psychiatric technician, came up to me to tell me that my sister was a sweetheart. That she had caused no trouble. I smiled at the nurse, wondering if she felt as trapped here as I did.

On 18 September 2016, I told my sister the news of our grandfather's passing. My mother's father died in São Paulo, Brazil, exactly a year to the day that my mom had died the year before. Our grandfather learned Japanese and trained to be a nurse for Japanese soldiers who had invaded Taiwan. Later, after he immigrated to Brazil, he was imprisoned for selling counterfeit watches. He survived two years in prison, the Brazilian dictatorship, great economic instability and a contentious relationship with our grandmother, who we suspect engaged in sex work to support their family. Our grandfather was a quiet, unassuming man. He had lived a long life.

Jessica did not react immediately to the news of his passing over, but I started crying in the ward's communal space. She held me as we sat on heavy, plastic, maroon chairs, weighed down so they could not be thrown. She missed him too, of course she did. But in that moment, she only saw me saddened by our loss of him, our mother's death, our precarious future. Her arms wrapped tightly around me, we sat next to a shatter-resistant, double-paned window and the sun set and turned the sky a soft pink and purple hue. Jessica said that she stared at the clouds quite a bit there, that they were some of the most beautiful clouds she had ever seen. A few days later, she would grow upset and distrustful of me for having committed her, but in that moment, we were together.

I picked her up from the hospital six days after she was admitted. She was relieved to be outside once more and upset with me that her stay had happened at all. She had little tolerance for so-called healing practices that involve intrusive bureaucracy and constant surveillance. Still, a couple days after she was discharged, I gathered together the paperwork with her to enter Houston's public mental health care system. The first day, I drove her from where she was staying; the next day I called her multiple times and waited nervously until she showed up, late, to our appointment. We spent four hours on two separate days wading through the red tape of the intake system. We saw a case manager, a social worker, a nurse, a psychiatrist, a pharmacy tech and a pharmacist. There should be a special circle of hell for people who devise these systems of paperwork that need to be filled out by someone who is still experiencing alternated mental states. Jessica reluctantly, angrily, signed forms she could not at the time comprehend. While I waited indoors for her name to be called, she sat outside doing yoga or meditating in a small patch of landscaped grass. The medication slowed her cognitive function. I felt like being with her slowed mine and wore down my patience too. It is not as though this system is particularly healing, but my sister's New Age community and all of their alternative healing practices have never adequately supported her either.

We walked out of the intake centre to the parking lot to go our separate ways. She turned to me after a long day and said: 'I did not feel suicidal until people started asking me if I was.' She wielded her words strategically, knowing they would wound me. If this was her way of resisting diagnosis, so be it. I wondered silently if her medications were making her worse – a common complaint among those who have experienced the full violence of the psychiatric system. I was at a loss for how to respond. She knew she had won this round. I retreated to my car and drove away in tears. Oppressor, oppressed – who knows who is who by now?

Train your college students to listen to others, to excavate the stories behind the ones that are on the surface. The affordable housing centre where they will collect oral histories will become a sanctuary for watching others' stories slowly becoming unearthed. This is the time to be present, to witness, to listen. It is precious and fleeting. Students with their coursework and residents with their many appointments, jobs and visitors have little time or energy to share. Value their labour. Remember the residents who have volunteered their presence to teach your students. The many misfortunes and fateful turns that have come to some are far worse to bear than your own burdens; the least you can do is help residents and students tell each other's stories well.

Grade liberally. You were not on top of your game this semester either.

Local history is important in contextualising one's place within it. So teach your students about Houston's history. About Juneteenth, about Reconstruction and Jim Crow. Remember Alva Braziel. Remember Sandra Bland (Shackleford, 2016). Hope that your students will learn from the past, embrace a community's capacity to build bridges, to come together in hard times. Profess your truth that the people united will never be defeated, even if you are not sure that is the case.

The era of the radical professor is over, an online journal declares (Nair, 2017). You stare at your laptop screen and nod your head in agreement. There is nothing radical about working a precarious position at an enterprising university. You find yourself turning bitter, just a few semesters after your own graduation.

On the night of 8 November 2016, Jessica and I sit on my porch as the election results trickle in. Unfortunate circumstances had brought us together that evening. We wonder what has become of a country that never seemed quite ours. Just a couple of miles away, petrochemical refineries along the Houston Ship Channel quietly emit toxins that contribute to disproportionate rates of childhood asthma and leukaemia in the neighboring Latino communities (Union for Concerned Scientists, 2016). The next morning, I wake up to the news that Trump has been elected president. Tears well up in my eyes. I greet my morning cultural anthropology class at the University of Houston. I am surprised that anyone has shown up. We watch Hilary Clinton's concession speech on a projector. We are all stunned. We are the second most diverse public university in the country and most of the student body will be directly affected by the xenophobia and travel bans and environmental deregulations that are to come.

Thanksgiving 2016 marks a shift for the better. My partner's family flies down to visit. I prepare a feast for them, my sister and my dad. We stare into the same fire for several hours; it's a cloudy night. Quiet conversations lapse into silence. There is much to consider. Jessica has returned to herself, it seems. If not that, her mind has settled somewhat from its restless state. She stopped taking her medication several weeks ago. Now it is easier to breathe. Even still, I know the threat of another breakdown is very real. It hangs heavy in the air. Jessica has other ways of interpreting what happened. I am not sure which she clings to the most but for her sake, I hope she can hold on to the multiple threads for as long as possible.

When the fall semester is over, and a gentle winter comes, breathe a sigh of relief. You and your blood have made it through the underworld once more. Your sister will move in with you and your partner. She will be wanted in your family. She will help you grow a herb garden, sweep the floors, talk of life and death, make tea and find beauty in the unexpected. Your stories will weave together.

In Spring 2017, I invite Jessica to teach Reiki in my Introduction to Social Medicine class. She talks about the practice earnestly, while I contextualise the history of its practice, describing its role and function in providing care and tensions between its legitimation through clinical experiments and the ineffable sense of care that escapes quantitative measure and scholarly interpretation. A pre-medical student plays the antagonist in the group. He asks about the evidence behind this practice, its limits in the face of disease. The others, mostly Brown students, understand that there is something else going on.

Jessica brings out pendulums to demonstrate energy sources. I lie on the floor in the classroom while she lays her hands over me, searching for cold and warm points in my chakras. My students laugh or stare in disbelief. One of them snapchats the demonstration on his iPhone. My sister's acts of care for me have a flair to them as well.

Ironically, if she had been in paid work, Jessica would have been billed several thousands of dollars for her hospital stay and for her use of other social services. Being indigent probably spurred her breakdown, but it also saved her from medical debt. What is more, Jessica's hospitalisation in the fall enabled her to enroll in an early intervention programme, complete with a case manager, a peer support specialist and counsellor who will meet her at our home, into which she has recently moved.

I ask her if I can do some family counselling with her. Jessica makes the necessary arrangements to switch counsellors to a woman who would be better suited for us both. In April 2017, her new counsellor comes over to our home. By this time, I have long given up hope of finding a counsellor without a two-month waiting list who is willing to take my health insurance. Jessica is still resistant to any form of social services. I am sceptical for other reasons. Nevertheless, over a few weeks, we let down our guards and accept what we can. Every visit, our assigned counsellor asks about the start of Jessica's health insurance coverage, which will signal the cut-off of her sessions with us. We are on a short timeline for 'recovery' – two months to be exact. We must heal quickly, even though none of us believe these things work in this way. We are all constrained.

Our counsellor does not understand Jessica's desire to live off the grid. How can I explain that Jessica has never wanted to work for the petrochemical industries and that her options, as an engineer, are very limited in Texas? Her critiques of capitalisms are not like mine, but they are deeply felt antagonisms to an industry that is surely speeding up global warming. There is no time to talk about climate change, only about behavioural changes.

Likewise, our counsellor does not understand my own preoccupation with community-based strategies to promote mental wellness (this is what I tell her is my work, instead of using the term 'Mad Studies scholar'). Her expression when I tell her I question my decision to send my sister into forced treatment at the hospital indicates her skepticism towards my defence of social justice perspectives within disability rights. I doubt myself too. I know not to bring up my critiques of sovereignty over minds and lands – how we all came to extract and dominate each other. I am not sure how I would define my research or intellectual stance now – my thoughts are muddled and I censor myself (Cresswell & Spandler, 2016). Even so, with this counsellor, I have found a sympathetic ear for my cause as a caregiver, a person to whom I can confide my fears. I have found validation of my responses to situations that were thrown at me. It feels good to vent about everything I felt I could not share with my sister or others. I use diagnostic labels, secretively. They roll off of my tongue liberally – an indulgence of sorts, far different from my talk of 'tricky spaces' and my clunky academic use of 'mental distress'. For this time, I grow less preoccupied with my critiques of the psy disciplines from Mad Studies. I want whatever help I can get.

------

14 May 2017 is the second Mother's Day since our mom died. I am feeling anxious and grumpy throughout the day. I have started a new hormonal birth control a few days ago and have been feeling more on edge than normal. I do not respond well to medicalisation either. Over the last few weeks, allergies have been getting the better of me, and I am finding it hard to sleep through the night; I wake up sneezing. I do chores about the house, clearing the dust from bookshelves and vacuuming the rugs. The time to clean is precious. I clean and wallow in self-pity that no one is helping me. It's a trivial concern, I know, but I still feel empty and over-extended, as though – after all of my efforts to help them – my family is not taking my health needs as seriously as I deserve.

In the evening, Jessica and I attempt to go to a Buddhist temple nearby our house, but it is closed. I drive us to a gas station to fill up for the week. She asks if she should pay, since she will be using the car for work over the next two weeks. It is a small gesture, but one that I appreciate. As I drive back to our home, she asks me what is on my mind. I tell her I am upset with my partner, although I'm really upset with both of them for not helping me with the chores. And, underneath that guise,

I am still reckoning with the shock of the last few months, and a deep fear that I will once again regress into my role as a caregiver. She starts off with some unhelpful advice, and then falls silent. She tells me, 'That must be difficult.' We drive the rest of the way back home in silence.

I give Jessica the keys to my car, which we are now sharing. Houston is a driving city, a city long averse to public transportation. If we did not share my car, she would have a two-hour commute one way on the bus, meandering slowly to her workplace through the urban sprawl and patchwork ethnic enclaves (Wingard, 2013). She goes off to another Buddhist temple nearby. I take a walk, feeling moody and altogether too womanly. I feel the weight of Jessica's precarious situation around me. She hates her job, but at least she has one. It is hard to imagine the world otherwise, when we are both struggling with the constant traffic and lack of city planning. I walk angrily towards the downtown, near where old Chinatown used to be. Tears breach the corners of my eyes.

When I come back home, Jessica has set up an altar of sorts on our dining room table. She has placed a bouquet of Gold Star Esperanza in a glass vase over a yellow table runner made of silk, a gift from Buddhist monks in thanks for her playing the violin at one of their events. A red candle is surrounded by obsidian Aztec figurines from one of my trips down to Mexico City. On the runner, she has placed a grapefruit, sandstone from a dried-up lake-bed in northern Texas – a souvenir from a trip she made several years ago. There is a small malachite box of coins, a matching pyramid that could fit on the palm of my hand and trinkets from our grandfather's travels to Central and South America. Two medium-sized bowls potted with aloe vera and burro's tail succulents are placed at either end of the silk runner. She lights the candle, a smudging stick of Palo Santo, incense and a bundle of dried white sage. She turns off the lights after dinner and sits in one of our mismatched dinner table chairs. Light from the candle flickers across her face. I look at her across the table. I avoid eye contact. Whatever bonds we share sometimes overwhelm us.

I sit at the table, the altar. Jessica says a few words to honour our mother's presence and to thank her and our grandmother for their existence. She tells them we are okay. I think of them, their many sacrifices, the many other futures that could have been. I feel their absence, their presence deeply. Jessica sits by me and wraps her arms around my shoulders. She keeps them there until my shudders subside. In this moment, Jessica's words ring true – we are all right.

A full year and a half have passed since Jessica's first breakdown. Her new job working at an engineering company for fire protection is one of the few engineering jobs not directly supporting oil and gas, a small miracle in Houston. The job gives her limited health benefits but does not cover any therapy.

We have just a few sessions left with our counsellor before her services will no longer be offered to us. Given Jessica's real need to purchase a car soon and fund other basic necessities, therapy seems to veer between charity and luxury. I contemplate paying $500 for five more sessions for Jessica after her health insurance takes our counsellor away from us. I ask the counsellor if I should contribute financially to my sister's therapy and she tells me I should recognise codependent thinking and set some personal boundaries. Fair enough, I suppose.

After two years at the University of Houston, I decide to accept a position at a research institute. A board member who made millions from investments in oil and gas has funded the position. I accept it gratefully. The job will keep me in Houston for two more years. This is where I need to be.

These days I cannot read the future; perhaps I never could. All I know is that my worst fears were manifested and I coped as best as I could. A Chicana friend who will begin her residency in psychiatry this summer tells me that she respects what I have done for my family. As she drives me home, she tells me, 'You are your family's matriarch now.' The thought never crossed my mind until then. I look at her and smile sadly. She cannot understand the small cruelties I have inflicted or the small acts of violence she will enact in her field – our complicities and burdens as caregivers.

What would it mean to move through these fears? On good days, I envision a life lived courageously, dangerously (Evans & Reid, 2014); I welcome my sister and the many conversations we will have. We garden, talk, cook together. We create a community. We become alongside the thunderous storms, pipes with traces of Chromium 6, the dioxin-rich floodwaters, looming hurricanes, the sweltering melancholy and other monstrous dreams that will come to Houston.

When my sister and I die again, bury us with wreaths of bluebonnets, sunflowers, pink evening primrose, magnolias, wild sage and a yellow rose. Bury us with remedies, the antidotes of our elders. Sing us a song of the Karankawa, in a language not our own, on land that was never ours, but on which we have found a home.

References

Anzaldúa G (2015). *Light in the Dark/Luz en lo Oscuro: rewriting identity, spirituality, reality* (AL Keating ed). Durham, NC: Duke University Press.

Anzaldúa G (2007). *Borderlands/La Frontera: the new Mestiza* (3rd ed). San Francisco, CA: Aunt Lute Books.

Behrouzan O (2016). *Prozak Diaries: psychiatry and generational memory in Iran.* Stanford, CA: Stanford University Press.

Burstow B, LeFrancois B (2014). Impassioned praxis: an introduction to theorizing resistance to psychiatry. In: Burstow B, LeFrancois B, Diamond S. *Psychiatry Disrupted: theorizing resistance and crafting the (r)evolution*. Montreal: McGill-Queen's University Press (pp3–15).

Cresswell M, Spandler H (2016). Solidarities and tensions in mental health politics: mad studies and psychopolitics. *Critical and Radical Social Work* 4(3): 1–23.

Cvetkovich A (2003). *An Archive of Feelings: trauma, sexuality, and lesbian public cultures*. Durham, NC: Duke University Press.

Evans B, Reid J (2014). *Resilient Life: the art of living dangerously*. Cambridge: Polity Press.

Fanon F (2008/1952). *Black Skin, White Masks*. London: Pluto Books.

Harper J (2004). Breathless in Houston: a political ecology of health approach to understanding environmental health concerns. *Medical Anthropology* 23(4): 295–326.

Hester RJ (2016). Culture in medicine: an argument against competence. In: Whitehead A, Woods A (eds). *The Edinburgh Companion to Critical Medical Humanities*. Edinburgh: Edinburgh University Press (pp541–558).

Icarus Project (2013). *Friends Make the Best Medicine: a guide to creating community mental health support networks* (2nd ed). New York, NY: The Icarus Project.

Jones N, Kelly T (2015). Inconvenient complications: on the heterogeneities of madness and their relationship to disability. In: Spandler H, Sapey B, Anderson J (eds). *Madness and the Politics of Disablement*. Cambridge: Polity Press (pp43–56).

Luhrmann T, Marrow J (eds) (2016). *Our Most Troubling Madness: case studies in schizophrenia across cultures*. Oakland, CA: University of California Press.

Mellody P, Miller AW, Miller JK (2003). Facing Codependence: what it is, where it comes from, how it sabotages our lives. San Francisco, CA: HarperCollins Publishers.

Metzl J (2009). *The Protest Psychosis: how schizophrenia became a black disease*. Boston, MA: Beacon Press.

Nair Y (2017). The dangerous academic is an extinct species. [Online.] *Current Affairs* 7 June. www.currentaffairs.org/2017/04/the-dangerous-academic-is-an-extinct-species (accessed 21 May 2017).

Nixon R (2013). *Slow Violence and the Environmentalism of the Poor*. Cambridge, MA: Harvard University Press.

Reid J (2014). Climate, migration, and sex: the biopolitics of climate-induced migration. *Critical Studies on Security* 2(2): 196–209.

Rodriguez CO (2017). How academia uses poverty, oppression, and pain for intellectual masturbation. [Online.]   *RaceBaitr*   6   April.   http://racebaitr.com/2017/04/06/how-academia-uses-poverty-oppression/# (accessed 21 May, 2017).

Rosenthal E (2016). When the hospital fires the bullet. [Online.] *New York Times* 12 February. www.nytimes.com/2016/02/14/us/hospital-guns-mental-health.html (accessed 25 May 2017).

Satija N, Collier K, Shaw A (2016). Boomtown, floodtown. *The Texas Tribune/ProPublica* 7 December. www.texastribune.org/boomtown-floodtown (accessed 24 May 2017).

Seikkula J, Olson ME (2003). The open dialogue approach to acute psychosis: its poetics and micropolitics. *Family Process* 42(3): 403–418.

Shackelford A (2016). We were never meant to survive: on considering suicide in a world designed to kill us. [Online.] *Wear Your Voice Magazine* 8 July. https://wearyourvoicemag.com/identities/race/

we-were-never-meant-to-survive-on-considering-suicide-in-a-world-designed-to-kill-us (accessed 21 May 2017).

Tamas S (2009). Writing and righting trauma: troubling the autoethnographic voice. *FQS: Forum Qualitative Social Research 10*(1): art 22. www.qualitative-research.net/index.php/fqs/article/view/1211/2642 (accessed 24 May 2017).

Tuana N (2008). Viscous porosity: witnessing Katrina. In: Alaimo S, Heckman S (eds). *Material Feminisms*. Bloomington, IN: Indiana University Press (pp188–213).

Union for Concerned Scientists and Texas Environmental Justice Advocacy Services (2016). *Double Jeopardy in Houston: acute and chronic chemical exposures pose disproportionate risks for marginalized communities*. Cambridge, MA: Union of Concerned Scientists. https://www.ucsusa.org/sites/default/files/attach/2016/10/ucs-double-jeopardy-in-houston-full-report-2016.pdf (accessed 24 May 2017).

Vimalassery M, Pegues JH, Goldstein A (2016). On colonial unknowing. *Theory & Event 19*(4): 1–13.

Wingard J (2013). Assembling Houston: writing and teaching the neoliberal city. *JAC 33*(3/4): 553–583.

13 | Mental health nursing as a therapy

Tony McSherry

This chapter is an attempt to indicate one way in which mental health nursing could define itself and function as a discipline separate from psychiatry. Pause here for a moment and really think why these two should be separated. Who cares? My responses are personal, and to separate the two reflects my own personal difficulty, which perhaps may throw light on others' experience and be of help. Stumbling into mental health nursing was like being given the wrong hotel address in the wrong destination. Offered shelter and a place to sleep, it was hard to notice the strangeness at first. Now, writing in the foyer, mental health nursing and psychiatry appear to run a strange establishment. Breathing the same recycled air, I am trying to find a place to open a window, but it's hard even to pull back the curtains. Perhaps some other mental health nurses, psychiatrists, psychologists and others feel the same way.

However, it could be that mental health nursing and psychiatry are inseparable, as the two disciplines are dependent on each other, although the latter dominates. There is the nagging suspicion that psychiatry will always generate its attendants, just like of old (Nolan, 1993), no matter what we call them. It is worth wondering whether the relationship between the two is symbiotic or mutually parasitic. Perhaps it is both. It seems to be particularly susceptible to the resentful conflict of the co-dependent, or the Master/Slave relationship (see Paley, 2002). Can we really imagine a place where mental health nurses can work therapeutically with people in extreme distress without the help of psychiatry? Can we really imagine that psychiatry could be therapeutic with those people without the help of mental health nursing? Perhaps we can imagine new places, and it's the place of mental health nursing that I will explore in this chapter.

I will try to make some sense through my own experience here, hoping it will let in some air and light on the experience of the reader who may be interested in the field of mental health nursing. What we cannot do in writing is speak, and this is a pity as it seems to me that true learning comes only through attempting to speak truthfully (see Heaton, 2010). Apart from poetry, the written word seems to eventually collapse into dogma. This makes me think that therapeutic mental health nursing has something to do with speaking, dialogue, openness to the other person, and little to do with the written word in dogmatic form. Indeed, it seems to me that therapeutic mental health nursing has little to do with 'prescription' of any kind.

Already you, the reader, may see a chasm opening up between psychiatry and what I envisage as mental health nursing if it were therapeutic. I am saying that, when something therapeutic happens between a mental health nurse and another person, it has little to do with 'mental health' or psychiatry or nursing. What happens appears to me to be like a conversation between two people, one of whom, hopefully, will be more prepared for that dialogue to be therapeutic.

I am trying not to 'use language' in a technical way in this chapter. Indeed, language often uses *us*. I refer to theory but intend it to be read like the signposts on a journey rather than set prescriptions for rule-making (after Wittgenstein, 2009). For example, I have read some of Lacan, and struggled to understand it, yet certain ideas captivated me and I wondered why. Does such captivation 'speak' a truth in some way, or is it more a way out of not facing experience? These questions are phenomenological in nature (Loewenthal, 2011) and it seems that we somehow need to be able to ask them freely or else we become like automata. The main threads of the therapeutic that I pick up are about freeing a person from being categorised or summed up and instead opening ourselves out into allowing a multiplicity of ways of being.

I will try to sketch how mental health nursing still seems to me to occupy a space that can allow for this 'freeing up', for the idiosyncrasies of being human, unlike the normalising categorisation of 'mental health' prevalent in mainstream psychiatry, mental health nursing and psychology. There seems to be a space where mental health nursing might come to define itself as a therapeutic endeavour in its own right. The space is like a plot of wasteland where wild plants and creatures can still survive. The only other social space I can see that allows this is that of *some* therapists' rooms, or in art (see Gadamer, 2004).

Phenomenology as description

The thinking in this chapter is rooted in a phenomenological research project whose method may not be hugely at odds with autoethnography, especially in view of Holman Jones, Adams and Ellis (2013: 23), who state that one is writing autoethnographically if 'aspects of experience illuminate more general cultural phenomena and/or show how the experience works to diminish, silence, or deny certain people and stories'. The stories in this chapter are those of patients in mental health services and those of some mental health nurses whose therapeutic potential is stymied by a system focused on audit and control (see Rose, 1999).

Phenomenology values experience while at the same time attempting to suspend assumptions that come 'naturally' about that experience, including those immersed in language (Zahavi, 2003).

Influenced by Franz Brentano, whose lectures Sigmund Freud also attended in Vienna, Edmund Husserl established phenomenology as a philosophical discipline. Husserl's aim was to provide a solid ground for understanding how anything can be known at all, a project he was never to complete. Husserl was not against science but saw that we had lost touch with our experience by only trusting results from scientific method (Husserl, 1970; Moran, 2000; see Rawlins, 2008). As Giorgi (2009) puts it:

> Husserl is respectful and trusting with respect to experience. It is not the case that experience cannot be illusory, it is just that illusions and others sorts of error are also corrected by experience. (p69)

Husserl also came to acknowledge how the matrix of cultural practices and language in which we are embedded informs what can be known. He was perhaps the single most influential philosopher of the last century, his most influential student being Martin Heidegger (Polt, 1999). Husserl also had a profound influence on Emmanuel Levinas, Maurice Merleau-Ponty, Jean Paul Sartre, Jacques Derrida and many others (Loewenthal & Snell, 2003). Although the basic phenomenological premise, to stay with experience while suspending one's 'natural attitude' (everyday assumptions) about that experience, sounds simple, it is deceptively difficult (Finlay, 2008).

If there is a 'method' to Husserl's phenomenology it is to describe how things appear, unflinchingly and without reserve. To simply say what appears can be extraordinarily difficult when there can be so much at stake – for example, for an individual's inhering and perhaps fundamental sense of self. And not to radically question how things appear would be antithetical to phenomenology.

At the same time, language is ubiquitous in that 'the whole landscape is overrun with words' (Merleau-Ponty, 1968: 155). What Merleau-Ponty means here is that the experience we speak of, which we try to describe unflinchingly, is already 'overrun with words'; language is at work in us in such a way that we cannot become entirely disentangled from its effects. For this reason, it is not easy to describe an experience of something in a way that is different to how it may have been already 'written' in ourselves. How do we know we are being therapeutic? Might we not just be imposing our own 'words' (views, ideas, entrenched ways of being) on the other person?

The diagnostic categories in psychiatry, for example, have become so embedded in common language that it is as if these *descriptions* have some real *substance*. If you believe they do, then it might be helpful to question this belief rigorously. This phenomenon of language informing being, and being enrolled in power relations, is not new, of course. For example, the language of psychoanalysis, along with the implicit meanings attached to it, has infiltrated much of Western society (Parker, 1997). The language of 'cognitive science' is now dominating 'mental health', giving a false impression that we are simply information processors rather than relational beings, subject to others (Loewenthal, 2011) and language (Parker, 2011).

Caught up in a context

In being 'overrun with words' in our own selves, we can only ever try to understand each other in a context. In attempting to be therapeutic, we make decisions that are rooted in our own context, in the ways we are already embedded in relationships and language, which sometimes emerges in tacit actions.

Tacit knowledge is acquired through the kind of learning involved in acquiring a craft – learning from the 'master' through a process of repetition and mimicry until one 'knows' (Gill, 2000). Polanyi's (1983) exploration of tacit knowledge shows the importance of focal and subsidiary awareness and embodiment. When one is focused on reading, for example, the focal activity is following the meaning of the words, while a myriad subsidiary activities makes this possible, which are embodied. Polanyi drew on the work of Merleau-Ponty, who in turn drew on Husserl (Gill, 2000). Polanyi (1983) named as *indwelling* the interaction of the body with the particulars of which one is subsidiarily aware. The key point is that one reacts as if one understands at first without fully understanding. Learning to speak one's mother tongue is an example of such a process (Gill, 2000).

This implies that a person may feel he is being therapeutic, based on a tacit way of being he has learned from others, when he may in fact be the opposite, without knowing it. Therefore, in order to practise in a more 'freed up' way with another person, it is probably necessary to have had some sort of incisive understanding as to how one's own personal landscape has been 'overrun with words'. There would then be less of a risk of mindlessly (even mindfully) imposing that landscape on others, or mapping it into their behaviours and actions.

Being caught up in one's own context is so complex, it is reasonable to suggest that it has resulted in the widely diverging types of 'therapies' in circulation (Heaton, 1999). However, certain ways of thinking have coalesced into a powerful, influential network, including psychiatry, termed the 'psy-complex' (Rose, 1985), which defines what it means to be 'normal', what is pathological and what treatments should be applied to rectify those pathological departures (Parker, 1997). Mental health nursing is part of the psy-complex but ironically seems to be held in such low regard that there is a certain amount of freedom within it for broader versions of the therapeutic to exist. Some would see such broadening as illicitly 'covert' and 'self-aggrandising' Morrall (1997: 57); I view it as emancipatory and counteracting 'totalising perspectives' (Holmes, Gastaldo & Perron, 2007: 85).

The key point appears to be that, if we feel certain we 'know' somebody, we are likely to be 'totalising' them: summing them up from within our own context, in a violent way. Think what it feels like when someone does this to you: 'He's rude';

'She's greedy'; 'They're all the same, those people.' There seems to be no release from the 'diagnosis'.

Fragments of my own context

My own career moves involved changes from science into mental health nursing via a life as a Franciscan friar. The steps from one sphere to another were not entirely foreseen. This trajectory accidentally threw light on something I found relevant to mental health nursing.

Being invisible

Phenomenologically, what I noticed was that, from working in science, I was used to my thoughts being taken seriously, my knowledge being significant or 'visible' to others. In the same way, my life as a Franciscan was recognised as indicating significant knowledge, including spirituality. The move from the Franciscans to mental health nursing, however, was disturbing, in the sense that my knowledge – and, indeed, my place in the world of others – no longer counted for much. The disturbing effects of such an experience made themselves known immediately and over several years, and included making me feel invisible within the landscape of psychiatric medicine and psychological dogma. I was particularly struck by the sense that I was immersed in a social structure and its framework of knowledge that marginalised the importance of mental health nurses' interactions with patients. Yet it appeared that many other nurses did not have this difficulty. The sense of the insignificance of mental health nursing has also been noted in other ways: for example, Happell (2004) regarding research, and Browne, Cashin and Graham (2012) in relation to not feeling entitled to recognition. The overall invisibility of nursing as a 'treatment' has been noticed and theorised by nurse academics, including Barker and colleagues (2005) and Bjorklund (2004). It is, indeed, a wonder that therapeutic mental health nurses can hang on in the system (Cutcliffe et al, 2015).

To get away from this experience, I trained in counselling and psychotherapy and worked as a nurse therapist, but the landscape still had not changed. My psychotherapeutic education introduced me to a way of articulating my own experience that was phenomenological but also looked theoretically at ideas on how culture and language intersect in one's own self (Loewenthal & Snell, 2003). Some ideas rang true for me, as if I already knew about them tacitly; some were totally new and drew me towards them, and some did not gain purchase. This process also involved the work of individual psychotherapy and group therapy.

Being decentred

My experience of acute mental health nursing left me with several questions, one of which was: 'What was I trying to distance myself from in leaving this occupation?' This question has taken me some time to answer adequately. In leaving the Franciscans, I wished to remain 'central' in the sense of taking control of my destiny through carrying over the spirituality of Francis of Assisi into everyday life. I believed it was possible to still be Franciscan but in a secular way, rather than from within the organisation of the Order of the Friars Minor. Mental health nursing seemed to offer a way through into something else, a stepping stone to becoming this 'secular Franciscan', living in a way that seemed the only way to live in the world at that time. I was influenced by having met a Franciscan in my training as a friar whom I regarded as inherently therapeutic, and he had previously worked as a nurse. But I did not realise that I could not just walk through the world of nursing as if I were an ambassador in a foreign country, adapting to the local customs for my own motives, and emerge unscathed. In this way, it became clear over time that one is 'subject to' something, and that the attempt to remain 'central' is thwarted by something else that 'decentres' our best intentions. This is a crucial point (Loewenthal & Snell, 2003), and I will approach this in different ways here.

Being 'decentred' can also be understood as the means whereby a person is 'interpellated' in an ideology (Althusser, 1964, cited in Parker, 1997: 221):

> Freud has discovered for us that the real subject, the individual in his unique essence, has not the form of an ego, centred on the 'ego', on 'consciousness', or on 'existence'… that the human subject is de-centred, constituted by a structure which has no 'centre' either, except in the imaginary misrecognition of the 'ego', ie. in the ideological formations in which it recognises itself.

Althusser is drawing on Lacan's ideas of the Symbolic (language in its broadest sense) and Imaginary (narcissistic infantile identifications) registers (Parker, 1997: 120–121). What appears important here for mental health nursing is that, in order to change, mental health nurses need a way of understanding the ideology to which they are subject and the influence of 'personal ideologies'.

Being 'subject to' – re-founding mental health nursing

For a principal source of thinking about being 'subject to', see Loewenthal and Snell (2003). In my work as a mental health nurse, there seemed to be something in play that created an overbearing weight, which was 'given' in the phenomenological sense (that is, *experienced*). It was present and had embodied effects that were disturbing. For example, it was expressed in the drive to be designated by some other word rather than 'nurse.' But this impetus was not always obvious. It was 'given' in an attitude, a resistance to something. But when one does not have the words, one is not able to articulate what is happening, although one can experience it. What I draw from this is that mental health nurses need to 'find the words' to articulate their own practice and experience.

Apart from therapy, what also helped me was reading, sometimes with others, and being open to my own experience (not an easy task). Being with others was important in an ordinary but also reflective sense, especially being with those who were able to listen in an attentive way rather than just seeing a conversation as a means of imposing an opinion.

Through this process, I realised that working as a mental health nurse was like moving through a 'field of significance' that was bigger than my own determination to be Franciscan in a secular way. Something bigger and far more 'powerful' was at work, 'de-centring' me, which Lacan would call the Other (Fink, 1995). Lacanian theory was helpful, therapeutic even, as a means to speak of something that was 'given' phenomenologically but was hard to express in words. For example, here is Lacan, on desire and recognition (showing Hegelian influences):

> Man's desire finds its meaning in the desire of the other, not so much because the other holds the key to the object desired as because its first object of desire is to be recognised by the other. (Lacan, 1977: 58, cited in Borch-Jacobsen, 1991: 132)

We need recognition from others, and this places us in a precarious situation in the world of others, as we are dependent on them. In working as a mental health nurse, I became 'subject to' the Other in a way which was unforeseen. I became subject to a field of feminine signifiers, created by culture and society. Such 'signifiers' were not 'just words' but carried with them embodied effects (McSherry, Loewenthal & Cayne, 2015).

Taking the above quote on recognition into account, it affects one's being to have one's experience and knowledge go unrecognised. There is an effect being experienced here (and phenomenology takes experience seriously) that indicates something of the 'imbrication' of 'language, the human and the material' (Lather & St Pierre, 2013: 630) – that is, how a field of signification (language), one's subjectivity (the human) and embodiment (the material) interdependently link together. Phenomenologically then, 'knowing and doing' involves 'being.'

Recognising the effects of this, the Other, in one's life might be a way into a different, critical training in mental health nursing. This might also be a way for mental health nursing to come to know itself as a discipline. I would see it as a way into mental health nursing beginning to become a discipline in its own right that is respectful of what psychiatry and psychology have to offer but respects experience first. In this way, a person may be less alienated from him- or herself. It is interesting that psychiatrists were once called alienists (Foucault, 1989). In becoming a mental health nurse, I alienated myself from what was important about Franciscanism to me. Coming to appreciate my own experience, with the help of others, showed this.

Returning to experience – the Apostle versus the Genius

Murray and Holmes (2013) have discussed this link between knowing and being by drawing on the work of Hannah Arendt (and Merleau-Ponty). Arendt (2005: 8, cited in Murray & Holmes, 2013: 343) shows that, since Plato, thinking has been regarded as 'a soundless dialogue between me and myself'. Following Arendt (2005), Murray and Holmes ask what happens when, for example:

> the mediating terms of one's self-understanding become increasingly narrow... The dilemma is that we can neither *know* nor *feel* with certainty that we are doing wrong... knowledge and feelings measure one's social conformity or non-conformity to received principles, rules, codes, behaviours and mores. These are always situated, social, historical, and bound up with the world in complex ways. (2013: 343–344)

This shows itself very clearly in Kierkegaard (2010: 73–75), where he contrasts the Genius and the Apostle. The latter is subject to the authority of 'the Other' and has become a vessel of the beliefs and doctrine of a 'Truth'; the Genius, however, struggles to discover within himself his own truth. It seems worth noting that Lacan would see Kierkegaard's Apostle as an example of the subject of the signifier or the Freudian unconscious (Žižek, 2006: 219). The Apostle is a channel of the authority of 'the Other'. He (it is often a 'he') already has his identity 'ready-made' (off the peg), while the Genius has to struggle with her own truth in her experience. Things change and are born through this struggle.

Changing a coat

Staying with Lacanian language for a moment, it appears that moving from being a Franciscan to being a nurse involved moving from a masculine signifying system to one that was feminine. The Order of the Friars Minor is a prominent religious order whose aim is to spread the Gospel through the charism of St Francis of Assisi. What is essential here, what makes this a 'masculine' pursuit, is its acknowledgement as such by the Other and, embedded in this, its central role to represent, and embody, 'The Word'. The 'Word' is masculine (phallic even) in that it comes from masculine culture and institutions (Lacan, 1977). Nursing perhaps had to do with something else that for me was linked to spirituality. While Lacanian theory here is seductive, phenomenologically the theory seemed to coincide with what my ordinary experiences were saying about my ongoing resistance to 'being a nurse'. The signifiers of nursing were feminine – for example, the call bell in the toilets had a figure of a woman in a skirt and nursing headgear; nursing was not recognised by the Other as a masculine role in society.

As Kierkegaard would say, one cannot simply put on another self like changing a coat (Kierkegaard, 1954: 186, in Friedman, 1999: 371), and it felt like this was what I had done precisely by opting for nursing. In the course of my research, I found a resistance in myself to continuing it that was linked to identifying myself as a nurse. The resistance was both 'within' me and 'outside' of me, showing how we are indeed subject to 'the Other'. It is as if we are swimming around in words, views and ideas of 'the Other', as a fish inhabits water. How such meanings form us seems to be idiosyncratic, which indicates that what I will argue is a crucial and critical feature of what some who work as mental health nurses may address – the quirkiness and strangeness of being a person.

Having understood some aspects of my own context, I returned to researching mental health nursing as a kind of 'outsider' to the discipline. It also makes me think that there is something about mental health nursing that will always be 'other' to me, to which I will have to remain open but which I may wish to get away from or dismiss, as well as elements that may be difficult for me to grasp. For example, it is hard for me sometimes to grasp the sheer kindness and hard work of some nurses in situations where they go unappreciated.

In this way too, 'theorising' about mental health nursing may be missing something uniquely individual about the therapeutic person. For example, think about sitting with someone during the night who has tried to strangle themselves, about trying to 'be with' that person. The therapeutic aspect in these hours and moments may have nothing to do with medication, diagnosis or psychological formulation and everything to do with the person of the mental health nurse and how she or he has come to be.

Against systematising the person

With the importance of idiosyncratic ways of being and living in the world in mind, I would like to illustrate this further with regard to 'science', with reference to Harré and Derrida. My aim here is to throw light on the impoverished culture of categorisation of people and 'therapy' in mainstream psychiatry and psychology, alongside which mental health nursing appears elided as a professional practice.

> Traditionally, philosophy starts with a sense of wonder. Then theory steps in
> with heavy tread to explain the sources and reasons of the glorious wonder.
> (Rabaté, 2002: 1)

It seems here that scientific views of being a person 'kill wonder' through imposing a technical explanation that alienates the 'personal' from the person. It seems that what makes us feel alive is always personal, or private, carrying meanings that belong to a sensual landscape of the individual person. Think of why you might miss a loved one, or a friend, for example. Is it because they are good at maths? The feelings, experience and landscape you find yourself in will be a sensual one, involving words imbued with meanings that are inseparable from that landscape, irreducible to the simple conveying of a meaning that the other can fully understand

(McSherry, 2018). In the attempt to explain, you may say things like, 'I miss my friend because I miss him.'

For this reason, it feels important not to embrace theory too vehemently, as it tends to have a narrowing effect so that experience comes to be understood through theory and nothing can be appreciated that is not subsumed in its terms.

A 'theory' of oneself

At the same time, however, it would appear that 'personal beings' are products of social influences from the very beginning, acquiring ideas about themselves as 'theories' through language, so in this sense one can never escape theory (Harré, 1983: 21). It is intuitively clear that one needs an identity in order to function among others, and this is what Harré means when he talks about the process of becoming a 'personal being'; it involves acquiring an identity that is, in effect, the same as acquiring a theory of oneself – a cohering sense of one's history, involving self-knowledge and agency (Harré, 1983).

My original training in science developed a 'natural attitude' that used to be that one can make assumptions about the world *and others*, test these through empirical data, and either confirm, change or refine one's assumptions. In the 'natural attitude' of the natural sciences, there is an assumption that there is a mind-independent reality that can be explored and understood objectively (Zahavi, 2003). This assumption certainly appears valid for most of the physical sciences, apart from quantum physics (Heaton, 1999). A difficulty arises when this view is applied to human subjectivity: can a person's experience of the world of others' experiences, and of himself, be examined in the same way as an object in the physical sciences? I argue it cannot, because a person's meanings belong in a sensual landscape (as noted above).

Applying physical scientific method and inquiry to human subjectivity is what mainstream academic psychology tends to do.

> Academic psychologists… make the implicit assumption that men, women and children are high-grade automata, the patterns of whose behaviour are thought to obey something very like natural laws… It is assumed that there are programmes which control action and the task of psychology is to discover the 'mechanisms' by which they are implemented. (Harré, 1983: 4)

A second image of human psychology for Harré is one in which:

> … all of those who have to deal in a practical way with human beings tend to think of people as agents struggling to maintain some sort of reasoned order in their lives against a background flux of emotions, inadequate information and the ever-present tides of social pressures. (1983: 4)

Either we are like automata, obeying our own mechanism, or we are agents struggling to manage. Harré (1983: 4) suggests that the differences in these two ways of thinking about human psychology are due to 'unexamined political and moral assumptions that show up in the choice of rhetoric, in morally and politically loaded ways of speaking, and… writing'. In summary, according to Harré (1983: 25), 'people create themselves and their patterns of interaction by virtue of the psychological and social theories to which they subscribe'.

Harré (1983: 24) highlights a critical detail about science and how we come to know anything, in that words, ideas, language, speech and thought are interleaved, so that the very concepts that are being 'tested' infiltrate the testing of those concepts. That the person cannot be understood as an object in the world, as other objects can, is also fundamental to Husserl (Zahavi, 2003: 48). For example, as discussed above, being a Lacanian may cause one to always see Lacanian concepts in how others are. Harré (1983: 20) describes this creation of patterns by the patterns themselves:

> The fundamental human reality is a conversation, effectively without beginning or end, to which, from time to time, individuals may make contributions. All that is personal in our mental and emotional lives is individually appropriated from the conversation going on around us and perhaps idiosyncratically transformed. The structure of our thinking and feeling will reflect, in various ways, the form and content of that conversation.

To 'interpret', to say 'Yes, I know what you mean', always comes from somewhere and we are always coming from somewhere.

This could also be shown in terms of Merleau-Ponty's operative intentionality (after Husserl), whereby one's grasp of the world is embodied and 'always already' active in any interpretation so that 'beneath' any interpretation is an original 'grip' on the world (Merleau-Ponty, 1962/2014: xxxii). How we grasp the world might show itself in how we relate to others, the 'results' we get or look for.

> We uncovered, beneath act or thetic intentionality – and in fact as its very condition of possibility – an operative intentionality already at work prior to every thesis and every judgement; we discovered a 'Logos of the aesthetic world' [after Husserl in Formal and Transcendental Logic (1969)] or a 'hidden art in the depths of the human soul' [after Kant in Critique of Pure Reason(1781/2007)] and that, like every art, only knows itself in its results (Merleau-Ponty, 1962/2014: 453/492).

Think of someone you don't like. This might show you how there is a 'hidden art' at work in how you have 'captured' that person you dislike in a certain 'grasp'. Why is it so difficult to speak of them differently? The conversation seems tightly closed off.

Psychology may find its results, and be known by its results, in such a way that the conversation becomes closed down. The terms it uses to understand others define what is understood or 'found'. In a similar way, psychiatry has become a dogma rather than the phenomenological exploration it once was (Walker, 1994) and so it too will 'find itself in its results'. Theory causes 'regurgitations' of sameness (Rabaté, 2002: 100). We get caught up in this.

Openness to something else

Is it not this 'closure', this 'repetition', that is found repeatedly in the 'mental health' monologue? And is it not one person's openness to another person, and her speaking, that breaks this monologue? I would argue that there still remains the space in mental health nursing – through openness to others – for a conversation to happen whereby the other person can come to find himself in his *own terms*.

Preventing a dogmatic monologue seems to be why Derrida reacted so surprisingly to a guide to his own works that he prepared with his friend, Geoffrey Bennington.

> GB would have liked to systematize JD's thought to the point of turning it into an interactive program, which, in spite of its difficulty, would in principle be accessible to any user. As what is at stake in JD's work is to show how any such system must remain essentially open, this undertaking was doomed to failure from the start… In order to demonstrate the ineluctable necessity of the failure, our contract stipulated that JD, having read GB's text, would write something escaping the proposed systematization, surprising it (Bennington & Derrida, 1991: 1, in Rabaté, 2002: 101).

The surprise was a text, *Circumfession (Circonfession)* (Derrida, 1991), arranged in 59 footnotes (Derrida was aged 59 when he wrote it), on the subject of circumcision and confession, including autobiographical details of Derrida's relationship with his mother and grandmother, and his 'private obsessions' with his own circumcision (Rabaté, 2002: 101). Derrida is here pushing 'theory elsewhere, to a private "beyond"' that the 'theoretician cannot totally disown', while at the same time developing 'new deconstructive strategies' (Rabaté, 2002: 101). Rabaté (2002: 101–102) asks whether this gesture of Derrida's could be repeated and answers emphatically in the negative. This is because Derrida's method cannot be taught but is more like a virtue in the Socratic sense, that arrives through (divine) inspiration that is peculiar to Derrida (Rabaté, 2002: 102). What is perhaps most important – signalled by Rabaté's (2002: 101–102) observation, 'One is sent back to one's private subjectivity in the end' that 'one cannot totally disown' – is that Derrida appeals to the idiosyncrasy of his own subjectivity to undermine the systematisation of his own thought. Thereby, I would say, he creates an 'openness' where other meanings and other ways of being can happen and be allowed. One difficulty here, however, is that some people (perhaps many) need dogma and monologue to feel secure in the world.

Some implications for mental health nursing

At least two aspects emerge from this milieu that are relevant to mental health nursing. First, if there is an essence to a meaning, or something that is trying to be communicated, then it is linked with something to do with a 'private subjectivity'. Second, if the therapeutic is viewed as making the right move or decision, then it may be linked to something that resists systematisation, something that is towards inspiration, to do with 'private subjectivity' and more of an art than a science, perhaps (see Gadamer, 2004). Systematisation leads to 'regurgitation'. Derrida's move was to both reveal something that systematisation could not have known and, thereby, open it to systematisation, and also indicate that it is important to resist systematisation, or all-encompassing theory. Mental health nursing appears to offer a space for this kind of non-systematising conversation to happen, which involves being with the other person. I would argue that learning to be in this anxiety-provoking space might be crucial for mental health nurses developing a discipline separate to psychiatry.

A vision for the future?

What is striking about the literature in mental health nursing is its overall lack of a commitment to a cohering theory such as, for example, the scientific method. The discipline itself resists systematisation, although there have been calls and attempts to do so, as Cutcliffe (2000: 633) indicates. These have generally been along the lines of the biomedical 'contain and fix' approach (for example, Gournay, 2000) versus the 'personal process' approach (for example, Barker & Reynolds, 1996). There is a plethora of different approaches between and beyond these, invoking numerous ways of thinking about the other person and involving varying emphases on theory, practice-based evidence, qualitative research, case studies and philosophical perspectives. It appears that, precisely because mental health nursing has not been systematised in the same way as psychiatry and psychology, those in the discipline who choose or are inclined to can allow the other person to speak from a place that resists categorisation, that gives precedence to the idiosyncratic ways of being human despite the pressure to conform to the demands of psychiatry or the psy-complex. This is something that is worth defending and developing – a field of 'enabling difference' at the heart of a system that is inherently narrowed and systematised. In my view, it indicates that the discipline has more to do with the humanities than medicine or psychology. Derrida escaped from the perils of systematisation by moving towards his own private subjectivity, and I argue that mental health nursing provides a space where this private subjectivity – being a person – can be allowed and valued.

Regarding therapeutic interactions with patients, the Nursing and Midwifery Council (2010; 2017) expects the mental health nurse to engage in the therapeutic use of self, as well as maintain therapeutic relationships using a range of interpersonal approaches and skills. The mental health nurse must herself be therapeutic through the 'therapeutic use of self' (Nursing and Midwifery Council, 2010: 18). At the same time, she must also be able to 'draw on a range of evidence-based psychological, psychosocial interventions and other complex therapeutic skills to provide person-centred support and care' (Nursing and Midwifery Council, 2010: 17–18).

It appears then that an ambiguity lies at the heart of mental health nursing about what it is that mental health nurses are there to do, in that the discipline is on the border between an academic pursuit (in the current dominant paradigm, this is a narrow, 'evidence-based' approach) and one that involves other ways of relating, using the 'self'. There is also an indication here, apparently tacit, that it is acknowledged in nursing that mental health nurses work therapeutically in idiosyncratic ways because their very selves are important in some way. Paradoxically, it appears that idiosyncrasy ('therapeutic use of self') is valued in a discipline that serves a psychiatric system that overwhelmingly systematises (Davies, 2013) what it is to be a person and what 'mentally well' may mean.

Rather than view this ambiguity negatively, I suggest that mental health nursing could address it as indicating the idiosyncrasy of being a person and define a new relation to this as a discipline, and perhaps a profession. This would involve mental health nurses getting to grips with their own idiosyncrasies throughout their lives and education. The academic literature indicates that this is already happening on a small scale, but that the discipline has not yet found the language and the political will to define itself differently.

I suggest here that, in order for the discipline to establish itself as critical and capable of agency, it needs to shed the title 'mental health nursing', as these words are too tied up with the suffocating relationship to medical and psychological technologies that imply that 'mental health' is something located in an 'autonomous brain', and we could all achieve it if only we could acquire the right skills or brain chemistry to do so (Davies, 2013; House, 2010; Kelly & Moloney, 2018).

Finding new words

Words are not easily found to replace 'mental health nurse'. I tentatively suggest 'social therapist', as it reflects something of how the Other informs and forms us, along with the healing aspects of the therapeutic that happens in relation with others.

What seems to be needed at the heart of a system that is capable of addressing the needs of those in 'mental distress' are people who are able and have the authority to thoughtfully reflect on and work with what it is and means to be a person among others. This would mean that mental health nursing would need to split from nursing as a discipline, as it is too tied to medicine (or biology). To protect and make room for a broader view of what it is to be a person, and therefore what a person's distress may signify, such a discipline would need to play a central role in developing an alternative to the current system, with its fixation on systematisation, risk and pharmacological interventions.

Perhaps this is an idealistic vision for the future but it is still one worth envisioning, as it would free up those doing mental health nursing to offer a more critical, thoughtful engagement with and availability to others. Of course, some mental health nurses are already doing this when they can, but in a milieu in which they are often invisible and under considerable distress (see Banks et al, 2013).

I want now to draw on an example from the literature to illustrate some of the difficulties of developing mental health nursing as a critical discipline 'of the person'. The following is part of Hem and Heggen's (2003) abridged version of an interview with a mental health nurse on her experience of working with a difficult patient. The nurse describes how '[it] seemed to be more and more difficult for me to be myself… my communication with him became more and more difficult'. The patient was, she says, 'psychotic and anxious… I managed to calm him and give him a sense of security'. Yet she also felt under attack: 'It was as if all of me was being closely observed, he was trying to find out who I was… and he yelled at me day after day… "Shut your mouth, you fucking cow". I was intensely rejected for days on end.'

> Every day all of this negativity directed towards me… He constantly demeaned me, and that was hard to take. I suppose he used me as a shock absorber. I tried not to let it get to me. I tried to just put up with it and act normally… It would have been easy for me just to trade insults with him. I felt I was being affected, I became insecure because I was continually provoked. My communication with him became unclear and incongruent. I was becoming more and more unclear… I felt that I was side-lined, and that I lost my grip over him and others. I experienced something of an identity crisis. (Hem & Heggen 2003: 103)

But sometimes their interactions were less difficult, they 'communicated very well… We told each other stories', and in those moments:

> I saw something in him, that he was a vulnerable boy who was carrying a lot of pain. I don't think that his parents ever really saw him. I don't think he could bear to sit alone with all that suffering… but he also said, 'We mustn't talk about it', 'I don't want to be looked at in that way while I'm here', 'Don't dig too deeply – I can't handle it.' He simply couldn't tolerate that we tried to pierce his defences. I said that this was alright, that it was enough… there was understanding and contact between us. (Hem & Heggen 2003: 103)

Hem and Heggen (2003) point out the paradoxical nature of the encounter, in that the mental health nurse sees the dignity of the person and, through her own vulnerability, gains insights into his problems, but she and her colleagues deem this unprofessional. She is uncertain what to do but, despite feeling like a 'shock absorber', retains a 'stubborn empathy' for the patient (p104). She thinks it is unprofessional to feel out of control with the patient, and to lose her perspective on what is happening, yet it is these characteristics that may have facilitated contact with him. Significantly, she is exposed to a situation where she is expected 'to be both intimate and distanced' (Hem & Heggen, 2003: 106).

Being open to the other person

It seems that the mental health nurse's *openness* here is the premise of any interaction with the patient. Openness and the ability to tolerate the 'inconclusiveness' this brings are demanding emotionally and intellectually (Eriksen et al, 2014: 715). But this nurse's openness also exposes her to an experience that erodes her sense of self and integrity. This may have resulted in the loss of her ability to communicate clearly, and she becomes unsure of what she wants to say; she becomes 'uncertain', 'unclear' and 'split'.

Later in this account, the nurse also describes how she felt isolated from her colleagues and others, as if she was misguided in how she was with this patient. Her colleagues are wary of her approach, perhaps with good reason, and encourage her to gain some distance from this patient. While she is the one who probably knows the patient best and has been working therapeutically with him, she is not included in discussions about him with the psychologist. It is highly likely that the latter would be coming from a conceptual position, following guidelines in the 'psy-complex', and so the nurse feels excluded and marginalised both by her colleagues and her patient.

Perhaps I am finding my own feelings in the account of her experience. But I imagine that it is precisely at this moment that it is revealed that she has had no grounding in her experience, or understanding of how she has come to be in relation to 'society', the Other. She is open enough to the other person to be affected by him and draws on a humanistic sense that at some level he is a wounded boy who can be healed. But professionally she may represent what is lost about mental health nursing in that her willingness to stay with the uncertainty, the difficulty, the distress of this man is not viewed by colleagues as leading anywhere. The 'doctors' come in and take over. Perhaps this was the right course of action in this case, but we are still left wondering what being a mental health nurse means. Surely, she was on to something in the struggle for dialogue that also put her own self under question?

In conclusion

Currently, mental health nurse training appears to be at its core a blind launch into an apprenticeship in learning dogma, psychiatric categories of thought and drug and electro-convulsive treatments. Even psychologically, the training is shot through with naïve, although well-meaning, possibly violent, humanistic (Rogers, 1961) thinking, and seemingly apolitical although ego-psychological (for example, Balint, 1950; Bentall, 2004; Fonagy 2004; cf. Parker, 2011) ideas about the person that position the 'master-clinician' as a model for normality, correcting 'faulty thinking' (for example, England, 2006: 735). From different perspectives, I have tried to indicate instead that what is therapeutic about mental health nursing has to do with speaking and 'the art of being a person', which seems implicit in how therapeutic mental health nurses relate to others. It seems then that the discipline belongs in the humanities, as its therapeutic activity has little to do with medicine and more to do with dialogue. A harsh truth may be that psychiatry generates mental health nursing as it needs attendants for its purposes.

Nevertheless, I have argued that one way in which mental health nursing may be able to define itself as a therapeutic discipline separate from psychiatry is through being open to how each person comes to be 'de-centred'. In this way, each 'nurse' could come to speak from a critical position in which aspects of the relation to the Other are understood, or at least from a facilitated critical process of unfolding. Training for this kind of discipline would also explore what has brought the person to want to embark on such a career. I have tentatively suggested a name change from mental health nurse to 'social therapist' to reflect the dialogue inherent to therapeutic nursing as well as how the Other both forms and informs us.

Acknowledgements

Thanks to Sean Walton, Teresa McClelland, Jonathan Gadsby and Pete Bull for helpful comments on earlier drafts of this chapter.

References

Althusser L (1964/1971). Freud and Lacan. In: Althusser L. *Lenin and Philosophy and Other Essays*. London: New Left Books.

Arendt H (2005). *Responsibility and Judgement*. New York, NY: Schocken.

Balint M (1950). On the termination of analysis. *International Journal of Psycho-Analysis* 31: 196-199.

Banks D, Clifton AV, Purdy MJ, Crawshaw P (2013). Mental health nursing and the problematic of supervision as a confessional act. *Journal of Psychiatric and Mental Health Nursing* 20(7): 595–600.

Barker P, Buchanan-Barker P, Rolfe G, Cutcliffe J (2005). Still invisible after all these years: mental health nursing on the margins. *Journal of Psychiatric and Mental Health Nursing* 12(2): 252–256.

Barker PJ, Reynolds B (1996). Rediscovering the proper focus of nursing: a critique of Gournay's position on nursing theory and models. *Journal of Psychiatric and Mental Health Nursing* 3(1): 76–80.

Bennington G, Derrida J (1991). *Jacques Derrida*. Chicago, IL: University of Chicago Press.

Bentall R (2004). *Madness Explained: psychosis and human nature*. London: Penguin.

Bjorklund P (2004). Invisibility, moral knowledge and nursing work in the writings of Joan Liaschenko and Patricia Rodney. *Nursing Ethics 11*(2): 110–121.

Borch-Jacobsen M (1991). *Lacan: the absolute master* (D Brick trans). Stanford, CA: Stanford University Press.

Browne G, Cashin A, Graham I (2012). The therapeutic relationship and mental health nursing: it is time to articulate what we do! *Journal of Psychiatric and Mental Health Nursing 19*(9): 839–843.

Cutcliffe JR (2000). Fit for purpose? Promoting the human side of mental health nursing? *British Journal of Nursing 9*(10): 632–637.

Cutcliffe JR, Santos JC, Kozel B, Taylor P, Lees D (2015). Raiders of the lost art: a review of published evaluations of inpatient mental health care experiences emanating from the United Kingdom, Portugal, Canada, Switzerland, Germany and Australia. *International Journal of Mental Health Nursing 24*(5): 375–385.

Davies J (2013). *Cracked: why psychiatry is doing more harm than good*. London: Icon Books.

Derrida J (1993/1991). Circumfession (G Bennington trans). In: Bennington G, Derrida J. *Jacques Derrida*. Chicago, IL: University of Chicago Press (pp3–315).

England M (2006). Cognitive intervention for voice hearers. *Issues in Mental Health Nursing 27*(7): 735–751.

Eriksen KÅ, Dahl H, Karlsson B, Arman M (2014). Strengthening practical wisdom: mental health workers' learning and development. *Nursing Ethics 21*(6): 707–719.

Fink B (1995). *The Lacanian Subject: between language and jouissance*. Princeton, NJ: Princeton University Press.

Finlay L (2008). A dance between the reduction and reflexivity: explicating the 'phenomenological psychological attitude'. *Journal of Phenomenological Psychology 39*(1): 1–32.

Fonagy P (2004). Psychotherapy meets neuroscience: a more focused future for psychotherapy research. *Psychiatric Bulletin 28*(10): 357–359.

Foucault M (1989). *Madness and Civilisation: a history of insanity in the age of reason* (R Howard trans). London: Routledge.

Friedman M (1999). *The Worlds of Existentialism: a critical reader*. New York, NY: Humanity Books.

Gadamer HG (2004). *Truth and Method* (2nd ed). London: Continuum.

Gill JH (2000). *The Tacit Mode: Michael Polanyi's postmodern philosophy*. Albany, NY: State University of New York Press.

Giorgi A (2009). *The Descriptive Phenomenological Method in Psychology: a modified Husserlian approach*. Pittsburgh, PA: Duquesne University Press.

Gournay K (2000). Commentaries and reflections on mental health nursing in the UK at the dawn of the new millennium: commentary 2. *Journal of Mental Health 9*(6): 621–623.

Happell B (2004). The Centre for Psychiatric Nursing Research and Practice: an innovative approach enhancing clinical nursing research in the psychiatric/mental health field. *Issues in Mental Health Nursing 25*(1): 47–60.

Harré R (1983). *Personal Being*. Oxford: Blackwell.

Heaton JM (2010). *The Talking Cure: Wittgenstein's therapeutic method for psychotherapy*. Basingstoke: Palgrave Macmillan.

Heaton JM (1999). Scepticism and psychotherapy: a Wittgensteinian approach. In: Mace C (ed). *Heart & Soul: the therapeutic face of philosophy*. London: Routledge (pp49–64).

Hem MH, Heggen K (2003). Rejection: a neglected phenomenon in psychiatric nursing. *Journal of Psychiatric and Mental Health Nursing 11*(1): 55–63.

Holman Jones S, Adams T, Ellis C (2013). Introduction: coming to know autoethnography as more than method. In: Jones H, Adams T, Ellis C (eds). *Handbook of Autoethnography*. Walnut Creek, CA: Left Coast Press (pp17–49).

Holmes D, Gastaldo D, Perron A (2007). Paranoid investments in nursing: a schizoanalysis of the evidence-based discourse. *Nursing Philosophy 8*(2): 85–91.

House R (2010). *In, Against and Beyond Therapy: critical essays towards a post-professional era*. Ross-on-Wye: PCCS Books.

Husserl E (1970). *The Crisis of European Sciences and Transcendental Phenomenology: an introduction to phenomenological philosophy* (D Carr trans). Evanston, IL: Northwestern University Press.

Husserl E (1969). *Formal and Transcendental Logic* (D Cairns trans). The Hague: Martinus Nijhoff.

Kant I (1781/2007). *Critique of Pure Reason* (M Weigelt trans & ed). London: Penguin Books.

Kelly P, Moloney P (2018). CBT is the Method: the object is to change the heart and soul. In: Loewenthal D, Proctor G (eds). *Why Not CBT? Against and for CBT Revisited* (2nd ed). Monmouth: PCCS Books (pp82–105).

Kierkegaard S (2010). *The Present Age: on the death of rebellion* (A Dru trans). New York, NY: Harper Collins.

Kierkegaard S (1954). *Fear and Trembling* and *The Sickness unto Death* (W Lowrie trans). New York, NY: Double Day/Anchor Books.

Lacan J (1977). *Écrits: a selection* (A Sheridan trans). London: Tavistock Publications.

Lather P, St Pierre EA (2013). Post-qualitative research. *International Journal of Qualitative Studies in Education 26*(6): 629–633.

Loewenthal D (2011). From existentialism (and post-modernism) to post-existentialism: from Buber to Levinas. In: D. Loewenthal (ed). *Post-Existentialism and the Psychological Therapies*. London: Karnac Books (pp19-30).

Loewenthal D, Snell R (2003). *Post-modernism for Psychotherapists: a critical reader*. Hove/New York, NY: Brunner-Routledge.

McSherry A (2018). *What is the need, if any, for therapeutic education in mental health nursing? An empirical phenomenological study of mental health nurses' responses to this question*. Unpublished PhD thesis. Roehampton: Roehampton University.

McSherry T, Loewenthal D, Cayne J (2015). The implications of Kristeva's notion of the abject in understanding the significance of therapeutic knowledge and practice in mental health nursing. *Journal of Psychiatric and Mental Health Nursing 22*(1): 82–88.

Merleau-Ponty M (1968). *The Visible and the Invisible*. Evanston, IL: North Western University Press.

Merleau-Ponty M (1962/2014). *Phenomenology of Perception* (C Smith trans). London: Routledge & Kegan Paul.

Moran D (2000). *Introduction to Phenomenology*. London: Routledge.

Morrall PA (1997). Lacking in rigour: a case-study of the professional practice of psychiatric nurses in four community mental health teams. *Journal of Mental Health 6*(2): 173–179.

Murray SJ, Holmes D (2013). Toward a critical ethical reflexivity: phenomenology and language in Merleau-Ponty. *Bioethics 27*(6): 341–347.

Nolan P (1993). *A History of Mental Health Nursing*. London: Chapman & Hall.

Nursing and Midwifery Council (2017). *Draft Standards of Proficiency for Registered Nurses*. London: NMC.

Nursing and Midwifery Council (2010). *Standards for Competence for Registered Nurses*. London: NMC.

Paley J (2002). Caring as a slave morality: Nietzschean themes in nursing ethics. *Journal of Advanced Nursing 40*(1): 25–35.

Parker I (2011). *Lacanian Psychoanalysis: revolutions in subjectivity*. London: Routledge.

Parker I (1997). *Psychoanalytic Culture: psychoanalytic discourse in Western society*. London: Sage Publications.

Polanyi M (1983). *The Tacit Dimension*. Gloucester, MA: Peter Smith.

Polt RFH (1999). *Heidegger: an introduction*. London: UCL Press.

Rabaté J (2002). *The Future of Theory*. Oxford: Blackwell Publishers.

Rawlins M (2008). Harveian Oration: *De testimonio*: on the evidence for decisions about the use of therapeutic interventions. *Lancet 372*(9656): 2152–2161.

Rogers C (1961). *On Becoming a Person: a therapist's view of psychotherapy*. London: Constable.

Rose N (1999). *Governing the Soul: the shaping of the private self*. London: Free Association Books.

Rose N (1985). *The Psychological Complex: psychology, politics and society in England, 1869–1939*. London: Routledge & Kegan Paul.

Walker C (1994). Karl Jaspers and Edmund Husserl: 1. the perceived convergence. *Philosophy, Psychiatry, & Psychology 1*(2): 117–134.

Wittgenstein L (2009). *Philosophical Investigations* (4th ed) (Schulte J, Hacker PMS eds). Oxford: Wiley-Blackwell.

Zahavi D (2003). *Husserl's Phenomenology*. Stanford, CA: Stanford University Press.

Žižek S (2006). Burned by the sun. In: Žižek S (ed). *Lacan: the silent partners*. London: Verso (pp217–230).

Contributors

Pete Bull
Pete spent six months as a day hospital outpatient in South London in 1997, when he was just 18, and this has shaped a lot of his understanding of life since that time. After attending several universities, dropping out, having over 40 jobs and travelling through Australia, Pete began training as an existential counsellor and psychotherapist in 2004, finally qualifying with an MA (and finishing his first BA) in 2010. Since then he has worked (and qualified) as a CBT therapist and registered mental health nurse. He has had a lot of psychotherapy. He has been in the NHS for over 12 years. He is currently a community mental health nurse in Brighton.

Anne Felton
As a mental health nurse, critical perspectives have underpinned Anne's practice as she maintained a commitment to finding different ways of working that challenge the power relationships within practice and the medicalisation of mental health care. Anne has carried these values into her academic role through the education of pre-registration mental health nurses and her research in the areas of decision-making, risk, co-production and recovery. Anne is currently Associate Professor and Academic Lead of the Mental Health and Learning Disabilities Nursing Team at the University of Nottingham.

Erica Fletcher
Erica Hua Fletcher holds a PhD in Medical Humanities from the University of Texas Medical Branch in Galveston, Texas. After graduating in August 2015, she served as the programme director for a community health service learning organisation for undergraduate students at the University of Houston's Honors College, where she taught classes in social medicine, anthropology and public health. In June 2017, she began a two-year postdoctoral research position as

the Zorich Fellow in Mental Health Policy at the Hope and Healing Center & Institute in Houston, Texas. Her research focuses on the roles of people with lived experience of mental health struggles in supporting each other's wellbeing through informal and institutional means. She also teaches part-time in the Department of Anthropology at the University of California, Los Angeles.

Jonathan Gadsby

Jonathan Gadsby qualified as a mental health nurse in Bristol in 2001. Critical elements of the course left him with a lot of good questions about mental health nursing and these only intensified through acute work and a number of community roles over the next 10 years. Then he did a Masters (Philosophy and Ethics of Mental Health) at Warwick, followed by a PhD at Birmingham City University, under the direction of Mervyn Morris and Marius Romme. Now he works as a teacher of mental health nurses and social workers at Birmingham City University. He was one of the founders of the Critical Mental Health Nurses' Network and has continued to contribute to their website as a writer and editor.

Benny Goodman

Benny Goodman is a lecturer in adult nursing in the School of Nursing and Midwifery at Plymouth University. He qualified as a registered general nurse in the 1980s, followed by a BSc in sociology and politics. He writes on topics such as sustainability, climate change and health but always within a socio-political framework. He is author and co-author of two books: *Collaborative Practice* and *Sociology and Psychology in Nursing*. Current interests include the socio-political role of the nurse.

Alec Grant

Alec Grant PhD is a social researcher who has worked as an independent scholar since his retirement from the University of Brighton in 2017, where he held the post of Reader in Narrative Mental Health. He is well published in the areas of autoethnography, mental health survival and critical mental health, in books, book chapters and journal articles. He co-originated and led/co-edited three of the *Our Encounters with...* series, published by PCCS Books, which promotes first hand, lived-experience narratives: *Our Encounters with Madness* (2011), *... with Suicide* (2013), and *... with Stalking* (2017). He also co-edited *Contemporary British Autoethnography* (with Nigel Short and Lydia Turner (2013)) and *International Perspectives on Autoethnographic Research and Practice* (with Short, Turner and Tony Adams (2018)). He originally trained as a mental health nurse in the mid-1970s, before moving into cognitive behavioural psychotherapy in the 1980s, and then into Higher Education in the 1990s. He is on the International Advisory Board of *Nurse Education Today*.

Mick McKeown

Mick is Professor of Democratic Mental Health in the School of Nursing, University of Central Lancashire, and trade union activist with Unison, supporting service user and carer involvement at the university and union strategising on nursing. He has taken a lead in making the case for union organising to extend to alliance formation with service users/survivors.

Tony McSherry

Tony McSherry began working in mental health nursing through a vocation as a Franciscan friar. His interests in the latter were principally in spirituality rather than religion. As a Franciscan, he studied in the Gregorian University in Rome, where he first became familiar with philosophy. Before this, his studies were in the sciences. He was educated in University College Dublin, and he worked as a geologist for some time. Alongside these activities, he became involved in counselling and psychotherapy, with a special interest in Lacanian psychoanalysis, existentialism and phenomenology. In 2018, he completed a PhD exploring what is therapeutic in any relation with another, in terms of healing. He is accredited through the UK Council for Psychotherapy as a psychotherapeutic counsellor, humanistic and integrative psychotherapist and existential-analytical psychotherapist. He works as a psychotherapist in the NHS and in private practice. He has published papers on the relevance of psychoanalysis to mental health nursing, and is currently working on the importance of phenomenology as research.

Darren Mills

Darren Mills is an occupational therapy lecturer at Te Kura Matatini ki Otago/ Otago Polytechnic. He also maintains clinical practice through a crisis assessment and intervention service. Darren completed a Master of Health Research in 2017, which explored the emergence of recovery as a guiding philosophy within Aotearoa New Zealand's mental health service provision.

Alastair Morgan

Alastair works as a senior lecturer in mental health nursing at the University of Manchester. His research interests are in critical theory (particularly the first generation of the Frankfurt School and the philosophy of TW Adorno), philosophy of psychiatry, critical neuroscience, critical medical humanities and ethics and values in mental health. He has written three books, published several contributions to edited books and published widely in peer-reviewed journals. Most recently, Alastair is the lead author (with Anne Felton and Bill Fulford) of a book entitled *Values and Ethics in Mental Health: an exploration for practice (2015).*

Steven Prosser

Steven Prosser is a Cornishman living in Yorkshire married to a Lancastrian, which is an enigma in itself. He has battled with addiction for 40 years and is happy to talk about his recovery. Steven didn't realise he has any form of mental health problems because no one told him. He thought he was just different and eccentric until his mental health deteriorated in the last 10 years, costing him a job and a period of depression which he attempted to hide. Steven believes in talking therapy as a means of helping to start recovery and also, since the Recovery College, WRAP. Steven is a keen gardener and at the moment experimenting with gardening as a form of therapy and mindfulness gardening as a holistic treatment for himself and others, as well as physical exercise and healthy eating. Steven is grandfather to Isaaq, with yet another grandchild due in the autumn of 2018.

Marc Roberts

Marc Roberts is a researcher, lecturer and author with extensive and varied experience in mental health practice and education. He has published widely in a variety of scholarly journals and is the author of two books, *Critical Thinking and Reflection for Mental Health Nursing Students* (2015) and *Understanding Mental Health Care: critical issues in practice* (2018). In addition to having clinical experience in mental health, he also has an academic background in philosophy. His work is therefore concerned with the way in which critical thinking, critical reflection and philosophy more generally can contribute to the theory and practice of contemporary mental health care.

Gary Sidley

Gary Sidley is a freelance writer, trainer, blogger and conference speaker. In 2013, he opted for early retirement from his post as professional lead/consultant clinical psychologist after 33 continuous years of employment in the UK's National Health Service. He is a vocal critic of bio-medical approaches to mental health, illustrating his concerns with anecdotes drawn from his extensive experience of working within the psychiatric system. His book, *Tales from the Madhouse: an insider critique of psychiatric services*, is published by PCCS Books (2015). Gary's NHS career began in 1980 as a psychiatric nurse, and he qualified as a clinical psychologist in 1989. In 2000, he obtained his PhD for a thesis exploring the psychological predictors of suicidal behaviour. His articles can be found on his blog at http://talesfromthemadhouse.com and at http://gsidley.hubpages.com/. He also regularly tweets about mental health issues at https://twitter.com/GarySidley

Tony Sparkes

Tony has over 28 years of experience, working largely within community mental health services, in a variety of roles for both the NHS and local authority social services in the north west of England. His interest in mental health recovery began in the late 1990s, during time spent managing a community mental health support team. Tony qualified as a social worker in 2005 and in 2009 was awarded an Economic and Social Research Council (ESRC) studentship to follow up his longstanding interest in recovery. He was awarded his PhD in 2013. Tony currently works as a social work tutor in the division of social work and social care at the University of Bradford. He is involved with undergraduate and postgraduate social work education and is Programme Director for the approved mental health professional (AMHP) programme. Tony is research active and is particularly interested in qualitative approaches to mental health recovery.

Gemma Stacey

Gemma Stacey is a mental health nurse and Associate Professor at the University of Nottingham. Her research and practice are underpinned by a critical consideration of the organisational, relational and professional factors that influence the expression of values in healthcare practice. She is committed to the premise of healthcare education as a vehicle to promote emancipatory practice and has developed a programme of educational scholarship focused on approaches that enable transformational learning.

Stephen Williams

Stephen Williams has been a lecturer-practitioner in mental health nursing at the University of Bradford for the past eight years, where he is currently the Field Lead in Mental Health, working with a small and dedicated team delivering the pre-registration mental health nurse education and contributing to the development of post-registration education. His specialist interest is in the development of psychological therapeutic interventions for people with psychosis, and in 2016 he authored the book *Recovering from Psychosis: empirical evidence and lived experience*. Stephen has mainly worked in a community mental health team as a nurse specialist in psychological therapy, but he has held posts as a lead nurse for high-functioning autism spectrum services and a research nurse exploring the complexities of different kinds of decision-making styles on service-user satisfaction in specialist secondary mental health services. Currently he is delivering a community education emotional health service at the University of Bradford called the Wellness Academy, offering emotional wellbeing-related interventions and education. He is a graduate psychologist, a registered mental health nurse and a Fellow of the Higher Education Academy and has a postgraduate qualification in higher education practice.

Name index

Subject index